国家卫生和计划生育委员会"十三五"规划教材
全国高等医药教材建设研究会"十三五"规划教材

全国高等学校药学类专业第八轮规划教材

供药学类专业用

药 学 英 语

（上 册）

第5版

U0386376

主　编　史志祥

副主编　龚长华　张予阳　唐　漫

主　审　裴　瑾

编　者（按姓氏笔画排序）

王　炜（湖南中医药大学）	张艳春（安徽中医药大学）
叶　慧（中国药科大学）	张维芬（潍坊医学院）
史志祥（中国药科大学）	侯　琳（郑州大学药学院）
刘　浩（蚌埠医学院）	姚　丽（哈尔滨医科大学）
孙　宏（牡丹江医学院）	郭　昊（徐州医科大学）
李　鹏（新乡医学院）	唐　漫（中国医科大学）
杨　静（南京医科大学）	黄　显（福建医科大学）
何永志（天津中医药大学）	黄　靓（大连医科大学）
张予阳（沈阳药科大学）	龚长华（广东药科大学）
张宇辉（中国药科大学）	符　垚（四川大学华西药学院）

编写秘书　陈　菁（中国药科大学）

人民卫生出版社

图书在版编目（CIP）数据

药学英语. 上册 / 史志祥主编. — 5 版. —北京：人民卫生
出版社，2016

　　ISBN 978-7-117-22728-5

　　Ⅰ. ①药…　Ⅱ. ①史…　Ⅲ. ①药物学－英语－医学院
校－教材　Ⅳ. ①R9-43

　　中国版本图书馆 CIP 数据核字（2016）第 191897 号

人卫社官网　www.pmph.com	出版物查询，在线购书
人卫医学网　www.ipmph.com	医学考试辅导，医学数据库服务，医学教育资源，大众健康资讯

药学英语（上册）

第 5 版

主　　编：史志祥
出版发行：人民卫生出版社（中继线 010-59780011）
地　　址：北京市朝阳区潘家园南里 19 号
邮　　编：100021
E - mail：pmph @ pmph.com
购书热线：010-59787592　010-59787584　010-65264830
印　　刷：北京铭成印刷有限公司
经　　销：新华书店
开　　本：850×1168　1/16　印张：14
字　　数：385 千字
版　　次：1986 年 6 月第 1 版　　2016 年 2 月第 5 版
　　　　　2023 年 6 月第 5 版第 11 次印刷（总第 52 次印刷）
标准书号：ISBN 978-7-117-22728-5/R·22729
定　　价：37.00 元
打击盗版举报电话：010-59787491　E-mail：WQ @ pmph.com
　　　（凡属印装质量问题请与本社市场营销中心联系退换）

　　全国高等学校药学类专业本科国家卫生和计划生育委员会规划教材是我国最权威的药学类专业教材,于1979年出版第1版,1987—2011年进行了6次修订,并于2011年出版了第七轮规划教材。第七轮规划教材主干教材31种,全部为原卫生部"十二五"规划教材,其中29种为"十二五"普通高等教育本科国家级规划教材;配套教材21种,全部为原卫生部"十二五"规划教材。本次修订出版的第八轮规划教材中主干教材共34种,其中修订第七轮规划教材31种;新编教材3种,《药学信息检索与利用》《药学服务概论》《医药市场营销学》;配套教材29种,其中修订24种,新编5种。同时,为满足院校双语教学的需求,本轮新编双语教材2种,《药理学》《药剂学》。全国高等学校药学类专业第八轮规划教材及其配套教材均为国家卫生和计划生育委员会"十三五"规划教材、全国高等医药教材建设研究会"十三五"规划教材,具体品种详见出版说明所附书目。

　　该套教材曾为全国高等学校药学类专业唯一一套统编教材,后更名为规划教材,具有较高的权威性和较强的影响力,为我国高等教育培养大批的药学类专业人才发挥了重要作用。随着我国高等教育体制改革的不断深入发展,药学类专业办学规模不断扩大,办学形式、专业种类、教学方式亦呈多样化发展,我国高等药学教育进入了一个新的时期。同时,随着药学行业相关法规政策、标准等的出台,以及2015年版《中华人民共和国药典》的颁布等,高等药学教育面临着新的要求和任务。为跟上时代发展的步伐,适应新时期我国高等药学教育改革和发展的要求,培养合格的药学专门人才,进一步做好药学类专业本科教材的组织规划和质量保障工作,全国高等学校药学类专业第五届教材评审委员会围绕药学类专业第七轮教材使用情况、药学教育现状、新时期药学人才培养模式等多个主题,进行了广泛、深入的调研,并对调研结果进行了反复、细致的分析论证。根据药学类专业教材评审委员会的意见和调研、论证的结果,全国高等医药教材建设研究会、人民卫生出版社决定组织全国专家对第七轮教材进行修订,并根据教学需要组织编写了部分新教材。

　　药学类专业第八轮规划教材的修订编写,坚持紧紧围绕全国高等学校药学类专业本科教育和人才培养目标要求,突出药学类专业特色,对接国家执业药师资格考试,按照国家卫生和计划生育委员会等相关部门及行业用人要求,在继承和巩固前七轮教材建设工作成果的基础上,提出了"继承创新""医教协同""教考融合""理实结合""纸数同步"的编写原则,使得本轮教材更加契合当前药学类专业人才培养的目标和需求,更加适应现阶段高等学校本科药学类人才的培养模式,从而进一步提升了教材的整体质量和水平。

　　为满足广大师生对教学内容数字化的需求,积极探索传统媒体与新媒体融合发展的新型整体教学解决方案,本轮教材同步启动了网络增值服务和数字教材的编写工作。34 种主干教材都将在纸质教材内容的基础上,集合视频、音频、动画、图片、拓展文本等多媒介、多形态、多用途、多层次的数字素材,完成教材数字化的转型升级。

需要特别说明的是,随着教育教学改革的发展和专家队伍的发展变化,根据教材建设工作的需要,在修订编写本轮规划教材之初,全国高等医药教材建设研究会、人民卫生出版社对第四届教材评审委员会进行了改选换届,成立了第五届教材评审委员会。无论新老评审委员,都为本轮教材建设做出了重要贡献,在此向他们表示衷心的谢意!

众多学术水平一流和教学经验丰富的专家教授以高度负责的态度积极踊跃和严谨认真地参与了本套教材的编写工作,付出了诸多心血,从而使教材的质量得到不断完善和提高,在此我们对长期支持本套教材修订编写的专家和教师及同学们表示诚挚的感谢!

本轮教材出版后,各位教师、学生在使用过程中,如发现问题请反馈给我们(renweiyaoxue@163.com),以便及时更正和修订完善。

全国高等医药教材建设研究会

人民卫生出版社

2016 年 1 月

国家卫生和计划生育委员会"十三五"规划教材
全国高等学校药学类专业第八轮规划教材书目

序号	教材名称	主编	单位
1	药学导论(第4版)	毕开顺	沈阳药科大学
2	高等数学(第6版)	顾作林	河北医科大学
	高等数学学习指导与习题集(第3版)	顾作林	河北医科大学
3	医药数理统计方法(第6版)	高祖新	中国药科大学
	医药数理统计方法学习指导与习题集(第2版)	高祖新	中国药科大学
4	物理学(第7版)	武 宏	山东大学物理学院
		章新友	江西中医药大学
	物理学学习指导与习题集(第3版)	武 宏	山东大学物理学院
	物理学实验指导★★★	王晨光	哈尔滨医科大学
		武 宏	山东大学物理学院
5	物理化学(第8版)	李三鸣	沈阳药科大学
	物理化学学习指导与习题集(第4版)	李三鸣	沈阳药科大学
	物理化学实验指导(第2版)(双语)	崔黎丽	第二军医大学
6	无机化学(第7版)	张天蓝	北京大学药学院
		姜凤超	华中科技大学同济药学院
	无机化学学习指导与习题集(第4版)	姜凤超	华中科技大学同济药学院
7	分析化学(第8版)	柴逸峰	第二军医大学
		邸 欣	沈阳药科大学
	分析化学学习指导与习题集(第4版)	柴逸峰	第二军医大学
	分析化学实验指导(第4版)	邸 欣	沈阳药科大学
8	有机化学(第8版)	陆 涛	中国药科大学
	有机化学学习指导与习题集(第4版)	陆 涛	中国药科大学
9	人体解剖生理学(第7版)	周 华	四川大学华西基础医学与法医学院
		崔慧先	河北医科大学
10	微生物学与免疫学(第8版)	沈关心	华中科技大学同济医学院
		徐 威	沈阳药科大学
	微生物学与免疫学学习指导与习题集★★★	苏 昕	沈阳药科大学
		尹丙姣	华中科技大学同济医学院
11	生物化学(第8版)	姚文兵	中国药科大学
	生物化学学习指导与习题集(第2版)	杨 红	广东药科大学

续表

序号	教材名称	主编	单位
12	药理学(第 8 版)	朱依谆	复旦大学药学院
		殷 明	上海交通大学药学院
	药理学(双语)★★	朱依谆	复旦大学药学院
		殷 明	上海交通大学药学院
	药理学学习指导与习题集(第 3 版)	程能能	复旦大学药学院
13	药物分析(第 8 版)	杭太俊	中国药科大学
	药物分析学习指导与习题集(第 2 版)	于治国	沈阳药科大学
	药物分析实验指导(第 2 版)	范国荣	第二军医大学
14	药用植物学(第 7 版)	黄宝康	第二军医大学
	药用植物学实践与学习指导(第 2 版)	黄宝康	第二军医大学
15	生药学(第 7 版)	蔡少青	北京大学药学院
		秦路平	第二军医大学
	生药学学习指导与习题集★★★	姬生国	广东药科大学
	生药学实验指导(第 3 版)	陈随清	河南中医药大学
16	药物毒理学(第 4 版)	楼宜嘉	浙江大学药学院
17	临床药物治疗学(第 4 版)	姜远英	第二军医大学
		文爱东	第四军医大学
18	药物化学(第 8 版)	尤启冬	中国药科大学
	药物化学学习指导与习题集(第 3 版)	孙铁民	沈阳药科大学
19	药剂学(第 8 版)	方 亮	沈阳药科大学
	药剂学(双语)★★	毛世瑞	沈阳药科大学
	药剂学学习指导与习题集(第 3 版)	王东凯	沈阳药科大学
	药剂学实验指导(第 4 版)	杨 丽	沈阳药科大学
20	天然药物化学(第 7 版)	裴月湖	沈阳药科大学
		娄红祥	山东大学药学院
	天然药物化学学习指导与习题集(第 4 版)	裴月湖	沈阳药科大学
	天然药物化学实验指导(第 4 版)	裴月湖	沈阳药科大学
21	中医药学概论(第 8 版)	王 建	成都中医药大学
22	药事管理学(第 6 版)	杨世民	西安交通大学药学院
	药事管理学学习指导与习题集(第 3 版)	杨世民	西安交通大学药学院
23	药学分子生物学(第 5 版)	张景海	沈阳药科大学
	药学分子生物学学习指导与习题集★★★	宋永波	沈阳药科大学
24	生物药剂学与药物动力学(第 5 版)	刘建平	中国药科大学
	生物药剂学与药物动力学学习指导与习题集(第 3 版)	张 娜	山东大学药学院

续表

序号	教材名称	主编	单位
25	药学英语(上册、下册)(第5版)	史志祥	中国药科大学
	药学英语学习指导(第3版)	史志祥	中国药科大学
26	药物设计学(第3版)	方　浩	山东大学药学院
	药物设计学学习指导与习题集(第2版)	杨晓虹	吉林大学药学院
27	制药工程原理与设备(第3版)	王志祥	中国药科大学
28	生物制药工艺学(第2版)	夏焕章	沈阳药科大学
29	生物技术制药(第3版)	王凤山	山东大学药学院
		邹全明	第三军医大学
	生物技术制药实验指导★★★	邹全明	第三军医大学
30	临床医学概论(第2版)	于　锋	中国药科大学
		闻德亮	中国医科大学
31	波谱解析(第2版)	孔令义	中国药科大学
32	药学信息检索与利用*	何　华	中国药科大学
33	药学服务概论*	丁选胜	中国药科大学
34	医药市场营销学*	陈玉文	沈阳药科大学

注:*为第八轮新编主干教材;**为第八轮新编双语教材;***为第八轮新编配套教材。

全国高等学校药学类专业第五届教材评审委员会名单

顾　　问　　吴晓明　中国药科大学

周福成　国家食品药品监督管理总局执业药师资格认证中心

主 任 委 员　毕开顺　沈阳药科大学

副主任委员　姚文兵　中国药科大学

郭　姣　广东药科大学

张志荣　四川大学华西药学院

委　　员（以姓氏笔画为序）

王凤山　山东大学药学院	陆　涛　中国药科大学
朱　珠　中国药学会医院药学专业委员会	周余来　吉林大学药学院
朱依谆　复旦大学药学院	胡　琴　南京医科大学
刘俊义　北京大学药学院	胡长平　中南大学药学院
孙建平　哈尔滨医科大学	姜远英　第二军医大学
李　高　华中科技大学同济药学院	夏焕章　沈阳药科大学
李晓波　上海交通大学药学院	黄　民　中山大学药学院
杨　波　浙江大学药学院	黄泽波　广东药科大学
杨世民　西安交通大学药学院	曹德英　河北医科大学
张振中　郑州大学药学院	彭代银　安徽中医药大学
张淑秋　山西医科大学	董　志　重庆医科大学

《药学英语》(上册、下册)第4版于2011年面世以来,全国医药院校和综合性大学药学院(系)积极采用,使本书先后印刷多次,发行量较大,得到了应有的社会效益。

为了确保本教材能更好地适应药学教育的新形势和各高校开设基础药学英语以及专业药学英语的需要,人民卫生出版社及本书编者在全国高校进行了广泛调研,使得第5版与第4版相比在许多方面有所改进。

第5版《药学英语》仍然由主干教材(上、下册)及《药学英语学习指导》组成;上册为基础药学英语部分,选课文28篇(按题材分成14个单元,每个单元两篇文章),单元体例为相关背景知识介绍、课文A(后附词汇、注释和习题)、课文B(后附词汇和注释)、医药科技英语构词知识介绍以及英汉翻译技巧等;下册为专业药学英语部分,选课文18篇(按专业学科领域分成9个单元,每个单元两篇文章),单元体例为相关学科介绍、课文A(后附词汇、注释和习题)、课文B(文章前附中文导读,文章后附词汇和注释)、汉英翻译技巧以及药学英语写作技巧等;《药学英语学习指导》除了提供主干教材上、下册练习答案及每个单元第一篇核心课文参考译文之外,还附有"药学英语分类词汇"。为了节省篇幅,第5版上、下册教材书后不再附词汇总表。总体来说,与前几版相比,本套教材增加了临床药学及制药工程等方面的内容,更加重视药学学科的完整性;与此同时,编者更加强调单元练习的多样性,强调学生英汉双向药学英语翻译、药学学术英语写作及药学英语词汇等方面能力的提高。

为了使本教材更好地适应当今药学英语教学改革的需要,本套教材将适时推出核心课文配套录音等材料作为增值服务内容。

本教材使用对象:上册可供各医药类院校药学类各专业本、专科生"通用药学英语"教学用,在注重药学英语能力提高的同时强调药学英语词汇和英汉翻译能力的提升;下册可供各医药类院校药学类各专业本科生和硕士研究生"专业药学英语"教学用,在注重药学专业英语水平提高的同时强调汉英药学英语翻译能力和药学英语学术写作能力的提升;《药学英语学习指导》与主干教材配套使用。

本套教材的编写由来自中国药科大学、沈阳药科大学、广东药科大学、中国医科大学、四川大学、郑州大学、南京医科大学、大连医科大学、哈尔滨医科大学、福建医科大学、徐州医科大学、天津中医药大学、湖南中医药大学、安徽中医药大学、新乡医学院、蚌埠医学院、牡丹江医学院、潍坊医学院等18所医药院校的22位专家、教授共同完成。编者中既有博通药学知识的英语专家,也有长期从事相关药学领域教学及研究且精通英语的药学专家。

　　全套教材除本人主编外,尚有广东药科大学龚长华教授、沈阳药科大学张予阳教授及中国医科大学的唐漫教授担任《药学英语》上、下册及《药学英语学习指导》副主编。本套教材第 4 版副主编、吉林大学药学院裴瑾教授抽出宝贵时间审阅了教材。另外,教材编委会还专门聘请了本书编者中国药科大学外语系药学英语教研室的陈菁老师担任本套教材上册编写秘书。

　　在编写过程中,所有编者除了完成自己分工的内容之外,还协助其他编者完成相关编写及译文审校工作;所有编者不辞辛劳,数次集中召开编写及定稿会议。在此谨对为本教材编写工作做出巨大贡献的各位编者致以衷心的感谢。

　　本人还要特别感谢中国药科大学相关领导及专家,特别是外语系主任张国申教授、中国药科大学工学院副院长王志祥教授、制药工程教研室主任黄德春副教授。没有他们的帮助,本教材难以顺利付梓。此外,我还要感谢中国药科大学药学英语教研室甘珏、张洁、林玲等老师以及苏州大学附属第一医院药学部易玲博士等所给予的帮助。

　　由于编者水平有限,不足之处在所难免,敬请各位专家及读者指正。同时,编者愿意和各高校同仁就"药学英语"的教学及本套教材的使用进行交流,欢迎与我们联系。

中国药科大学　史志祥

shizhixiang@cpu.edu.cn

2016 年 2 月

Contents

Unit One Physiology and Pathology

Stated most simply and broadly, physiology is the study of how living organisms work. As applied to human beings, its scope is extremely broad. At one end of the spectrum, it includes the study of individual molecules-for example, how a particular protein's shape and electrical properties allow it to function as a channel for sodium ions to move into or out of a cell. At the other end, it is concerned with complex processes that depend on the interplay of many widely separated organs in the body-for example, how the brain, heart, and several glands all work together to cause the excretion of more sodium in the urine when a person has eaten salty food.

Pathology is the science of diseases, which deals with the studies of etiology, pathogenesis, morphologic structures, changes in functions and metabolism in the living organisms by means of natural science. It illustrates the discipline of the development and the evolution of diseases and the essence of diseases to provide a theoretical basis for the treatment and prevention of varied types of diseases.

Pathophysiology is the study of functional changes in the body which occur in response to diseases or injuries. The field of pathophysiology is designed to help people study the progress of diseases so that they can quickly identify diseases and consider various treatments. One of the major issues in pathophysiology is that every human body is different. What may be normal in one person could be abnormal in another, and diseases will not always behave in the same way. For this reason, it is critical for the researchers in this field to be exposed to a diversity of patients and disease manifestations, so that they see real-world examples of physiological and pathological differences.

简明而广义地讲, 生理学是研究生物体如何工作的学科。应用于人类, 生理学研究范畴就更为广泛, 其一方面研究的是单个分子, 如特定的蛋白质的形状和电生理特性如何发挥传运通道的作用使钠离子进出细胞; 而另一方面研究的是在人体中广泛分布的各个器官如何相互作用的复杂过程, 如大脑、心脏和各种腺体在人体摄入含盐食物后如何协调工作, 使更多的钠分泌到尿液中。

病理学是研究疾病的科学, 是用自然科学的方法研究生物体发病的病因、发病机制、形态结构、功能和代谢等方面的改变。病理学用来阐明疾病发生和发展的规律, 揭示疾病的本质, 从而为各种疾病的防治提供理论基础。

病理生理学研究的是机体对疾病或损伤产生的应答而引起的功能性改变。该领域的研究有助于人们研究疾病的进展, 以便快速鉴别疾病, 考虑选择不同的治疗方案。病理生理学关注的主要问题之一是个体是有差异的, 在某个体身上属于正常的范畴, 而在另一个体就可能是异常, 疾病的表现不会总是一样。正因为如此, 这一领域的研究人员非常有必要接触各种患者, 了解疾病的表现, 这样才能理解实践中生理学和病理学的差异。

笔记

1

Text A
Introduction to Physiology

Introduction

Physiology is the study of the functions of living matter. It is concerned with *how* an organism performs its varied activities: how it feeds, how it moves, how it adapts to changing circumstances, how it spawns new generations. The subject is vast and embraces the whole of life. The success of physiology in explaining how organisms perform their daily tasks is based on the notion that they are intricate and exquisite machines whose operation is governed by the laws of physics and chemistry.

Although some processes are similar across the whole spectrum of biology–the replication of the genetic code for example–many are specific to particular groups of organisms. For this reason it is necessary to divide the subject into various parts such as bacterial physiology, plant physiology, and animal physiology.

To study how an animal works it is first necessary to know how it is built. A full appreciation of the physiology of an organism must, therefore, be based on a sound knowledge of its anatomy. Experiments can then be carried out to establish how particular parts perform their functions. Although there have been many important physiological investigations on human volunteers, the need for precise control over the experimental conditions has meant that much of our present physiological knowledge has been derived from studies on other animals such as frogs, rabbits, cats, and dogs. When it is clear that a specific physiological process has a common basis in a wide variety of animal species, it is reasonable to assume that the same principles will apply to humans. The knowledge gained from this approach has given us an insight into human physiology and endowed us with a solid foundation for the effective treatment of many diseases.

The building blocks of the body are the cells, which are grouped together to form tissues. The principal types of tissue are epithelial, connective, nervous, and muscular, each with its own characteristics. Many connective tissues have relatively few cells but have an extensive extracellular matrix. In contrast, smooth muscle consists of densely packed layers of muscle cells linked together via specific cell junctions. Organs such as brain, heart, lungs, intestines and liver are formed by the aggregation of different kinds of tissues. The organs themselves are parts of distinct physiological systems. The heart and blood vessels form the cardiovascular system; the lungs, trachea, and bronchi together with the chest wall and diaphragm form the respiratory system; the skeleton and skeletal muscles form the musculoskeletal system; the brain, spinal cord, autonomic nerves and ganglia, and peripheral somatic nerves form the nervous system, and so on.

Cells differ widely in form and function but they all have certain common characteristics. Firstly, they are bounded by a limiting membrane, the plasma membrane. Secondly, they have the ability to break down large molecules to smaller ones to liberate energy for their activities. Thirdly, they possess a nucleus which contains genetic information in the form of deoxyribonucleic acid (DNA) at some point in their life history.

Living cells continually transform materials. They break down glucose and fats to provide energy for other activities such as motility and the synthesis of proteins for growth and repair. These chemical changes are collectively called metabolism. The breakdown of large molecules to smaller

笔记

ones is called catabolism and the synthesis of large molecules from smaller ones anabolism.

In the course of evolution, cells began to differentiate to serve different functions. Some developed the ability to contract (muscle cells), others to conduct electrical signals (nerve cells). A further group developed the ability to secrete different substances such as hormones (endocrine cells) or enzymes. During embryological development, this process of differentiation is re-enacted as many different types of cells are formed from the fertilized egg.

Most tissues contain a mixture of cell types. For example, blood consists of red cells, white cells, and platelets. Red cells transport oxygen around the body. The white cells play an important role in defending against infection and the platelets are vital components in the process of blood clotting. There are a number of different types of connective tissue but all are characterized by having cells distributed within an extensive noncellular matrix. Nerve tissue contains nerve cells and glial cells.

The Principal Organ Systems

The cardiovascular system

The cells of large multicellular animals cannot derive the oxygen and nutrients they need directly from the external environment. The oxygen and nutrients must be transported to the cells. This is one of the principal functions of the blood, which circulates within blood vessels by virtue of the pumping action of the heart. The heart, blood vessels and associated tissues form the cardiovascular system.

The heart consists of four chambers, two atria and two ventricles, which form a pair of pumps arranged side by side. The right ventricle pumps deoxygenated blood to the lungs where it absorbs oxygen from the air, while the left ventricle pumps oxygenated blood returning from the lungs to the rest of body to supply the tissues. Physiologists are concerned with establishing the factors responsible for the heartbeat, how the heart pumps the blood around the circulation, and how it is distributed to perfuse the tissues according to their needs. Fluid exchanged between the blood plasma and the tissues passes into the lymphatic system, which eventually drains back into the blood.

The respiratory system

The energy required for performing the various activities of the body is ultimately derived from respiration. This process involves the oxidation of foodstuffs to release the energy they contain. The oxygen needed for this process is absorbed from the air in the lungs and carried to the tissues by the blood. The carbon dioxide produced by the respiratory activity of the tissues is carried to the lungs by the blood in the pulmonary artery where it is excreted in the expired air. The basic questions to be answered include the following: How is the air moved in and out of the lungs? How is the volume of air breathed adjusted to meet the requirements of the body? What limits the rate of oxygen uptake in the lungs?

The digestive system

The nutrients needed by the body are derived from the diet. Food is taken in by the mouth and broken down into its component parts by enzymes in the gastrointestinal tract. The digestive products are then absorbed into the blood across the wall of the intestine and pass to the liver via the portal vein. The liver makes nutrients available to the tissues for their growth and repair and for the production of energy. In the case of the digestive system, key physiological questions are: How is food ingested? How is it broken down and digested? How are the individual nutrients absorbed? How is the food moved through the gut? How are the indigestible remains eliminated from the body?

笔记

The kidneys and urinary tract

The chief function of the kidneys is to control the composition of the extracellular fluid. In the course of this process, they also eliminate non-volatile waste products from the blood. To perform these functions, the kidneys produce urine of variable composition which is temporarily stored in the bladder before voiding. The key physiological questions in this case are: how do the kidneys regulate the composition of the blood? How do they eliminate toxic waste? How do they respond to stresses such as dehydration? What mechanisms allow the storage and elimination of the urine?

The reproductive system

Reproduction is one of the fundamental characteristics of living organisms. The gonads produce specialized sex cells known as gametes. At the core of sexual reproduction is the creation and fusion of the male and female gametes, the sperm and ova (eggs), with the result that the genetic characteristics of two separate individuals are mixed to produce offspring that differ genetically from their parents.

The musculoskeletal system

This consists of the bones of the skeleton, skeletal muscles, joints, and their associated tissues. Its primary function is to provide a means of movement, which is required for locomotion, for the maintenance of posture, and for breathing. It also provides physical support for the internal organs. Here the mechanism of muscle contraction is a central issue.

The endocrine and nervous systems

The activities of the different organ systems need to be coordinated and regulated so that they act together to meet the needs of the body. Two coordinating systems have evolved: the nervous system and the endocrine system. The nervous system uses electrical signals to transmit information very rapidly to specific cells. Thus the nerves pass electrical signals to the skeletal muscles to control their contraction. The endocrine system secretes chemical agents, hormones, which travel in the bloodstream to the cells upon which they exert a regulatory effect. Hormones play a major role in the regulation of many different organs and are particularly important in the regulation of the menstrual cycle and other aspects of reproduction.

The immune system provides the body's defenses against infection both by killing invading organisms and by eliminating diseased or damaged cells.

Although it is helpful to study how each organ performs its functions, it is essential to recognize that the activity of the body as a whole is dependent on the intricate interactions between the various organ systems. If one part fails, the consequences are found in other organ systems throughout the whole body. For example, if the kidneys begin to fail, the regulation of the internal environment is impaired which in turn leads to disorders of function elsewhere.

Homeostasis

Complex mechanisms are at work to regulate the composition of the extracellular fluid and individual cells have their own mechanisms for regulating their internal composition. The regulatory mechanisms stabilize the internal environment despite variations in both the external world and the activity of the animal. The process of stabilization of the internal environment is called homeostasis and is essential if the cells of the body are to function normally.

Taking one example, the beating of the heart depends on the rhythmical contractions of cardiac muscle cells. This activity depends on electrical signals which, in turn, depend on the concentration

笔记

of sodium and potassium ions in the extracellular and intracellular fluids. If there is an excess of potassium in the extracellular fluid, the cardiac muscle cells become too excitable and may contract at inappropriate times rather than in a coordinated manner. Consequently, the concentration of potassium in the extracellular fluid must be kept within a narrow range if the heart is to beat normally.

How Does the Body Regulate Its Own Composition?

The concept of balance

In the course of a day, an adult consumes approximately 1 kg of food and drinks 2-3 liters of fluid. In a month, this is equivalent to around 30 kg of food and 60-90 liters of fluid. Yet, in general, body weight remains remarkably constant. Such individuals are said to be in balance; the intake of food and drink matches the amounts used to generate energy for normal bodily activities plus the losses in urine and feces. In some circumstances, such as starvation, intake does not match the needs of the body and muscle tissue is broken down to provide glucose for the generation of energy. Here, the intake of protein is less than the rate of breakdown and the individual is said to have a *negative nitrogen* balance. Equally, if the body tissues are being built up, as is the case for growing children, pregnant women and athletes in the early stages of training, the daily intake of protein is greater than the normal body turnover and the individual is in *positive nitrogen* balance.

This concept of balance can be applied to any of the body constituents including water and salt and is important in considering how the body regulates its own composition. Intake must match requirements and any excess must be excreted for balance to be maintained. Additionally, for each chemical constituent of the body there is a desirable concentration range, which the control mechanisms are adapted to maintain. For example, the concentration of glucose in the plasma is about 4-5mmol/L between meals. Shortly after a meal, plasma glucose rises above this level and this stimulates the secretion of the hormone insulin by the pancreas, which acts to bring the concentration down. As the concentration of glucose falls, so does the secretion of insulin. In each case, the changes in the circulating level of insulin act to maintain the plasma glucose at an appropriate level. This type of regulation is known as negative feedback. During the period of insulin secretion, the glucose is being stored as either glycogen or fat.

A negative feedback loop is a control system that acts to maintain the level of some variables within a given range following a disturbance. Although the example given above refers to plasma glucose, the basic principle can be applied to other physiological variables such as body temperature, blood pressure, and the osmolality of the plasma. A negative feedback loop[1] requires a sensor of some kind that responds to the variable in question but not to other physiological variables.[2] Thus an osmoreceptor should respond to changes in osmolality of the body fluids but not to changes in body temperature or blood pressure. The information from the sensor must be compared in some way with the desired level by some form of comparator. If the two do not match, an error signal is transmitted to an effector, a system that can act to restore the variable to its desired level. These features of negative feedback can be appreciated by examining a simple heating system. The controlled variable is room temperature, which is sensed by a thermostat. The effector is a heater of some kind. When the room temperature falls below the set point, the temperature difference is detected by the thermostat which switches on the heater. This heats the room until the temperature reaches the pre-set level whereupon the heater is switched off.

To summarize, the body is actually a social order of about 100 trillion cells organized into different functional structures, some of which are called organs. Each functional structure contributes

笔记

its share to the maintenance of homeostatic conditions in the extracellular fluid, which is called the internal environment. As long as normal conditions are maintained in this internal environment, the cells of the body continue to live and function properly. Each cell benefits from homeostasis, and in turn, each cell contributes its share toward the maintenance of homeostasis. This reciprocal interplay provides continuous automaticity of the body until one or more functional systems lose their ability to contribute their share of function. When this happens, all the cells of the body suffer. Extreme dysfunction leads to death; moderate dysfunction leads to sickness.

Word Study

1. anabolism [ə'næbəlizəm] *n.* 合成代谢, 同化, 同化作用
2. catabolism [kə'tæbəlizəm] *n.* 分解代谢, 异化, 异化作用
3. comparator ['kɔmpəreitə] *n.* 精密度测量器, 比较仪
4. deoxygenate [di'ɔksidʒəneit] *vt.* 除去氧气; 脱氧
5. deoxyribonucleic [di:ɔksi:raibəunu:'kli:ik] *adj.* 脱氧核糖核的
6. differentiate [difə'renʃieit] *vt.&vi.* 分化, 区分, 区别, 产生差别
7. embryo ['embriəu] *n.* 胚胎, 萌芽
8. embryological [ˌembriə'lɔdʒikl] *adj.* 胚胎学的
9. endow [in'dau] *vt.* 捐助, 赋予, 使具有某种品质
10. epithelial [epi'θi:liəl] *adj.* 上皮的
11. exquisite ['ekskwizit] *adj.* 精挑细选的, 精致的, 细腻的, 强烈的
12. extracellular [ekstrə'seljulə] *adj.* 细胞外的
13. fertilized ['fə:tilaizd] *adj.* 已受精的
14. gamete ['gæmi:t] *n.* [生理] 配子, 接合体
15. ganglia ['gæŋgliə] *n.* [解剖] 神经节
16. glial ['glaiəl] *adj.* [解剖] 神经胶质的
17. glucagon ['glu:kəgən] *n.* 胰高血糖素
18. glucose ['glu:kəus] *n.* 葡萄糖
19. gonad ['gɔnæd] *n.* [解剖] 性腺; [解剖] 生殖腺
20. homeostasis [həumiə'steisis] *n.* 自动平衡, 体内平衡, 内稳态
21. hormone ['hɔ:məun] *n.* 激素
22. insulin ['insəlin] *n.* 胰岛素
23. locomotion [ləukə'məuʃ ən] *n.* 运动, 移动, 转位, 移位
24. matrix ['meitriks] *n.* [细胞] 基质, 原料
25. metabolism [me'tæbəlizəm] *n.* 新陈代谢
26. nitrogen ['naitrədʒən] *n.* 氮
27. non-volatile ['nʌn 'vɔlətail] *n. & adj.* 不易挥发物, 不易挥发的
28. osmolality [ɔsmə'læliti] *n.* 渗透浓度
29. osmoreceptor [ɔzməuri'septə] *n.* 渗透压感受器
30. potassium [pə'tæsiəm] *n.* 钾
31. reciprocal [ri'siprəkəl] *adj.* 互补的, 相互的, 相反的
32. re-enact ['ri:i'nækt, ri:in'ækt] *vt.* 再次扮演, 再次展现, 重新制定
33. sodium ['səudiəm] *n.* 钠
34. spawn [spɔ:n] *v.* 产卵, 种菌丝, 产生, 造成

Notes

1. A negative feedback loop：负反馈环是一个控制系统，生物体正常新陈代谢的必要条件是体内相对的稳态，所以需要负反馈来减弱或者阻止远离稳态的变化。简单地说，负反馈就是防止变化。负反馈调节的主要意义在于维持机体内环境的稳态。

2. A negative feedback loop requires a sensor of some kind that responds to the variable in question but not to other physiological variables. 译为：负反馈环需要某种感受器对不确定的变量产生应答，而不是对其他生理变量产生应答。句中"that"引导定语从句；"in question"在这里表示不确定的。

Exercises

1. Decide whether the following statements are true (T) or false (F) according to the passage.

(1) Much of our present physiological knowledge has been found from the experiments and studies on human beings.

(2) Living cells break down glucose and fats to provide energy for other activities, which is called catabolism.

(3) The right atrial pumps deoxygenated blood to the lungs where it absorbs oxygen from the air.

(4) The nervous system uses electrical signals to transmit information very rapidly to specific cells.

(5) With the level of sodium increasing in the extracellular fluid, the cardiac muscle cells become too excitable and may contract.

(6) A negative feedback loop is a control system that acts to maintain the level of some variables within a given range following a disturbance.

2. Questions for oral discussion.

(1) What does physiology deal with?

(2) What are the common characteristics of different forms of cells?

(3) How do you understand the concept of balance in the human body?

(4) What are the two coordinating systems and how do they perform their functions?

3. Choose the best answer to each of the following questions.

(1) Which of the following descriptions about the characteristics of physiology is wrong?

   A. It is the study of how living organisms work.

   B. It illustrates the discipline of the development and the evolution of disease and the essence of disease.

   C. It is to study the living phenomena and the function activities of living organs.

   D. It is to explain how they are regulated and integrated.

(2) Which of the following are specialized in producing force and movement?

   A. muscle cells   B. connective tissues

   C. nerve cells   D. epithelial cells

(3) The fluid environment surrounding each cell is called the _____.

   A. intracellular fluid   B. infracellular fluid

   C. internal environment   D. external environment

(4) Which of the following is not the fundamental characteristic of living organisms?

   A. metabolism   B. adaption

   C. reproduction   D. passive diffusion

(5) Which of the following is a physiological process with negative feedback?

笔记

A. blood coagulation   B. process of passing urine

C. sino-aortic baroreceptor reflex   D. process of parturition

(6) Which of the following is not the characteristic of regulation by hormone?

A. diffuse in nature   B. longer in duration

C. accurate in action   D. action in overcorrection

(7) Which of the following is not the characteristic of cells?

A. They are bound by the plasma membrane.

B. They have the ability to break down large molecules to smaller ones to liberate energy for their activities.

C. They possess a nucleus which contains genetic information in the form of deoxyribonucleic acid (DNA).

D. Living cells can not transform materials.

(8) The breakdown of large molecules to smaller ones is called _____.

A. respiration   B. anabolism

C. catabolism   D. absorption

(9) Which of the following descriptions about the characteristics of nervous regulation is wrong?

A. It responds fast.   B. It acts exactly.

C. It responds slowly.   D. Duration is short.

(10) Which of the following descriptions about the control of body function is wrong?

A. Homeostasis is kept by feedback control.

B. Negative feedback minimizes the changes, leading to stability.

C. Positive feedback is not useful.

D. Feed-forward makes human body foresee and adapt itself to the environment promptly.

4. Write down each word in the box before its corresponding definition.

> anabolism, excitability, homeostasis, hormones, internal environment, kidney, metabolism, pathology, physiology, right ventricle

(1) _____ The study of how living organisms work, the goal is to study the normal functions and their regular patterns of organs or organ systems of living organism.

(2) _____ It illustrates the discipline of the development and the evolution of disease.

(3) _____ It means all the chemical reactions in all the cells of the body, and includes all material and energy transformations that occur in the body.

(4) _____ The synthesis of large molecules from smaller ones.

(5) _____ It is the environment that all cells of the body live in the extracellular fluid.

(6) _____ It pumps deoxygenated blood to the lungs where it absorbs oxygen from the air

(7) _____ The chief function is to control the composition of the extracellular fluid.

(8) _____ Which play a major role in the regulation of many different organs and are particularly important in the regulation of the menstrual cycle and other aspects of reproduction.

(9) _____ The state maintenance of a constancy and balance in one's internal environment.

(10) _____ It is the ability of certain kinds of cells (excitable cells) to make response to the stimulus. Essentially, it is the ability of cells to generate action potential.

5. Translate the following sentences and paragraphs into Chinese.

(1) The success of physiology in explaining how organisms perform their daily tasks is based on the

笔记

notion that they are intricate and exquisite machines whose operation is governed by the laws of physics and chemistry.

(2) Metabolism, excitability, adaptability and reproduction are the basic characteristics of life activity.

(3) If there is an excess of potassium in the extracellular fluid, the cardiac muscle cells become too excitable and may contract at inappropriate times rather than in a coordinated manner.

(4) Signal transduction refers to the processes by which intercellular messengers (such as neurotransmitters, hormones and cytokines) which bind to specific receptors on or in the target cell, and are converted into biochemical and/or electrical signals within that cell.

(5) A negative feedback loop requires a sensor of some kind that responds to the variable in question but not to other physiological variables.

(6) All cells of the body are surrounded by extracellular fluid and so extracellular fluid forms the internal environment of the body. A stable internal environment is necessary for normal cell function and survival of the living organs. Homeostasis is the maintenance of a steady states in the body by coordinated physiological mechanism.

(7) Usually, a constancy of physiological variable requires a feedback mechanism that feeds the output information back to the control system so as to modify the nature of control. Negative feedback system work to restore the normal value of a variable and thus exert a stabilizing influence; while positive feedback amplifies the changes in order to finish the certain physiological process. Feedforward control mechanisms often sense a disturbance and can therefore take corrective action that anticipates changes.

Text B
General Pathology

Pathology is the science or study of disease. In its broadest sense, pathology is literally abnormal biology, the study of individuals who are ill or disordered. As a basic biologic science, pathology includes fields such as plant pathology, insect pathology, comparative pathology, as well as human pathology.

Pathology, in the context of human medicine, is not only a basic or theoretical science, but also a clinical medical specialty. Pathologists specialize in laboratory medicine; they consult with other physicians, thereby assisting in the diagnosis and treatment of disease. The scope of laboratory medicine includes all of the studies performed on patient samples, including samples of tissues, blood and other body fluids. Laboratory studies involve anatomic pathology study and assess morphologic alterations in cells and tissues. Surgical pathology, cytopathology, and autopsy pathology are included in this category. Many studies are performed using other means. These areas of clinical pathology include clinical chemistry, microbiology, hematology, immunology and immunohematology. Pathophysiology deals with the dynamic aspects of the disease process. It is the study of disordered or altered functions, for example, the physiologic changes caused by disease in a living organism.

Concept of Normalcy

Most people have some notion of normal and would define disease or illness as a deviation from or an absence of that normal state. However, on closer scrutiny, the concept of normalcy turns out to be complex and can not be defined simply; correspondingly, the concept of disease is far from simple.

笔记

Any parameter of measurement applied to an individual or group of individuals has some sort of average value that is considered normal. Average values for height, weight, and blood pressure are derived from observations on many individuals and include a certain amount of variation.

Variations in normal values occur for several reasons. First, individuals differ from one another in their genetic makeup. Thus, no two individuals in the world, except those derived from the same fertilized ovum, have exactly the same genes. Second, individuals differ in their life experiences and in their interaction with the environment. Third, in every individual there are variations in physiologic parameters because of the way in which the control mechanisms of the body function. For instance, blood glucose concentrations in a healthy person vary significantly at different times during the day, depending on food intake, activities of the individual, and so forth. These variations generally occur within a certain range. The situation is somewhat analogous to a thermostatically controlled room. The temperature may dip slightly below the desired level before such a drop is sensed by the thermostat. The corrective action triggered by the thermostat may, in turn, overshoot the ideal slightly before the heat input is halted. Indeed, such variations in body temperature, even in the normal state, occur in all individuals. Finally, for physiologic parameters measured by fairly intricate means, a significant amount of variation in observed values may result from error or imprecision inherent in the measurement process itself.

Because of these considerations, determining a normal range of variation from an average value is a complex matter. This complexity includes knowing the degree of physiologic oscillation of a particular measurement, accounting for the degree of variation among normal individuals even under baseline conditions, and figuring the precision of the measurement method.[1] Finally, the biologic significance of the measurement must be estimated. Single measurements, observations or laboratory results that seem to indicate abnormality must always be judged in the context of the entire individual. A single reading of elevated blood pressure does not make an individual hypertensive; a single slightly elevated blood glucose level does not mean that the individual is diabetic; and a single hemoglobin value lower than average does not necessarily indicate anemia.

To place the above considerations in perspective, concepts of normalcy and even of disease are, to an extent, arbitrary and influenced by cultural values as well as by biologic realities. For example, in our culture a defect of a central nervous system function may produce a significant reading disability and would be an abnormality, whereas the same defect might never be noted in a primitive culture. Furthermore, a trait that might be average and thus normal in one population might be considered distinctly abnormal in another. Consider, for instance, how a "normal" person from our population would be viewed by a group of central African pygmies[2]; or conversely, how an infant from a primitive culture, with the "normal" chronic diarrhea and poor weight gain, might be viewed in one of our well-baby clinics.

Concept of Disease

Disease can be defined as changes in individuals that cause their health parameters to fall outside the normal range. The most useful biologic yardstick for normalcy relates to the individual's ability to meet the demands placed on the body and to adapt to these demands or changes in the external environment so as to maintain reasonable constancy of the internal environment. All cells in the body need a certain amount of oxygen and nutrients for their continuing survival and function, and they also require an environment that provides narrow ranges of temperature, water content, acidity

笔记

and salt concentration. Thus, the maintenance of internal conditions within fairly narrow limits is an essential feature of the normal body. When some of the structures and functions of the body deviate from the norm to the point where the ability to maintain homeostasis is destroyed or threatened or where the individual can no longer meet environmental challenges, disease is said to exist. A person's subjective perception of disease is related to impairment of the ability to carry on daily activities comfortably.

Disease does not involve the development of a completely new form of life but rather is an extension or distortion of the normal life processes presented in the individual. Even in the case of an obviously infectious disease, where the body is literally invaded, the infectious agent itself does not constitute the disease but only evokes the changes that ultimately are manifested as disease. Thus, disease is actually the sum of the physiologic processes that have been distorted. To understand and adequately treat the disease, the identity of the normal processes interfered with, the character of the disturbances and the secondary effects of such disturbances on other vital processes must be taken into account.

A theme that will recur, with variations, throughout this volume is that disease above all is part and parcel of the patient. Normal and abnormal processes represent different points on the same continuous spectrum. In fact, the seeds of disease often lie within the adaptive mechanisms of the body itself, mechanisms that constitute a potential two-edged sword. For instance, the very same mechanism that allows us to become immune to certain infections evokes reactions such as hay fever and asthma when some of us are challenged by particular environmental agents. Similarly, the mechanism of cellular proliferation that allows us to repair wounds and constantly renew cell populations in various tissues may run amok, giving rise to cancer.

Development of Disease

Etiology

Etiology, in its most general definition, is the assignment of causes or reasons for phenomena. A description of the cause of a disease includes the identification of those factors that provoke the particular disease. Thus, the tubercle bacillus is designated as the etiologic agent of tuberculosis. Other etiologic factors in the development of tuberculosis include age, nutritional status, and even the occupation of the individual. Even in the case of an infectious disease, such as tuberculosis, the agent itself does not constitute the disease. Instead, all of the resulting responses to that agent, all the perversions of biologic processes taken together, constitute the disease.

Pathogenesis

Pathogenesis of a disease refers to the development or evolution of the disease. To continue with the above example, the pathogenesis of tuberculosis would include the mechanisms whereby the invasion of the body by the tubercle bacillus ultimately leads to the observed abnormalities.

Such an analysis would relate the proliferation and spread of tubercle bacilli to the evolving inflammatory responses, to the immunologic defenses of the body, and to the destruction of cells and tissues. The pattern and extent of the tissue damage would be ultimately related to the overt manifestations of disease. Pathogenesis also takes into account the sequential occurrence of certain phenomena and the temporal aspects of the evolving disease. A given disease is not static, but it is a dynamic phenomenon with a rhythm and natural history of its own. In the diagnostic evaluation of patients and the assessment of therapy, it is essential to keep in mind this concept of natural history

笔记

and the range of variation among different diseases with respect to their natural history. Some diseases characteristically have a rapid onset, whereas others have a long prodrome. Some diseases are self-limited, that is, they clear up spontaneously in a brief time. Others become chronic, and still others are subject to frequent remissions and exacerbations.

When considering the totality of human disease, the number of etiologic factors and the number of separately named diseases seem to be endless. However, the situation is not as difficult as indicated by sheer numbers. The response mechanisms of the body are finite. Therefore, disease A differs from disease B because it varies somewhat in terms of this or that pathogenetic mechanism being exaggerated. Thus, understanding a manageable number of pathogenetic mechanisms and their evolution permits understanding of a large number of seemingly different diseases.

Manifestations

Early in the development of a disease, the etiologic agent or agents may provoke a number of changes in biologic processes that can be detected by laboratory analysis even though there are no subjective symptoms. Thus, many diseases have a subclinical stage, during which the patient functions normally even though the disease processes are well established. The structure and function of many organs provide a large reserve or safety margin, and functional impairment may become evident only when the disease has become quite advanced. For example, chronic renal disease could completely destroy one kidney and partly destroy the other before any symptoms related to decreased renal function would be perceived. However, some diseases seem to begin as functional derangements and actually become clinically evident although no anatomic abnormalities can be detected at the time. Such functional illnesses may lead to secondary structural abnormalities.

As certain biologic processes are encroached on, the patient begins to feel subjectively that something is wrong. These subjective feelings are called symptoms of disease. By definition, symptoms are subjective and can be reported only by the patient to an observer. However, when manifestations of the disease can be objectively identified by an observer, these are termed signs of the disease. Nausea, malaise, and pain are symptoms, whereas fever, reddening of the skin, and a palpable mass are signs of disease. A demonstrable structural change produced in the course of a disease is referred to as a lesion. Lesions may be evident at a gross and/or a microscopic level. The outcome of a disease is sometimes referred to as a sequel. For example, the sequel to an inflammatory process in a given tissue might be a scar in that tissue. The sequel to acute rheumatic inflammation of the heart might be scarred, deformed cardiac valves. A complication of a disease is a new or separate process that may arise secondarily because of sonic change produced by the original entity. For example, bacterial pneumonia may be a complication of viral infection of the respiratory tract. Fortunately, many diseases can also undergo what is termed resolution, and the host returns to a completely normal state, without sequelae or complications. Resolution can occur spontaneously, that is, owing to body defenses, or it can result from successful therapy.

Finally, it is essential to reemphasize that disease is dynamic rather than static. The manifestations of disease in a given patient may change from day to day as biologic equilibria shift or as compensatory mechanisms are brought into play. Environmental influences brought to bear on the patient will also affect the disease. Therefore, every disease has a range of manifestations and a spectrum of expressions that may vary from patient to patient.

笔记

Word Study

1. amok [ə'mɔk] *adv.* 狂乱地
2. analogous [ə'næləgəs] *adj.* 类似的，相似的，可比拟的
3. compensatory [kəm'pensətəri] *adj.* 代偿的，补偿的
4. constancy ['kɔnstənsi] *n.* 恒定状态
5. chronic ['krɔnik] *adj.* 慢性的
6. cytopathology [saitəupə'θɔlədʒi] *n.* 细胞病理学
7. deformed [di'fɔ:md] *adj.* 畸形的
8. diabetic [ˌdaiə'betik] *adj.* 糖尿病的；*n.* 糖尿病患者
9. encroach [in'krəutʃ] *v.* 侵犯，侵占，侵害
10. equilibrium [ˌi:kwi'libriəm] *n.* 均衡，平衡
11. etiology [ˌi:ti'ɔlədʒi] *n.* 病因学
12. exacerbation [igzæsə'beiʃən] *n.* 恶化，加重
13. hematology ['hi:mə'tɔlədʒi] *n.* 血液学
14. hemoglobin [ˌhi:məu'gləubin] *n.* 血红蛋白
15. immunohematology [ˌimjunəuˌhi:mə'tɔlədʒi] *n.* 免疫血液学
16. malaise [mæ'leiz] *n.* 不适
17. morphologic [ˌmɔ:fə'lɔdʒik] *adj.* 形态学的
18. oscillation [ˌɔsi'leiʃən] *n.* 摆动，振动
19. overt ['əuvə:t] *adj.* 显性的，公开的
20. parameter [pə'ræmitə] *n.* 参数，参量
21. pathogenesis [ˌpæθə'dʒenisis] *n.* 发病机制
22. perversion [pə'və:ʃən] *n.* 变态，倒错，反常
23. prodrome ['prəudrəum] *n.* 前驱症状；先兆
24. remission [ri'miʃən] *n.* 缓解，减轻，弛张
25. sequel ['si:kwəl] *n.* 后遗症，后果，继续
26. static ['stætik] *adj.* 静止的，静位的，不动的
27. subclinical [sʌb'klinikl] *adj.* 临床症状不显的，亚临床的
28. temporal ['tempərəl] *adj.* 暂时的，当时的
29. thermostat ['θə:məstæt] *n.* 恒温器，自动调温器，温度调节装置
30. trigger ['trigə] *v.* 触发，使运行

Notes

1. This complexity includes knowing the degree of physiologic oscillation of a particular measurement, accounting for the degree of variation among normal individuals even under baseline conditions, and figuring the precision of the measurement method. 译为：这种复杂性包括了解一个特定测量工具在生理学上的摆动值，计算出正常个体在基线条件下的变化值，并且计算出测量方法的精确度。该句的结构是主＋谓＋宾，宾语部分由三个动名词短语"knowing, accounting for, figuring"构成并列结构。

2. central African pygmies：俾格米人，分布在非洲中部以及亚洲的安达曼群岛、马来半岛、菲律宾和大洋洲某些岛屿。俾格米人的体质特征是身材矮小，头大腿短，皮肤暗黑，鼻宽唇薄，头发卷曲，体毛发达。依靠狩猎采集为生，处于比较原始的状态。非洲俾格米人又称尼格利

笔记

罗人,亚洲俾格米人又称尼格利陀人,两词皆出自西班牙文。

Supplementary Parts

1.   Medical and Pharmaceutical Terms Made Easier (1)

(1)   How to Build your Medical and Pharmaceutical English Vocabulary

1)   英语词汇构成基础知识:英语和其他语言一样,其词汇是由词素(morpheme)结合而构成的,词素是语言中最小的包含有意义的单位,是不能再分的最小的语言结构单位。

英语词素按其功能可分为变词词素和构词词素,前者指那些语法范畴中表示语法作用的构形词缀,后者根据其在构词过程中的作用可分为词根词素和附加词素,词根词素是词汇意义的基本组成部分,附加词素是指那些依附于词根(或词干)的词素,词根(root)是构词的主要部分,是词的核心部分,附加成分是词的辅助部分,叫做构词词缀(affix)。

词素按其构词性质可以分为自由词素(free morpheme)及黏着词素(bound morpheme),前者指那些可以作为有独特意义的词来使用的词素,如 act、quick 等,它们可以单词形式单独出现,也可以和各种构词词素自由结合,而后者指那些不能作为一个有独立意义的词来使用的词素,如 reject 中的"re-"和"-ject",英语单词中的派生词和合成词是以这两种类型的词素作为构词成分的。

2)   英语词汇的构成方法:在现代英语中,词汇结构主要有四种类型,即:①根词(简单词);②派生词;③复合词和结合词;④缩略词。

从构词方法上来看有派生法(derivation 或 affixation);转化法(conversion);合成法(或合词法)(composition);缩略法(shortening);逆生法(back-formation)等。在科技英语中,还经常会见到从人名、地名、神名、星座名等造词的现象。

下面分别介绍几种常见的构词法:

A.   派生法(derivation):在一个词根或词干上增加构词词缀,从而构成新词。

如:electron(电子)+-ics → electronics 电子学

infra(外、超出)+red(红)→ infrared 红外线

pleur(肋膜、胸膜)+-itis(炎症)→ pleuritis 胸膜炎

总体上讲,构词词缀(前后缀)相对数量较少,因而较易掌握,而能否记住大量的词根便成了词汇识记的关键,尤其是在科技词汇中,涉及大量的学科名词术语,需要记忆大量的相关词根,难易显而易见,然而世上无难事,只怕有心人,只要我们用心去记去学,在掌握规律性方法的前提之下,记忆大量的专业术语词根,这样我们完全可以真正提高专业英语词汇的数量及记忆效果。

B.   转化法(conversion):这主要是指词类的转化,而且一般涉及比较简单的词,因此掌握起来比较容易,但切记不要创造性地使用词汇,否则会闹出一些笑话,比如将 instead 错用作动词等。

C.   合成法(composition):把两个或两个以上的单词(词干或词根)组合起来构成新词,在英语词汇构成中是一种很常见的方法,如 weekend、workload、spaceship 等,这种方法可以构成不同词类的合成词。

D.   缩略法(shortening):随着现代英语词汇的不断发展,缩略法被广泛用来构成一些含义丰富的词和略语,科技英语中尤其如此。缩略词就结构而言可以分为紧缩词(或拼缀词)(blends)、音节缩略词(clipping)及字母缩略词(acronyms)三大类,下面分别举例:

①紧缩词(blends)

brunch = breakfast + lunch

motel = motor + hotel

smog = smoke + fog

笔记

heliport = helicopter + airport

newscast = news + broadcast

travelog = travel + catalog

②音节缩略词（clipping）

advertisement → ad 或 advert

examination → exam

laboratory → lab

memorandum → memo

microphone → mike

photograph → photo

public house → pub

telephone → phone

aeroplane → plane

influenza → flu

refrigerator → fridge

③字母缩略词（acronyms）

AIDS → acquired immune deficiency syndrome

Laser → light amplification by stimulated emission of radiation

Radar → radio detecting and ranging

UFO → unidentified flying objects

CNS → central nervous system

HSLC → high speed liquid chromatography

UVL → ultraviolet light

E.　逆生法（back-formation）: 这是指删除派生词词缀的构词法。

television → televise *v.* 播放电视

laser → lase *v.* 放射激光

diagnosis → diagnose *v.* 诊断

burglar → burgle *v.* 撬门而入

editor → edit *v.* 编辑

以上介绍了几种常见的构词法，结合医药英语词汇的特点，以及中高级英语学习的特点，建议大家重点关注如何通过识记一定量的词素来达到识记并牢记大量词汇而展开。

3)　如何学习医药科技英语词汇：在医药英语词汇课程的教学中特别重视培养学生的医药英语的词汇能力，而不仅仅是向学生介绍大量的科技词汇。在现代英语中，词汇结构主要有四种类型，即根词（简单词）、派生词、复合词和结合词以及缩略词，因此整个课程的教学往往从英语构词法入手，介绍派生法（derivation 或 affixation）、转化法（conversion）、合成法（或合词法）(composition)、缩略法（shortening）以及逆生法（back-formation）等。

分析医药英语词汇的特点之后我们不难发现，它们主要有四种形式：

A. 基础词汇型：指基础英语词汇在科技英语中被赋予新的含义，如 addition 加成、lead 铅等；

B. 科技缩略型：指用首字母将由两个以上词汇或词根组成的术语用缩略字母来代表，如 AIDS 代表 acquired immune deficiency syndrome 艾滋病、HPLC 代表 high performance liquid chromatography 高效液相色谱、DNA 代表 deoxyribonucleic acid 脱氧核糖核酸等；

C. 专业术语型：指一般不用缩略、在某些专业领域使用的词汇，如 leukocyte 白细胞、hypercalcemia 高钙血（症）；

笔记

D. 专有名词型：指由人名、地名、神名、星座名等造词的现象来表达的术语，如 volt 伏特是由意大利物理学家 Alessandro Volt(1745－1827) 的姓氏而来，polonium 钋是由居里夫人的祖国波兰(Poland)得名的。

除了以上四种类型词汇之外，大多数科技英语词汇均可用现代英语构词法来进行解释，所以现代英语构词法对医药英语词汇的学习同样具有实际指导意义。

(2)   Common Morphemes in Terms of English for Physiology and Pathology

Morpheme	Meaning	Example
acus	听觉	paracusis 听觉倒错，错听
alg	疼痛	analgia 痛觉缺乏，无痛
anaphyl	过敏	anaphylatoxin 过敏毒素
ancyl, ankyl	弯曲	ankylosis 关节强硬，关节强直
anomal	异常	anomalous 异常的
asthen	无力，衰弱	asthenia 无力，虚弱
atel	发育不全	atelectasis 肺不张
carcin	癌	carcinoma 癌
choler	霍乱	cholera 霍乱
copr	粪	coprology 粪便学
crin	分泌	endocrine 内分泌
crypt	隐	cryptitis 隐窝炎
dacry	泪	dacryagogue 催泪剂
diabet	糖尿病	diabetes 糖尿病，多尿症
digest	消化	digestion 消化
diphther	白喉	diphtheria 白喉
ectas	扩张	ectasia 扩张，膨胀
edem	水肿	edema 水肿
emes, emet	呕吐	emesis 呕吐
emia	血症	anoxemia 缺氧血症
epidem	流行病	epidemic 流行性的，流行病
esthes, esthet	感觉	esthesia 感觉，知觉
fert	生育	fertility 生育力；多产，肥沃
galact	乳	galactagogue 催乳剂
gen	原	antigen 抗原
genit	生殖	generation 生殖，世代
gest	妊娠	progesterone 孕酮，黄体酮
gon	生殖；精液；淋病	gonosome 性染色体；gonococcus 淋球菌
gravid	妊娠	unigravida 初孕妇
hallucin	幻觉	hallucinogen 致幻剂
helc	溃疡	helcoid 溃疡状的
hemat	血	hematology 血液学
hered	遗传	heredity 遗传
hidr	汗	hidrosis 多汗
hormon	激素	parahormone 副激素
hypn	睡眠	hypnagogic 催眠的
hyster	癔症	hysteria 癔病，歇斯底里
immun	免疫	immunology 免疫学
kines	运动	kinematics 运动学
lacrim	泪	lacrimator 催泪的
lact	乳	lacteal 乳状的；lactate 乳酸
lymph	淋巴	lymphadenitis 淋巴结炎

续表

Morpheme	Meaning	Example
malac	软	malacia 软化症
man	疯狂	monomania 偏狂
meno	月经	menopause 绝经
menstru	月经	menstruation 月经
ment	精神	amentia 精神错乱
morb	病	morbid 病态的, 疾病的
muc	黏液	mucoid 黏液样的
narc	睡眠, 麻醉	narcolepsy 发作性睡眠病; narcotic analgesic 麻醉性镇痛药
nat	分娩、生产	neonatal 新生的
nos	病	nosology 疾病分类学
nutr	营养	nutrient 营养的, 营养物
odyn	疼痛	odynophagia 吞咽痛
onc	肿瘤	oncology 肿瘤学
osm	嗅觉	osmoreceptor 嗅觉感受器
oz	臭	ozena 臭鼻症
par	分娩	primipara 初产妇
part	分娩	parturifacient 催产的, 催产剂
path	情感	empathy 移情
path	病	pathology 病理学
pector	痰	expectoration 痰, 咳痰
pept, peps	消化	dyspepsia 消化不良
phag	吞噬	phagosome 吞噬体
phor	隐斜视	heterophoria 隐斜视
phren	精神	phrenic 精神的, 膈的
physi	生理	physiology 生理学
phyt	生长	exophytic 外部生长的
plas	发育	metaplasia（组织）化生
pleg	麻痹	diplegia 双瘫
pnea	呼吸	eupnea 正常呼吸（平静呼吸）
prax	运动	apraxia 运用不能症
pregn	妊娠	pregnancy 妊娠, 怀孕
psych	精神	psychiatry 精神病学
pyo-	脓	pyemia 脓血症
rheumat	风湿	rheumatic 风湿性的
rig	硬	rigid 刚硬的, 刚性的
saliv	唾液	salivation 流涎, 多涎
sanguin	血	exsanguinate 放血, 使无血
schist, schiz	裂	diaschisis 神经机能联系不能
scler	硬	sclerema 硬化病
secret	分泌	secretory 分泌的
semin	精液	semen 精液, 种子
sens	情感	sensation 感觉, 知觉
seps, sept	腐烂	septic 腐败性的, 败血病的
sequestr	死骨	sequestrum 死骨
ser	血清	serology 血清学
skat	粪	skatology 粪便学
somn	睡眠	somnambulism 梦游症
sorb, sorpt	吸收	absorption 吸收

笔记

续表

Morpheme	Meaning	Example
spasm	痉挛	spasmolysis 解痉作用
sphygm	脉搏	sphygmomanometer 血压计
spir	呼吸	spirograph 呼吸描记器
sten	狭窄	stenosis 狭窄
steril	不育	sterilizaton 绝育，灭菌
stimul	刺激	stimulation 刺激，兴奋
stip	便秘	constipation 便秘
syphil	梅毒	syphilis 梅毒
terat	畸形，畸胎	teratology 畸形学，畸胎学
tetan	破伤风	tetanus 破伤风；强直
thromb	血栓	thrombus 血栓
thromb	血小板	thrombocyte 血小板
traumat	外伤，创伤	trauma 外伤，创伤
trop	斜视	esotropia 内斜视
trophy	营养	amyotrophy 肌萎缩
tubercul	结核，结节	tuberculin 卷曲霉素
tum	肿，瘤	tumefaction 肿胀，肿大
typh	伤寒	typhoid 伤寒
typhl	盲	typhlosis 盲，视觉缺乏
ulcer	溃疡	ulceration 溃疡形成
urin	尿	urination 排尿
varic	曲张	varicocele 精索静脉曲张
varicell	水痘	varicelloid 水痘样的
venere	性	venereology 性病学

(3)　Fill in the blanks with the missing word root, prefix or suffix.

1)　an_____ia 痛觉缺乏

2)　_____ectasis 肺不张

3)　_____atoxin 过敏毒素

4)　endo_____ 内分泌

5)　_____osis 关节强硬

6)　_____ambulism 梦游症

7)　pro_____erone 孕酮，黄体酮

8)　_____agogue 催乳剂

9)　_____oid 溃疡状的

10)　_____ology 血液学

11)　_____ema 硬化病

12)　_____olepsy 发作性睡眠病

(4)　Word-matching.

1) ectasia	A. 副激素
2) anoxemia	B. 正常呼吸
3) parahormone	C. 感觉，知觉
4) menopause	D. 缺氧血症
5) dyspepsia	E. 血小板
6) eupnea	F. 解痉作用

续表

7) thrombocyte	G. 消化不良
8) exsanguinate	H. 扩张，膨胀
9) sensation	I. 外部生长的
10) spasmolysis	J. 血栓
11) thrombus	K. 绝经
12) exophytic	L. 放血，使无血

2. English-Chinese Translation Skills: 药学英语词汇特点与翻译

药学英语属于科技英语，具有科技英语的特点。药学英语词汇一般主要有四个特点：专业术语多；两栖词汇多；隐喻性词汇；首字母缩略词汇多。

(1) 专业术语多：药学英语涉及范围广，关联学科多，不仅含有药学领域专业词汇，还有很多相关领域词汇，包括：生理学、病理学、微生物学等。药学英语专业词汇数量虽多，但是语义固定，绝大多数可以通过专业词典找到汉语完全对等词，直译即可。如果词典中找不到对应词，可以采用以下三种办法：①分析原词的组成结构，拆分词根，造出对应的汉语表达。如：glycerol phenylbutyrate 可以译为"苯丁酸甘油酯"，因为 glycerol 意思是"甘油"，而 phenylbutyrate 是"丁酸苯酯"，再根据汉语表达习惯将化合物的译名顺序稍加调整就可以了。②如果在语义上难以造出对应的新词，可以考虑音译法。例如：viagra（伟哥、万艾可）。③意译与音译相结合。例如：carbidopa-levodopa 中的 levo 有"左旋的"的意思，该词可译为"卡比多巴-左旋多巴"（一种延迟释放制剂）。同理，hydrocodone 可译为"含氢可酮"。

(2) 两栖词汇是指那些既可以用于普通领域，又可以用于专业领域的词汇。药学英语中很多普通英语词汇被赋予了专业含义。翻译这类词汇，要结合上下文语境，参考专业词典或查阅相关资料。例如，administration 在普通英语中表示"行政管理""管理层"等意思，但在医药领域则是"给药""用药"的意思。其动词形式是 administer。有些两栖词汇在医药学不同学科内的意思也有差别，如 develop 在普通英语中意思是"发展"，在薄层色谱法中表示"显色"，而在描述微生物概念时则表示"生长"；formulation 在普通英语中意思是"规划，制定"，表示药物配方时可译为"处方"，表示药物制品时则应译为"制剂"。

(3) 药学英语中也有一些词汇存在隐喻现象，在翻译中应该采用直译还是意译要根据具体情况具体分析。如 orphan drugs 可以直接翻译成"孤儿药"，这种药物是指用于治疗罕见病的药物，适用人群少，销量有限，大部分医药公司不愿意投资研发，就好像"孤儿"一样无人照管，这种直译可保留原词的隐喻义，也为业界普遍接受。但是，隐喻性药学专业名词也不都采用直译法翻译，如，sandwich ELISA（夹心 ELISA）是用于测量抗原量的酶联免疫吸附法，在该测定法中被测量的抗原需要与上下两层抗体相结合，恰如汉堡的结构，由此得名。但如果直译为"汉堡 ELISA"则感觉缺乏科学的严谨性，因此意译为"夹心 ELISA"。同样，sandwiched osmotic tablet system 可译为"三层渗透泵片"。

(4) 首字母缩略词是指把构成术语的多个单词用它们各自开头字母大写缩略而成的特殊单词，医药英语中大量使用首字母缩略词。例如：BPC(bulk pharmaceutical chemicals, 原料药)、CFU(colony forming unit, 菌落形成单位)、USP(United States Pharmacopoeia, 美国药典)、OTC(over the counter, 非处方药品)、BBB (blood brain barrier, 血脑屏障)、QSAR (quantitative structure-activity relationship, 定量构效关系)等。这些缩略词都有规范译法，直接采用即可。有些缩略词可以分别表示不同术语意思，例如，TDD 既可以表示 transdermal delivery system（透皮给药系统）又可以表示 targeted delivery system(靶向给药系统)，要根据具体语境选择正确词义进行翻译。

笔记

Unit Two Microbiology

Life on earth is impossible without microorganisms, which are the ancestors of all living systems. Microbiology encompasses the whole of studying microscopic organisms, such as bacteria, protozoa, fungi, some types of algae and viruses. It has made contributions to many fields of human beings' life, including pharmacy. Pharmaceutical microbiology is one of the many facets of applied microbiology, having a special bearing on pharmacy in all its aspects. This will range from the manufacture and quality control of pharmaceutical products to an understanding of the mode of action of antibiotics. The further study of microbiology may help us understand some of the mysteries of living things and their greater applications will be available.

地球上的生命不可能离开微生物而存在，它们是所有生物系统的祖先。微生物学涉及所有的微生物研究，如细菌、原生动物、真菌、各种藻类和病毒，在人类生活中的很多方面做出了贡献，其中包括药学。药学微生物学是应用微生物学中的许多学科之一，在药学领域具有特殊意义。涉及范围从药品生产及其质量控制到了解抗生素的作用机制，进一步深入研究微生物学会有助于我们了解生物的奥秘并使其得到更广泛的应用。

笔记

Text A
The History of Microbiology

Microbiology is a broad term which includes virology, mycology, parasitology, bacteriology and other branches. A microbiologist is a specialist in microbiology and these other topics. The studies of microbes are conducted actively, and the field is advancing continually. It is estimated only about one percent of all of the microbe species on earth have been studied. Although microbes were directly observed over three hundred years ago, the field of microbiology can be said to be in its infancy relative to older biological disciplines such as zoology and botany.

In ancient times, the existence of microorganisms was hypothesized for many centuries before their actual discovery. Jainism postulated the existence of unseen microbiological life as early as 6th century BC. Mahavira[1](540−486 BC), one of the founders of Jainism, asserted existence of unseen microbiological creatures living in earth, water, and air. Jain scriptures also describe the microscopic creatures living in large clusters and having a very short life, which are said to pervade each and every part of the universe, even in tissues of plants and flesh of animals. Marcus Terentius Varro[2] (116−27 BC), made references to microbes when he warned against locating a homestead in the vicinity of swamps "because there are bred certain minute creatures which cannot be seen by the eyes, which float in the air and enter the body through the mouth and nose and which cause serious diseases." [3] In 1546, Girolamo Fracastoro[4] put forward the view that diseases were caused by particles too small to be seen, which could transmit infection by direct or indirect contact, or even without contact over long distances. He named the responsible agent a *contagium vivum*. However, early claims about the existence of microorganisms were speculative, and not based on any data or observation. Actual observation and discovery of microbes had to await the invention of the microscope in the 17th century.

Athanasius Kircher[5], a Jesuit priest scholar, using simple lenses of low magnification in 1671, stated that he observed peculiar "worms" in the blood of persons suffering from plague and considered these were the agents responsible for the disease. One of his books contains a chapter in Latin, which reads in translation: "Concerning the wonderful structure of things in nature, investigated by Microscope." Here, he wrote "who would believe that vinegar and milk abound with an innumerable multitude of worms." He also noted that putrid material is full of innumerable creeping animalcule. After Kircher's observation, Antonie van Leeuwenhoek[6], a Dutch draper whose hobby was the preparation of lenses, observed in 1676 bacteria and other microorganisms, using a single-lens microscope of his own design.

Bacteriology, a subdiscipline of microbiology later, was founded in the 19th century by Ferdinand Cohn[7], a botanist whose studies on algae and photosynthetic bacteria led him to describe several bacteria including bacillus and beggiatoa. Cohn was also the first to formulate a scheme for the taxonomic classification of bacteria and discover spores. Louis Pasteur[8] and Robert Koch[9] were contemporaries of Cohn's and are often considered to be the father of microbiology and medical microbiology, respectively. Pasteur is most famous for his series of experiments designed to disprove the then widely held theory of spontaneous generation, thereby solidifying microbiology's identity as a biological science. Pasteur also designed methods for food preservation and vaccines against several diseases such as anthrax, fowl cholera and rabies. Koch is best known for his contributions to the germ theory of disease, proving that specific diseases were caused by specific pathogenic microorganisms. He developed a series of criteria that have become known as the Koch's postulates. Koch was one of the first scientists to focus on the isolation of bacteria in pure culture resulting in his description of several novel bacteria including *Mycobacterium tuberculosis*, the causative agent of tuberculosis.

While Pasteur and Koch are often considered the founders of microbiology, their work did not accurately reflect the true diversity of the microbial world because of their exclusive focus on microorganisms having direct medical relevance. It was not until the late 19th century and the work of Martinus Beijerinck[10] and Sergei Winogradsky[11], the founders of general microbiology (an older term encompassing aspects of microbial physiology, diversity and ecology), that the true breadth of microbiology was revealed. Beijerinck made two major contributions to microbiology: the discovery of viruses and the development of enrichment culture techniques. While his work on the Tobacco Mosaic Virus established the basic principles of virology, it was his development of enrichment culturing that had the most immediate impact on microbiology by allowing for the cultivation of a wide range of microbes with wildly different physiologies. Winogradsky was the first to develop the concept of chemolithotrophy and to thereby reveal the essential role played by microorganisms in geochemical processes. He was responsible for the first isolation and description of both nitrifying and nitrogen-fixing bacteria.

Microorganisms affect the well-being of people in a great many ways and occur in large numbers in most natural environments. They may be tiny, but the relatively new science of microbiology is huge! Prokaryotic bacteria, eukaryotic fungi, and nonliving viruses are just some of the microbes that have much effect on our health and environment. The field of microbiology can be generally divided into several subdisciplines, such as microbial physiology, microbial genetics, cellular microbiology, veterinary microbiology, environmental microbiology, evolutionary microbiology, industrial microbiology, food microbiology, agricultural microbiology, medical microbiology, pharmaceutical microbiology, etc.

Some microbes are beneficial and others are detrimental. While there are undoubtedly some who fear all microbes due to the association of some microbes with various human illnesses, many microbes are actually also responsible for numerous beneficial processes such as industrial fermentation (e.g. the production of alcohol, vinegar and dairy products), antibiotic production and as vehicles for cloning in higher organisms such as plants. Scientists have also exploited their knowledge of microbes to produce biotechnologically important enzymes, such as Taq polymerase, reporter genes for use in other genetic systems and novel molecular biology techniques.

A variety of biopolymers, such as polysaccharides, polyesters and polyamides, are produced by microorganisms. Microorganisms are used for the biotechnological production of biopolymers with tailored properties suitable for high-value medical application such as tissue engineering and drug delivery. Microorganisms are used for the biosynthesis of xanthan, alginate, cellulose, cyanophycin, levan, hyaluronic acid, organic acids, etc.

Microorganisms are also beneficial for microbial biodegradation or bioremediation of domestic, agricultural and industrial wastes and subsurface pollution in soils, sediments and marine environments. The ability of each microorganism to degrade toxic waste depends on the nature of each contaminant. Since sites typically have multiple pollutant types, the most effective approach to microbial biodegradation is to use a mixture of bacterial species and strains, each specific to the

笔记

biodegradation of one or more types of contaminants.

Although there are various claims concerning the contributions to human and animal health by consuming probiotics, the bacteria potentially beneficial to the digestive system, and/or prebiotics, the substances consumed to promote the growth of probiotic microorganisms, their health benefits are numerous. Probiotics have been proven to help relieve symptoms of lactose intolerance, boost the immune system, and prevent diarrhea and colon cancer. Prebiotics have been shown to relieve constipation and diarrhea, and reduce the chances of osteoporosis and Type 2 diabetes.

Microbiology has not only made important contributions to many disciplines but also affected both medicine and pharmacy a lot. Medical microbiology is the study of the pathogenic microbes and the role of microbes in human illness, which includes the study of microbial pathogenesis and epidemiology and is related to the study of disease pathology and immunology. Pharmaceutical microbiology is considered the part of industrial microbiology that is responsible for creating medications. Microorganisms are used to produce human or animal biologicals such as insulin, growth hormone, and antibodies. Diagnostic assays that use monoclonal antibody, DNA probe technology or real-time PCR are used as rapid tests for pathogenic organisms in the clinical laboratory.

Recent research has suggested that microorganisms could be useful in the treatment of diseases, such as cancer. Research shows that clostridia can selectively target cancer cells. Various strains of non-pathogenic clostridia have been shown to infiltrate and replicate within solid tumors. Clostridia therefore have the potential to deliver therapeutic proteins to tumors. Lactobacillus and other lactic acid bacteria possess numerous potential therapeutic properties including anti-inflammatory and anti-cancer activities.

Vaccines are used to combat infectious diseases, however, the last decade has witnessed a revolution in the approach to vaccine design and development. Sophisticated technologies such as genomics, proteomics, functional genomics, and synthetic chemistry can be used for the rational identification of antigens, the synthesis of complex glycans, and the generation of engineered carrier proteins.

Members of the streptomyces genus are among the most prolific microorganisms producing secondary metabolites with wide uses in medicine and in agriculture. These organisms have a complex secondary metabolism producing antibiotic compounds and other metabolites with medicinal properties. Genomic studies, genomic mining and biotechnological approaches are being employed in the search for new antibiotics and other drugs in streptomyces.

What stated above demonstrates how applied microbiology is intertwined with human history. In the modern era, the potential applications for microorganisms and their products are vast and include the generation of high-value products such as drugs, chemicals, fuels and even electricity. Furthermore, recent advances in systems biology and synthetic biology now make it possible to engineer desirable characteristics in a microorganism, allowing them to be tailored to a specific task.

Word Study

1. algae ['ældʒiː] *n.* 藻类
2. alginate ['ældʒineit] *n.* 藻朊酸盐，藻酸盐
3. animalcule [ˌæni'mælkjuːl] *n.* 微生物，微小动物
4. anthrax ['ænθræks] *n.* 炭疽病
5. bacillus [bə'siləs] *n.* (复数 bacilli) 杆菌，芽胞杆菌，细菌

笔记

6. beggiatoa [beˈdʒiætəuə] *n.* 贝日阿托菌

7. biopolymer [ˌbaiəuˈpɔlimə] *n.* 生物聚合物，生物高分子

8. contaminant [kənˈtæminənt] *n.* 污染物，杂质

9. cellulose [ˈseljuləus] *n.* 纤维素；（植物的）细胞膜质

10. chemolithotrophy [keməliˈθɔtrəfi] *n.* 矿质化学营养，无机化能营养

11. cholera [ˈkɔlərə] *n.* 霍乱

12. clostridia [klɔsˈtridiə] *n.* （单数 clostridium）梭状芽孢杆菌

13. contagium vivum [ˌkənˈteidʒiəm ˈvaivəm] *n.* 接触传染物，活传染源

14. cyanophycin [ˌsaiənəuˈfaisin] *n.* 藻青素

15. detrimental [ˌdetriˈmentl] *adj.* 不利的，有害的

16. diarrhea [ˌdaiəˈriə] *n.* 腹泻，痢疾

17. eukaryotic [juːˌkæriˈɔtik] *adj.* 真核的，真核生物的

18. fermentation [ˌfəːmenˈteiʃən] *n.* 发酵

19. fowl [faul] *n.* 家禽，鸟，禽；*vi.* 打鸟，捕野禽

20. fungi [ˈfʌŋgai, ˈfʌŋgiː] *n.* （单数 fungus）真菌，菌类，蘑菇

21. glycan [ˈglaikæn] *n.* 聚糖，多糖

22. hyaluronic acid [ˈhaiəljuˈrɔnik ˈæsid] [生化] 透明质酸，玻璃酸

23. Jainism [ˈdʒainizm] *n.* 印度耆那教

24. lactobacillus [ˌlæktəubəˈsiləs] *n.* 乳酸菌；乳杆菌属

25. lactose [ˈlæktəus] *n.* 乳糖

26. levan [ˈlevæn] *n.* 果聚糖；无酵母面团

27. mycobacterium [ˌmaikəubækˈtiəriəm] *n.* 分枝杆菌

28. mycology [maiˈkɔlədʒi] *n.* 真菌学，霉菌学

29. nitrifying [ˈnaitrifaiiŋ] *adj.* 硝化的

30. nitrogen-fixing [ˈnaitrədʒən ˈfiksiŋ] *adj.* 固氮的

31. osteoporosis [ˌɔstiəupəˈrəusis] *n.* 骨质疏松症

32. parasitology [ˌpærəsiˈtɔlədʒi] *n.* 寄生虫学，寄生物学

33. polyamide [ˌpɔliˈæmaid] *n.* 聚酰胺，尼龙

34. polyester [ˌpɔliˈestə] *n.* 聚酯，涤纶

35. polysaccharide [ˌpɔliˈsækəraid] *n.* 多糖

36. probiotics [ˌprəbaiˈɔtiks] *n.* 益生菌，原生菌

37. prokaryotic [prəukæriˈɔtik] *adj.* 原核的

38. protozoa [ˌprəutəˈzəuə] *n.* 原生生物（单数 protozoan）

39. putrid [ˈpjuːtrid] *adj.* 〔动植物〕腐烂的

40. rabies [ˈreibiːz] *n.* 狂犬病

41. real-time PCR (polymerase chain reaction 的缩写) 实时聚合酶链反应

42. sophisticated [səˈfistikeitid] *adj.* 复杂的，精致的

43. sediment [ˈsedimənt] *n.* 沉积物，沉淀物；*v.* 沉积

44. spontaneous generation [spɔnˈteiniəs ˌdʒenəˈreiʃn] *n.* 无生源说；自然发生说

45. spore [spɔː] *n.* 孢子

46. streptomyces [streptəuˈmaisiːz] *n.* （单复同）链霉菌属

47. taxonomic [ˌtæksəˈnɔmik] *adj.* [生物] 分类（学）的

笔记

48. Tobacco Mosaic Virus [təˈbækəu məˈzeiik ˈvairəs] *n.* 烟草花叶病病毒

49. tuberculosis [tjuːˌbəːkjuˈləusis] *n.* 结核病

50. veterinary [ˈvetərinəri] *n.* 兽医；*adj.* 兽医的

51. vicinity [viˈsiniti] *n.* 附近，邻近（地区），近处

52. xanthan [ˈzænθən] *n.* 黄原胶

Notes

1. Mahavira(540—486 BC)：摩诃毗罗，印度耆那教的创始人之一。

2. Marcus Terentius Varro (116—27 BC)：马库斯•特伦修斯•瓦罗，罗马学者、作家。

3. Marcus Terentius Varro (116—27 BC), made references to microbes when he warned against locating a homestead in the vicinity of swamps "because there are bred certain minute creatures which cannot be seen by the eyes, which float in the air and enter the body through the mouth and nose and which cause serious diseases". 马库斯•特伦修斯•瓦罗告诫人们不要在沼泽附近建立家园时提到了微生物，"因为此处繁殖一些肉眼看不见的微小生物，它们浮在空气中，通过口鼻进入人体，由此引发严重的疾病"。句中"there are bred certain minute creatures…"是由 there 引导的倒装句。

4. Girolamo Fracastoro (1478—1553)：吉罗拉摩•弗拉卡斯特罗，意大利医师、科学家、诗人。

5. Athanasius Kircher (1602—1680)：阿塔纳斯•珂雪，德国耶稣会教士、学者。

6. Antonie van Leeuwenhoek (1632—1723)：安东尼•万•列文虎克，荷兰显微镜学家、微生物学开拓者。

7. Ferdinand Cohn (1828—1898)：费迪南•科恩，德国微生物学家、植物学家。

8. Louis Pasteur (1822—1895)：路易斯•巴斯德，法国化学家及微生物学家。

9. Robert Koch(1843—1910)：罗伯特•柯赫，德国医生、细菌学家。

10. Martinus Beijerinck (1851—1931)：马丁乌斯•贝杰林克，荷兰微生物学家和植物学家。

11. Sergei Winogradsky(1856—1953)：谢尔盖•维诺格拉斯基，俄国微生物学家，生态学家和土壤学家。

Exercises

1. **Decide whether each of the following statements is true (T) or false (F) according to the Text.**

(1) The existence of microorganisms was observed and discovered in earth, water, air and fire as early as the 6th century BC.

(2) Marcus Terentius Varro put forward the view that minute living bodies could cause diseases.

(3) Ferdinand Cohn established the science of bacteriology and discovered spores.

(4) Many microbes are widely used in various fields although all of them are associated with various human diseases.

(5) Medical microbiology is not only the study of the pathogenic microbes and the role of microbes in human illness, but also responsible for creating medications.

(6) Genomic studies, genomic mining and biotechnology are being employed in the research for new antibiotics and other drugs in streptomyces.

2. **Questions for oral discussion.**

(1) Is the study of microbiology at the initial stage relative to older biological disciplines such as zoology and botany? Why?

(2) Who established general microbiology? And what are their contributions to this field?

(3) What is the usefulness of microorganisms suggested by recent research?

笔记

(4) Has microbiology been accompanied by the history of human beings? please Illustrate your opinion with examples.

3. Choose the best answer to each of the following questions.

(1) Why does the author consider that the existence of microorganisms was pure speculation before their actual discovery in ancient times?

　A. They were not discovered until early 6th century BC.

　B. They were not observed until the invention of the microscope in the 17th century.

　C. They were not assumed to live in earth, water and air by Mahavira.

　D. They were not described by Marcus Terentius Varro as to how diseases could be caused.

(2) Who observed microorganisms with their simple lense microscopes in the 17th century?

　A. Athanasius Kircher and Antonie van Leeuwenhoek.

　B. Girolamo Fracastoro and Antonie van Leeuwenhoek.

　C. Athanasius Kircher and Girolamo Fracastoro.

　D. Marcus Terentius Varro and Girolamo Fracastoro.

(3) Why are Pasteur and Koch often considered to be the father of microbiology and medical microbiology, respectively?

　A. They focused on reflecting the true diversity of the microbial world and microorganisms with direct medical relevance.

　B. They disproved the theory of spontaneous generation and solidified microbiology's identity as a biological science.

　C. They proved that specific diseases were caused by specific pathogenic microorganisms.

　D. They discovered the methods of food preservation and vaccines against several diseases and contributed to the germ theory of disease.

(4) When was the breadth of microbiology revealed?

　A. It was not until the 17th century.

　B. It was not until the late 17th century.

　C. It was not until the 19th century.

　D. It was not until the late 19th century.

(5) What do you infer from "the relatively new science of microbiology is huge"?

　A. Microorganisms affect our health and environment in a great many ways.

　B. Microorganisms exist in large numbers in most natural environments.

　C. Microbiology contains the subdisciplines concerning many fields such as food, medicine, veterinarian, genetics, pharmacy, environment, industry, agriculture, etc.

　D. Microbiology has made important contributions to many disciplines such as the study of microbial pathogenesis and epidemiology, pathology and immunology.

(6) Why do some people fear microbes?

　A. Because they exist everywhere in the world.

　B. Because all human diseases are caused by microbes.

　C. Because some of microbes are associated with various human diseases.

　D. Because they are not only beneficial but also detrimental.

(7) Which of the following statements is the most efficient method of microbial biodegradation?

　A. Bacterial species and strains are mixed.

　B. Biopolymers, such as polysaccharides, polyesters and polyamides are mixed.

C. Each species of bacterium is used to degrade one type of contaminant.

D. Each species of bacterium is used to degrade more types of contaminants.

(8) What is beneficial to human and animal health by consuming probiotics?

A. It helps relieve symptoms of lactose intolerance, and reduce the chances of diarrhea and colon cancer.

B. It helps relieve symptoms of lactose intolerance, boost the immune system and prevent diarrhea and colon cancer.

C. It helps relieve constipation and diarrhea, and reduce the chances of lactose intolerance and colon cancer.

D. It helps relieve constipation and diarrhea, boost the immune system and prevent lactose intolerance and colon cancer.

(9) Why is pharmaceutical microbiology regarded as the part of industrial microbiology?

A. Microorganisms are used in the production of medications.

B. Microorganisms are used in diagnostic assays.

C. Microorganisms are used in the clinical laboratory.

D. Microorganisms are used in degradation of industrial wastes.

(10) What are the high-value products made from microbes?

A. Diagnostic assays, medications, chemicals and fuels.

B. Medications, chemicals, fuels and electricity.

C. Chemicals, electricity, fuels and antibiotics.

D. Fuels, electricity, chemicals and metabolites.

4.   Fill in the blanks with the words given below.

> contaminant, diversity, microorganisms, estimate, applications biologicals, associated, metabolism, probiotics, detrimental

(1) The speculations about the existence of _____ and their causation of diseases contribute to the development of bacteriology.

(2) Consumption of _____, the bacteria potentially beneficial to the digestive system, contributes a lot to human and animal health.

(3) Scientists _____ that about 99% of the microbes existing on earth have not yet been studied.

(4) Further study of microbiology may help us understand some of the mysteries of living things and their greater _____ will be available.

(5) Pasteur and Koch did not reveal the true _____ of the microbial world due to their exclusive focus on microorganisms having direct medical relevance.

(6) Microorganisms are used to produce human or animal _____, such as insulin, growth hormone and antibody.

(7) The nature of each _____ determines the ability of each microorganism to degrade toxic waste.

(8) Members of Streptomyces genus have a complex secondary _____ producing antibiotic compounds and other metabolites with medical properties.

(9) Pharmaceutical Microbiology involves the study of microorganisms _____ with the manufacture of pharmaceuticals.

(10) He always stays up so late that lack of sleep is _____ to his health.

笔记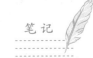

5. Translate the following sentences and paragraphs into Chinese.

(1) Although the existence of microbes was determined almost three hundred years ago, the study of microbiology is only getting started compared with zoology and botany.

(2) In ancient times, the existence of microbes was hypothesized and they might be the responsible agent of diseases, which was pure speculation as there was no microscope at the time.

(3) The first one who suggested taxonomic classification of bacteria and discovered spores was Ferdinand Cohn, a botanist and the founder of bacteriology.

(4) Microbes may be tiny, but the field of microbiology is relatively huge, which encompasses many subdisciplines affecting peoples' life and health a lot.

(5) Some microbes may cause diseases but not all of them are detrimental. Some of them are used in industrial fermentation to make wine and vinegar.

(6) The existence of microorganisms was hypothesized for many centuries before their actual discovery. They were supposed to live in earth, water, and air, and cause serious diseases. It was not until the 17th century that they were observed and discovered under simple microscopes. The study of microscopic, unicellular, and cell-cluster organisms, including eukaryotes and prokaryotes, is microbiology which typically includes the study of the immune system and viruses. Generally, immune systems interact with pathogenic microbes; these two disciplines often intersect which is why many colleges offer a paired degree such as "Microbiology and Immunology".

(7) Microbiology has not only made important contributions to many disciplines but also affected both medicine and pharmacy a lot. Medical microbiology is the study of the pathogenic microbes and the role of microbes in human illness, which includes the study of microbial pathogenesis and epidemiology and is related to the study of disease pathology and immunology. Pharmaceutical microbiology is considered the part of industrial microbiology that is responsible for creating medications. Microorganisms are used to produce human or animal biologicals such as insulin, growth hormone, and antibodies. Diagnostic assays that use monoclonal antibody, DNA probe technology or real-time PCR are used as rapid tests for pathogenic organisms in the clinical laboratory.

Text B
The Other Side of Antibiotics

Antibiotics have eliminated or controlled so many infectious diseases that virtually everyone has benefited from their use at one time or another. Even without such personal experience, however, one would have to be isolated indeed to be unaware of the virtues, real and speculative, of these "miracle" drugs.[1] The American press, radio, and television have done a good job of reporting the truly remarkable story of successes in the chemical war on germs. What's more, any shortcomings on their part have been more than made up for by the aggressive public relations activity of the pharmaceutical companies which manufacture and sell antibiotics.

In comparison, the inadequacies and potential dangers of these remarkable drugs are much less widely known. And the lack of such knowledge can be bad, especially if it leads patients to pressure their doctors into prescribing antibiotics when such medication isn't really needed, or leads them to switch doctors until they find one who is, so to speak, antibiotics-minded.[2]

Because the good side of the antibiotics story is well-known, there seems more point here to a review of some of the immediate and long-range problems that can come from today's casual use of these drugs. It should be made clear in advance that calamities from the use of antibiotics are rare in relation to the enormous amounts of the drugs administered. But the potential hazards, so little touched on generally, do need a clear statement. The antibiotics are not, strictly speaking, exclusively prescription drugs. A number of them are permitted in such over-the-counter products as nasal sprays, lozenges, troches, creams, and ointments. Even if these products do no harm, there is no point whatsoever in using them. If you have an infection serious enough to warrant the launching of chemical warfare, you need much bigger doses of the antibiotics than any of the non-prescription products are allowed to contain.

Over-the-counter products, however, account for only a small percentage of total antibiotics production. It is the prescription dosages that give people trouble. These drugs—even allowing for the diverse abilities of the many narrow-spectrum ones and the versatility of the broad-spectrum ones— are not the cure-alls, they often are billed as being. There are wide gaps in their ability to master contagious diseases. Such important infections as mumps, measles, common colds, influenza, and infectious hepatitis still await conquest. All are virus infections and despite intense efforts, very little progress has been made in chemotherapy against viruses. Only small progress has been achieved against fungi. Many strains of bacteria and fungi are naturally resistant to all currently available antibiotics and other chemotherapeutic drugs. Some microorganisms originally sensitive to the action of antibiotics, especially staphylococcus, have developed resistant strains. This acquired resistance imposes on the long range value of the drugs a very important limitation, which is not adequately met by the frequent introduction of new antimicrobial agents to combat the problem.[3]

It has been pretty well established that the increase in strains of bacteria resistant to an antibiotic correlates directly with the duration and extent of use of that antibiotic in a given location. In one hospital a survey showed that, before erythromycin had been widely used there, all strains of staphylococci taken from patients and personnel were sensitive to its action. When the hospital started extensive use of erythromycin, however, resistant staphylococcus strains began to appear.

The development of bacterial resistance can be minimized by a more discriminating use of antibiotics,[4] and the person taking the drug can help here. When an antibiotic must be used, the best way to prevent the development of resistance is to wipe out the infection as rapidly and thoroughly as possible. Ideally, this requires a bactericidal drug, which destroys, rather than a bacteriostatic drug, which inhibits. And the drug must be taken in adequate dosage for as long as it is necessary to eradicate the infection completely. The doctor, of course, must choose the drug, but patients can help by being sure to take the full course of treatment recommended by the doctor, even though symptoms seem to disappear before all the pills are gone. In rare instances the emergence of resistance can be delayed or reduced by combinations of antibiotics. Treatment of tuberculosis with streptomycin alone results in a high degree of resistance, but if para-aminosalicylic acid or isoniazid is used with streptomycin the possibility that this complication will arise is greatly reduced.

In hospital treatment of severe infections, the sensitivity of the infecting organism to appropriate antibiotics is determined in the laboratory before treatment is started. This enables the doctor to select the most effective drug or drugs; it determines whether the antibiotic is bactericidal or bacteriostatic for the germs at hand; and it suggests the amount needed to destroy the growth of the bacteria completely.[5] In either hospital or home, aseptic measures can help to reduce the prevalence of resistant strains of germs by preventing cross infection and the resultant spreading of organisms.

Every one of the antibiotics is potentially dangerous for some people. Several serious reactions may result from their use. One is a severe, sometimes fatal, shock-like anaphylactic action, which may strike people who have become sensitized to penicillin. Anaphylactic reaction happens less frequently and is less severe when the antibiotic is given by mouth. It is most apt to occur in people with a history of allergy, or a record of sensitivity to penicillin. Very small amounts of penicillin, even the traces which get into the milk of cows for a few days after they are treated with the antibiotic for mastitis, may be sufficient to sensitize; hence, the strong campaign by food and drug officials keeps such milk off the market.[6]

To minimize the risk of anaphylactic shock in illnesses where injections of penicillin are the preferred treatment, a careful doctor will question the patient carefully about allergies and previous reactions. In case of doubt another antibiotic will be substituted[7] if feasible, or other precautionary measures will be taken before the injection is given.

Other untoward reactions to antibiotics are gastrointestinal disorders—such as sore mouth, cramps, diarrhea, or anal itch—which occur most frequently after use of the tetracycline group but have also been encountered after use of penicillin and streptomycin. These reactions may result from suppression by the antibiotic of bacteria normally found in the gastrointestinal tract. With their competition removed, antibiotic-resistant staphylococci or fungi, which are also normally present, are free to flourish and cause what is called a super-infection. Such infections can be extremely difficult to cure.

A few antibiotics have such toxic effects that their usefulness is strictly limited. They include streptomycin and dihydro-streptomycin, which sometimes cause deafness, and chloramphenicol, which may injure the bone marrow. Drugs with such serious potential dangers as these should be used only if life is threatened and nothing else will work. All the possible troubles that can result from antibiotic treatment should not keep anyone from using one of these drugs when it is clearly indicated. Nor should they discourage certain preventive uses of antibiotics which have proved extremely valuable.

Word Study

1. anal ['einl] *adj.* 肛门的

2. anaphylactic [,ænəfi'læktik] *adj.* 过敏的

3. antimicrobial [,æntimai'krəubiəl] *adj.* 抗菌的；杀菌的；*n.* 抗菌剂

4. aseptic [ei'septik] *adj.* 无（病）菌的，防腐的

5. bactericidal [bæk,tiəri'saidl] *adj.* 杀菌的

6. bacteriostatic [bæk,tiriəs'tætik] *adj.* 抑菌的 *n.* 抑菌剂

7. dihydro-streptomycin [diː'haidrəu 'streptə'maisin] *n.* 双氢链霉素

8. eradicate [i'rædikeit] *vt.* 根除，消灭，歼灭

9. erythromycin [i,riθrə'maisin] *n.* 红霉素

10. hepatitis [hepə'taitis] *n.* 肝炎

11. isoniazid [aisəu'naiəzid] *n.* 异烟肼（一种抗结核药）

12. itch [itʃ] *n.* 痒；*v.* 发痒

13. lozenge ['lɔzindʒ] *n.* 锭剂，糖锭（用于治咳嗽或喉病，常作菱形）

14. mastitis [mæ'staitis] *n.* 乳腺炎

笔记

15. measles ['miːzlz] *n.* 麻疹

16. mumps [mʌmps] *n.* 腮腺炎

17. ointment ['ɔintmənt] *n.* 油膏，软膏，药膏

18. para-aminosalicylic acid ['pærə ə'miːnəu,sæli'silik 'æsid] *n.* 对氨基水杨酸

19. precautionary [pri'kɔːʃənəri] *adj.* 预先警告的

20. prevalence ['prevələns] *n.* 普遍，流行

21. sensitize ['sensətaiz] *v.* （使）敏感

22. speculative ['spekjələtiv] *adj.* 纯理论的，推测的

23. staphylococcus [stæfilə'kɔkəs] ([复]cocci ['kɔksai]) *n.* 葡萄球菌

24. super-infection ['suːpərinf'ekʃn] *n.* 双重感染，继发感染

25. suppression [sə'preʃn] *n.* 压抑，封闭

26. troche [trəuʃ] *n.* 糖锭，锭剂

27. untoward [,ʌntə'wɔːd] *adj.* 不幸的，不适当的

28. warfare ['wɔːfɛə] *n.* 战争，竞争

Notes

1. Even without such personal…of these "miracle" drugs: 但是如果一个人没有这样的亲身经历，他必定是离群所居才能不知道这些"神奇药物"的真实或推测的优点。"real and speculative"是"virtue"的后置定语。

2. …or leads them to switch…antibiotics-minded: or when the lack of such knowledge leads patients to change doctors until they find one (doctor) who is antibiotics-minded, as you can say.

3. This acquired resistance imposes on the long range value of the drugs a very important limitation, which is not adequately met by the frequent introduction of new antimicrobial agents to combat the problem. 译为：这种获得耐药性使药物的长期使用价值受到极大的限制，频繁使用新的抗菌药剂也不能完全解决这个问题。"which is not adequately met by…"译为：得不到满足。

4. The development of bacterial resistance can be minimized by a more discriminating use of antibiotics,…. 译为：较为辩证地使用抗生素会极大地降低抗药性的发生。

5. In hospital treatment of severe infections, the sensitivity of the infecting organism to appropriate antibiotics is determined in the laboratory before treatment is started. This enables the doctor to select the most effective drug or drugs; it determines whether the antibiotic is bactericidal or bacteriostatic for the germs at hand; and it suggests the amount needed to destroy the growth of the bacteria completely. 译为：在医院治疗严重感染时，感染菌对抗生素的敏感性在治疗前已在实验室确定，这样可以使医生选择最有效的药物，决定使用杀菌还是抑菌的抗生素来应对目前的细菌，对能完全破坏细菌生长所需的用量给出建议。"the amount needed"means"the amount of antibiotics needed in the treatment".

6. Very small amounts of penicillin, even the traces which get into the milk of cows for a few days after they are treated with the antibiotic for mastitis, may be sufficient to sensitize; hence, the strong campaign by food and drug officials keeps such milk off the market. 译为：抗生素治疗患乳腺炎的奶牛几天后，牛奶中带入的极少量甚至痕量的青霉素也可能引起过敏，所以食品药品监督员采取强有力的措施防止这种牛奶进入市场。"traces" 痕量：化学上指极小的量，少得只有一点儿痕迹。

7. In case of doubt another antibiotic will be substituted: If the patient's allergic history is not clear, the doctor will prescribe another antibiotic for him.

笔记

Supplementary Parts

1. Medical and Pharmaceutical Terms Made Easier (2): Common Morphemes in Terms of English for Microbiology

Morpheme	Meaning	Example
acar	螨虫	acaricide 杀螨的，杀螨剂
ameb	阿米巴	ameba 阿米巴，变形虫
aspergill	曲霉	aspergillus 曲霉病
bacill	杆菌	.bacillus 杆菌属，芽孢杆菌属
bacteri	细菌	bacteriology 细菌学
brucell	布鲁菌	brucella 布鲁菌属
coccidioid	球孢子菌	coccidioides 球孢子菌属
coccus	球菌	coccobacillus 球杆菌
ferment	发酵	ferment 酶，酵素；发酵
fung	真菌	fungus 真菌，霉菌
germ	病菌	germicide 杀菌剂
monil	念珠菌	monilia 念珠菌属
myc	霉菌	mycelium 菌丝体
nematod	线虫	nematode 线虫
parasit	寄生虫	parasite 寄生虫，寄生物
penicill	青霉	penicillin 青霉素
spirochaet	螺旋体	spirochaeta 螺旋体属
staphyl	葡萄	staphylococcus 葡萄球菌
strept	链	streptobacillus 链球杆菌属
virus	病毒	arbovirus 虫媒病毒
zym	发酵	zymogenic 引起发酵的

(1) Decompose the following words and translate them into Chinese.

1) actinomycetales　　　　　　　　＿＿＿＿＿＿＿＿＿＿＿＿＿
　　sample: actino - mycetales 放线菌目

2) bacteriology　　　　　　　　　　＿＿＿＿＿＿＿＿＿＿＿＿＿

3) colicin　　　　　　　　　　　　　＿＿＿＿＿＿＿＿＿＿＿＿＿

4) chlamydosis　　　　　　　　　　＿＿＿＿＿＿＿＿＿＿＿＿＿

5) microbiota　　　　　　　　　　　＿＿＿＿＿＿＿＿＿＿＿＿＿

6) mycobacteriology　　　　　　　＿＿＿＿＿＿＿＿＿＿＿＿＿

7) mycoplsamal　　　　　　　　　　＿＿＿＿＿＿＿＿＿＿＿＿＿

8) salmonellosis　　　　　　　　　＿＿＿＿＿＿＿＿＿＿＿＿＿

9) septicemia　　　　　　　　　　　＿＿＿＿＿＿＿＿＿＿＿＿＿

10) sporocyst　　　　　　　　　　　＿＿＿＿＿＿＿＿＿＿＿＿＿

11) immunotoxin　　　　　　　　　＿＿＿＿＿＿＿＿＿＿＿＿＿

12) vibriosis　　　　　　　　　　　　＿＿＿＿＿＿＿＿＿＿＿＿＿

(2) Word-matching.

1) fungus	A. 虫媒病毒
2) monilia	B. 曲霉病
3) penicillin	C. 念珠菌属

续表

4) arbovirus	D. 引起发酵的
5) staphylococcus	E. 线虫
6) zymogenic	F. 酶,酵素;发酵
7) nematode	G. 真菌,霉菌
8) coccobacillus	H. 杆菌属,芽孢
9) aspergillus	I. 杀螨的,杀螨剂
10) acaricide	J. 球杆菌
11) bacillus	K. 青霉素
12) ferment	L. 葡萄球菌

2.　English-Chinese Translation Skills: 药学英语句式特点与翻译

药学英语在句式上最显著的特点体现在句子主语上,一般有两种情况:使用无灵主语;使用名词化动词做主语。

(1)　跟其他科技英语类一样,药学英语经常使用无灵主语,把动作发出者隐退,强调动作和结果本身,表现在整个句子结构上就是被动语态,动作发出者有时候省略,有时候通过介词短语保留。

例 1: Bacteriology, a subdiscipline of microbiology later, was founded in the 19th century by Ferdinand Cohn, a botanist whose studies on algae and photosynthetic bacteria led him to describe several bacteria including bacillus and beggiatoa.

参考译文:19 世纪,费迪南·科恩创建了细菌学(后来成为微生物学的一个分支学科),这位植物学家对藻类和光合细菌进行了研究,描述了包括杆菌和贝日阿托氏菌在内的一些细菌。

说明:在翻译被动语态句子时,要不要加上动作发出者做主语,要看情况而定,上面这个例句,由于这个动作发出者是专有名词,就必须保留,译文改成了主动句,而且这个主语以不同方式重复了三次:"费迪南·科恩""这位植物学家"和"他"。而原文主语只有一个 bacteriology,在以 whose 引导的定语从句的主语是 studies。

药学语篇通常描述药物、药剂等专业内容或者有关药物性质、作用等客观现象,这些内容或现象经常出现在句子主语位置,这也是药学英语使用无灵主语多的另外一种情况,对于这类句子,直接翻译就可以。如:

例 2: Calcium ion plays a critical role in coupling surface membrane depolarization to muscle contraction.

参考译文:钙离子在偶联表面膜去极化和肌肉收缩方面起到关键作用。

例 3: Vaccines are used to combat infectious diseases, however, the last decade has witnessed a revolution in the approach to vaccine design and development. Sophisticated technologies such as genomics, proteomics, functional genomics, and synthetic chemistry can be used for the rational identification of antigens, the synthesis of complex glycans, and the generation of engineered carrier proteins.

参考译文:疫苗用来抵御传染病,然而过去的十年里彻底改变了疫苗设计和开发方法,高端技术如基因组学、蛋白质组学、功能基因组学和合成化学能用于合理地识别抗原、复杂的多聚糖合成,以及工程载体蛋白质的生成。

说明:在上面例句中,三个主语都是无灵主语:vaccines、the last decade、sophisticated technologies,在翻译时都采取了不同的策略。第一句是被动结构,翻译时没有刻意译成被动结构;第二句是一个隐喻结构,时间 the last decade 做主语,连接动词 witness(见证),如果按照原文结构翻译"过去 10 年见证了……",这类语言表达结构不太适合汉语科技文章;第三句就是按

笔记

照原文的结构自然译成,也符合汉语表达结构。

　　翻译药学英语使用无灵主语的句子,需要根据不同语境采用不同策略,这些在以后的章节中会分别讲解,这里不过多介绍。

(2)　名词化就是将动词转换成名词,名词化动词可以做主语、宾语等,这种结构可以使行文简洁,内容确切,将动作发出者退出主语位置,把动作本身作为信息点突显出来。药学英语语篇中大量使用名词化动词做主语。

　　例4: Absorption of moisture by the core and subsequent swelling leads to the release of drugs.

　　参考译文:片芯吸收水分并且随后膨胀从而导致药物释放。

　　说明:在上面例句中有三个名词性动词:absorption、swelling 和 release,在翻译中三个名词性动词的处理方式不一样:absorption 和 release 都译成了动词形式,swelling 保留了名词形式,这样的表达符合汉语语言习惯。

　　例5: While his work on the Tobacco Mosaic Virus established the basic principles of virology, it was his development of enrichment culturing that had the most immediate impact on microbiology by allowing for the cultivation of a wide range of microbes with wildly different physiologies.

　　参考译文:他研究烟草花叶病病毒的成果确立了病毒学的基本原理,与此同时,他发展的富集培养技术,可以大量培养具有不同生理的微生物,对微生物学产生直接影响。

　　说明:上面例句中主句和从句都是名词化动词做主语,这样的表达结构相对弱化动作发出者而突出动作本身,在翻译名词化动词做主语时,要注意英汉语言差别。汉语中一般都由动作发出者做主语,要适当改变原文结构。在该例句中,his work on… 和 his development of… 分别译成"他研究……的成果"和"他发展的……技术"都对原主语进行了适当的改变,符合汉语表达习惯。

　　翻译名词化结构做主语不能仅停留在表层结构上,要理解深层次的语义,名词化动词可以翻译成动词结构,也可以翻译成名词词组,这取决于具体语境。

Unit Three Biochemistry

Biochemistry, sometimes abbreviated as "BioChem", is the study of chemical processes in living organisms. Biochemistry governs all living organisms and living processes. By controlling information flow through biochemical signaling and the flow of chemical energy through metabolism, biochemical processes give rise to the seemingly magical phenomenon of life. Much of biochemistry deals with the structures and functions of cellular components such as proteins, carbohydrates, lipids, nucleic acids and other biomolecules, although increasingly processes rather than individual molecules are the main focus. Over the last 40 years biochemistry has become so successful at explaining living processes that now almost all areas of the life sciences from botany to medicine are engaged in biochemical research. Today the main focus of pure biochemistry is in understanding how biological molecules give rise to the processes that occur within living cells which in turn greatly relates to the study and understanding of whole organisms.

生物化学，有时缩写为"BioChem"，是研究生命体内化学过程的学科。生物化学掌控所有生命体和生命过程。通过控制生化信号转导通路的信息流和新陈代谢的化学能流动，生物化学过程引发各种神奇的生命现象。尽管生物化学的研究焦点逐渐从单个的分子转移到生命过程，生物化学更多地仍是研究细胞组成成分的结构和功能，例如蛋白质、糖类、脂类、核酸和其他生物分子。在过去的 40 年中，生物化学非常成功地解释了生命过程，以至于目前从植物学到医药学几乎所有生命科学领域都涉及生物化学研究。当前生物化学的主要研究焦点是了解生物分子是如何在活细胞中参与生命过程，而这又与进一步研究和了解整个有机体密切相关。

笔记

Text A
Foundation of Biochemistry

Biochemistry Seeks to Explain Life in Chemical Terms

The molecules of which living organisms are composed conform to all the familiar laws of chemistry, but they also interact with each other in accordance with another set of principles, which we shall refer to collectively as the molecular logic of life.[1] These principles do not involve new or yet undiscovered physical laws or forces. Instead, they are a set of relationships characterizing the nature, function, and interactions of biomolecules.

If living organisms are composed of molecules that are intrinsically inanimate, how do these molecules confer the remarkable combination of characteristics we call life? How is it that a living organism appears to be more than the sum of its inanimate parts? Philosophers once answered that living organisms are endowed with a mysterious and divine life force, but this doctrine (vitalism) has been firmly rejected by modern science. The basic goal of the science of biochemistry is to determine how the collections of inanimate molecules that constitute living organisms interact with each other to maintain and perpetuate life. Although biochemistry yields important insights and practical applications in medicine, agriculture, nutrition, and industry, it is ultimately concerned with the wonder of life itself.

All Macromolecules are Constructed from a Few Simple Compounds

Most of the molecular constituents of living systems are composed of carbon atoms covalently joined with other carbon atoms and with hydrogen, oxygen, or nitrogen. The special bonding properties of carbon permit the formation of a great variety of molecules. Organic compounds of molecular weight (MW) less than about 500, such as amino acids, nucleotides, and monosaccharides, serve as monomeric subunits of proteins, nucleic acids, and polysaccharides, respectively. A single protein molecule may have 1,000 or more amino acids, and deoxyribonucleic acid has millions of nucleotides.

Each cell of the bacterium *Escherichia coli* (*E. coli*)contains more than 6,000 different kinds of organic compounds, including about 3,000 different proteins and a similar number of different nucleic acid molecules. In humans there may be tens of thousands of different kinds of proteins, as well as many types of polysaccharides (chains of simple sugars), a variety of lipids, and many other compounds with lower molecular weight.

To purify and to characterize thoroughly all of these molecules would be an insuperable task, it were not for the fact that each class of macromolecules (proteins, nucleic acids, polysaccharides) is composed of a small, common set of monomeric subunits. These monomeric subunits can be covalently linked in a virtually limitless variety of sequences, just as the 26 letters of the English alphabet can be arranged into a limitless number of words, sentences, or books.

Deoxyribonucleic acids (DNA) are constructed from only four different kinds of simple monomeric subunits, the deoxyribonucleotides, and ribonucleic acids (RNA) are composed of just four types of ribonucleotides. Proteins are composed of 20 different kinds of amino acids. The eight kinds of nucleotides from which all nucleic acids are built and the 20 different kinds of amino acids from which all proteins are built are identical in all living organisms.[2]

Most of the monomeric subunits from which all macromolecules are constructed serve more than one function in living cells. The nucleotides serve not only as subunits of nucleic acids, but also as energy-carrying molecules. The amino acids are subunits of protein molecules, and also precursors of hormones, neurotransmitters, pigments, and many other kinds of biomolecules.

From these considerations we can now set out some of the principles in the molecular logic of life: all living organisms have the same kinds of monomeric subunits. There are underlying patterns in the structure of biological macromolecules. The identity of each organism is preserved by its possession of distinctive sets of nucleic acids and of proteins.

ATP Is the Universal Carrier of Metabolic Energy, Linking Catabolism and Anabolism

Cells capture, store, and transport free energy in a chemical form. Adenosine triphosphate (ATP) functions as the major carrier of chemical energy in all cells. ATP carries energy among metabolic pathways by serving as the shared intermediate that couples endergonic reactions to exergonic ones. The terminal phosphate group of ATP is transferred to a variety of acceptor molecules, which are thereby activated for further chemical transformation. The adenosine diphosphate (ADP) that remains after the phosphate transfer is recycled to become ATP, at the expense of either chemical energy (during oxidative phosphorylation) or solar energy in photosynthetic cells (by the process of photophosphorylation). ATP is the major connecting link (the shared intermediate) between the catabolic and anabolic networks of enzyme-catalyzed reactions in the cell. These linked networks of enzyme-catalyzed reactions are virtually identical in all living organisms.

Genetic Continuity Is Vested in DNA Molecules

Perhaps the most remarkable of all the properties of living cells and organisms is their ability to reproduce themselves with nearly perfect fidelity for countless generations. This continuity of inherited traits implies constancy, over thousands or millions of years, in the structure of the molecules that contain the genetic information. Very few historical records of civilization, even those etched in copper or carved in stone, have survived for a thousand years. But there is good evidence that the genetic instructions in living organisms have remained nearly unchanged over much longer periods; many bacteria have nearly the same size, shape, and internal structure and contain the same kinds of precursor molecules and enzymes as those that lived a billion years ago.

Hereditary information is preserved in DNA, a long, thin organic polymer so fragile that it will fragment from the shear forces arising in a solution that is stirred or pipetted. A human sperm or egg, carrying the accumulated hereditary information of millions of years of evolution, transmits these instructions in the form of DNA molecules, in which the linear sequence of covalently linked nucleotide subunits encodes the genetic message. Genetic information is encoded in the linear sequence of four kinds of subunits of DNA. The double-helical DNA molecule has an internal template for its own replication and repair.

The Structure of DNA Allows for Its Repair and Replication with Near-Perfect Fidelity

The capacity of living cells to preserve their genetic material and to duplicate it for the next

笔记

generation results from the structural complementarity between the two halves of the DNA molecule. The basic unit of DNA is a linear polymer of four different monomeric subunits, deoxyribonucleotides, arranged in a precise linear sequence. It is this linear sequence that encodes the genetic information. Two of these polymeric strands are twisted with each other to form the DNA double helix, where each monomeric subunit in one strand pairs specifically with the complementary subunit in the opposite strand. In the enzymatic replication or repair of DNA, one of the two strands serves as a template for the assembly of another, structurally complementary DNA strand. Before a cell divides, the two DNA strands separate and each serves as a template for the synthesis of a complementary strand, generating two identical double-helical molecules, one for each daughter cell. If one strand is damaged, continuity of information is assured by the information present on the other strand.

The Linear Sequence in DNA Encodes Proteins with Three-Dimensional Structures

The information in DNA is encoded as a linear (one-dimensional) sequence of the nucleotide units of DNA, but the expression of this information results in a three-dimensional cell. This change from one to three dimensions occurs in two phases. A linear sequence of deoxyribonucleotides in DNA codes (through the intermediary, RNA) for the production of a protein with a corresponding linear sequence of amino acids. The protein folds itself into a particular three-dimensional shape, dictated by its amino acid sequence. The precise three-dimensional structure (native conformation) is crucial to the protein's function as either catalyst or structural element. This principle emerges:

The linear sequence of amino acids in a protein leads to the acquisition of a unique three-dimensional structure by a self-assembly procession.

Once a protein has folded into its native conformation, it may associate noncovalently with other proteins, or with nucleic acids or lipids, to form supramolecular complexes such as chromosomes, ribosomes, and membranes. These complexes are in many cases self-assembling. The individual molecules of these complexes have specific, high-affinity binding sites for each other, and within the cell they spontaneously form functional complexes. Individual macromolecules with specific affinity for other macromolecules self-assemble into supramolecular complexes.

Noncovalent Interactions Stabilize Three-Dimensional Structures

The forces that provide stability and specificity to the three-dimensional structures of macromolecules and supramolecular complexes are mostly noncovalent interactions. These interactions, individually weak but collectively strong, include hydrogen bonds, ionic interactions among charged groups, van der Waals interactions, and hydrophobic interactions among nonpolar groups. These weak interactions are transient; individually they form and break in small fractions of a second. The transient nature of noncovalent interactions confers a flexibility on macromolecules that is critical to their function. Furthermore, the large numbers of noncovalent interactions in a single macromolecule makes it unlikely that at any given moment all the interactions will be broken. Thus, macromolecular structures are stable over time.

Three-Dimensional Biological Structures Combine the Properties of Flexibility and Stability

The flexibility and stability of the double-helical structure of DNA are due to the

笔记

complementarity of its two strands and many weak interactions between them. The flexibility of these interactions allows strand separation during DNA replication; the complementarity of the double helix is essential to genetic continuity.

Noncovalent interactions are also central to the specificity and catalytic efficiency of enzymes. Enzymes bind transition-state intermediates through numerous weak but precisely oriented interactions. Because the weak interactions are flexible, the complex survives the structural distortions as the reactant is converted into product.

The formation of noncovalent interactions provides the energy for self-assembly of macromolecules by stabilizing native conformations relative to unfolded, random forms. The native conformation of a protein is that in which the energetic advantages of forming weak interactions counterbalance the tendency of the protein chain to assume random forms. Given a specific linear sequence of amino acids and a specific set of conditions (temperature, ionic conditions, pH), a protein will assume its native conformation spontaneously, without a template or scaffold to direct the folding.[3]

The Physical Roots of the Biochemical World

We can now summarize the various principles of the molecular logic of life:

A living cell is a self-contained, self-assembling, self-adjusting, self-perpetuating isothermal system of molecules that extracts free energy and raw materials from its environment.

The cell carries out many consecutive reactions promoted by specific catalysts, called enzymes, which it produces itself.

The cell maintains itself in a dynamic steady state, far from equilibrium with its surroundings. There is great economy of parts and processes, achieved by regulation of the catalytic activity of key enzymes.[4]

Self-replication through many generations is ensured by the self-repairing, linear information-coding system. Genetic information encoded as sequences of nucleotide subunits in DNA and RNA specifies the sequence of amine acids in each distinct protein, which ultimately determines the three-dimensional structure and function of each protein.

Many weak (noncovalent) interactions, acting cooperatively, stabilize the three-dimensional structures of biomolecules and supramolecular complexes.

Word Study

1. adenosine [əˈdenəsiːn] *n.* 腺苷，腺嘌呤核苷
2. amino [əˈmiːnəu] *adj.* 氨基的
3. anabolic [əˈnæbəlik] *adj.* 合成代谢的
4. biomolecule [baiɔməuˈlekjuːl] *n.* 生物分子
5. capture [ˈkæptʃə] *vt.* 俘虏，捕获，占领，吸引；*n.* 夺获，俘获
6. catalyze [ˈkætəlaiz] *vt.* 催化
7. chromosome [ˈkrəuməsəum] *n.* 染色体
8. complementary [ˌkɔmpliˈmentəri] *adj.* 互补的，补充的
9. counterbalance [ˌkauntəˈbæləns] *n.* 平衡，平衡力；*vt.* 使平衡，抵消
10. covalently [kəuˈveiləntli] *adv.* 共价地
11. deoxyribonucleic acid [diːˌɔksiːraibəunuːˈkliːik ˈæsid] *n.* 脱氧核糖核酸（DNA）

笔记

12. diphosphate [dai'fɔsfeit] *n.* 二磷酸盐

13. doctrine ['dɔktrin] *n.* 学说，主义，正式声明

14. duplicate ['dju:plikit] *n.* 副本，复本，复制品；*adj.* 复制的，二重的；*v.* 复制

15. endergonic [ˌendə'gɔnik] *adj.* 需要能量的，吸能的

16. *Escherichia coli* [ˌeʃə'rikiə, 'kəulai] *n.* 大肠杆菌，大肠埃希菌

17. etch [etʃ] *v.* 蚀刻，铭刻

18. exergonic [ˌeksə'gɔnik] *adj.* 产生能量的，放能的

19. fidelity [fi'deliti] *n.* 忠诚，正确，精确，逼真度，保真度

20. fragile ['frædʒail] *adj.* 易碎的，脆的，易损坏的，虚弱的

21. hereditary [hi'reditəri] *adj.* 遗传的，遗传性的，世袭的

22. hydrogen ['haidrədʒən] *n.* 氢

23. inanimate [in'ænimit] *adj.* 无生命的，无生机的

24. insuperable [in'sju:pərəbl] *adj.* 难以克服的，不可逾越的

25. intermediary [ˌintə'mi:diəri] *adj.* 中介的，中间的；*n.* 媒介物，调解人，中间人

26. intrinsically [in'trinsikəli] *adv.* 内在地，固有地

27. isothermal ['aisəu'θə:məl] *adj.* 等温的，等温线的；*n.* 等温线

28. macromolecule [ˌmækrə'mɔləkju:l] *n.* 巨大分子，高分子

29. metabolic [ˌmetə'bɔlik] *adj.* 新陈代谢的

30. monomeric [ˌmɔnə'merik] *adj.* 单体的

31. monosaccharide [ˌmɔnə'sækəraid] *n.* 单糖

32. neurotransmitter [ˌnjuərəu'trænsmitə] *n.* 神经递质

33. noncovalently ['nɔn kəu'veiləntli] *adv.* 非共价地

34. nonpolar ['nɔn'pəulə] *adj.* 非极性的

35. nucleotidase [nju:kliə'taideis] *n.* 核苷酸酶

36. perpetuate [pə'petjueit] *vt.* 使永存，使不朽

37. phosphate ['fɔsfeit] *n.* 磷酸盐，磷肥

38. photophosphorylation [ˌfəutəufɔsfəri'leiʃn] *n.* 光磷酸化作用，光合磷酸化

39. photosynthetic [ˌfəutəusin'θetik] *adj.* 光合的

40. pigment ['pigmənt] *n.* 天然色素，色料

41. pipette [pi'pet] *n.* 吸量管，移液管

42. precursor [pri:'kə:sə] *n.* 先驱，先兆，前体，产物母体

43. random ['rændəm] *adj.* 任意的，随机的

44. ribonucleic [ˌraibənju:'kli:ik] *adj.* 核糖核酸的

45. ribonucleotide [ˌraibəu'nu:kliətaid] *n.* 核糖核苷酸

46. ribosome ['raibəsəum] *n.* 核糖体

47. scaffold ['skæfəuld] *n.* 鹰架，脚手架

48. sperm [spə:m] *n.* 精液，精子

49. spontaneously [spɔn'teiniəsli] *adv.* 自发地，自生地

50. supramolecular [ˌsju:prəmə'lekjulə] *adj.* 超分子的，由一个以上分子组成的

51. template ['templit] *n.* 模板，样板

52. triphosphate [trai'fɔsfeit] *n.* 三磷酸盐，三磷酸根

53. vest [vest] *n.* 背心；*v.* 授予，赋予

54. vitalism ['vaitəlizəm] *n.* 活力论，生机说

笔记

Notes

1. The molecules of which living organisms are composed conform to all the familiar laws of chemistry, but they also interact with each other in accordance with another set of principles, which we shall refer to collectively as the molecular logic of life. 译为：组成生命体的分子都遵循相似的化学规律，但是这些分子同时也遵循另外一套原理发生相互作用，我们将这些原理统称为生命的分子逻辑。句中"in accordance with"意思是"与……一致"。

2. The eight kinds of nucleotides from which all nucleic acids are built and the 20 different kinds of amino acids from which all proteins are built are identical in all living organisms. 译为：构成核酸的 8 种核苷酸和构成蛋白质的 20 种不同种类的氨基酸在所有活体生物中都是完全相同的。句中"living organisms"意思是有"生命的有机体，即活体"。

3. Given a specific linear sequence of amino acids and a specific set of conditions (temperature, ionic conditions, pH), a protein will assume its native conformation spontaneously, without a template or scaffold to direct the folding. 译为：在给定的氨基酸特定线性序列和特定的一系列条件下（温度、离子条件、pH），一种蛋白质将自发地形成其天然构象，无需模板或支架去指导其折叠。句中"sequence of amino acids"意思是"氨基酸（排列）顺序"。

4. There is great economy of parts and processes, achieved by regulation of the catalytic activity of key enzymes. 译为：通过关键酶催化活性的调控可以节约很多反应部分和反应过程。句中"key enzymes"意思是"关键酶"。

Exercises

1. Decide whether each of the following statements is true (T) or false (F) according to the passage.

(1) Living organisms are such complex systems that are governed by some new and even undiscovered physical laws or forces.

(2) Macromolecules in living organisms are constructed from monomeric subunits and serve various functions.

(3) Generation of ATP from ADP is an energy-liberating process.

(4) The most remarkable of all the properties of living cells and organisms is their ability to reproduce themselves with nearly perfect fidelity for countless generations.

(5) If one strand of DNA molecule is damaged, continuity of information will be damaged.

(6) The forces that provide stability and specificity to the three-dimensional structures of macromolecules and supramolecular complexes are mostly covalent interactions.

2. Questions for oral discussion.

(1) Why would the purification and thorough characterization of macromolecules be an insuperable task?

(2) How does ATP link catabolism and anabolism?

(3) How does DNA preserve genetic information?

(4) How to understand "one-dimensional sequence of DNA is translated into three dimensional proteins"?

3. Choose the best answer to each of the following questions.

(1) Biochemistry is to determine_____.

A. the intrinsic inanimateness of molecules in living organisms

笔记

B. undiscovered physical laws and forces that govern living organisms

C. application of living organisms in medicine, agriculture, nutrition and industry

D. how the collections of inanimate molecules that constitute living organisms interact with each other to maintain and perpetuate life

(2) All macromolecules are constructed from_____.

A.carbon atoms

B.monomeric subunits

C.precursors of hormones, neurotransmitters and pigments

D.many different types of simple compounds

(3) What is the function of ATP ?

A. ATP is an intermediate in catabolism but not in anabolism.

B. It carries chemical energy in all cells.

C. It is the connecting link for enzyme-catalyzed reactions in the cell.

D. It releases energy by accepting a phosphate group.

(4) Why can DNA repair and replicate with high fidelity?

A. Genetic information is encoded in the linear sequence of four kinds of subunits of DNA.

B. The continuity of inherited traits has been preserved in the structure of DNA for millions of years.

C. The structure of DNA is rigid enough to resist any damage and error during repair and replication.

D. DNA double helix contains two complementary strands, one serves as a template for the synthesis of the other.

(5) The three-dimensional structures of macromolecules and supramolecular complexes are stabilized by_____.

A. noncovalent interactions that are individually weak but collectively strong

B. noncovalent interactions conferring rigidity on macromolecules

C. transient covalent binding

D. hydrogen bonds and ionic interactions among charged groups

(6) The assembly of macromolecules into their native conformations needs_____.

A. a template

B. a scaffold to direct the folding

C. energy provided by the formation of noncovalent interactions

D. assuming random forms

(7) The molecular logic of life includes all the followings except_____.

A. A living cell extracts free energy and raw materials from its environment

B. Various enzymatic reactions are carried out by cells

C. Genetic information encoded as sequences of nucleotide subunits determines the three-dimensional structure and function of each protein

D. The cell maintains itself in a constantly steady state

(8) How to understand the underlined part in "The cell carries out many consecutive reactions promoted by specific catalysts, called enzymes, which it produces by itself"?

A. Catalysts produce enzymes by themselves.

B. Reactions can produce enzymes by themselves.

笔记

C. Cells produce enzymes by themselves.

D. Enzymes are produced by themselves.

(9) How to understand the sentence "A living organism appears to be more than the sum of its inanimate parts"?

A. A living organisms is in a larger size than the sum of its inanimate parts.

B. The number of living organisms is larger than that of inanimate parts.

C. A living organism is not only the accumulation of its inanimate parts.

D. There are more inanimate parts than living organisms.

(10) The monomeric subunits of macromolecules_____.

A. have a molecular weight (MW) larger than about 500

B. can be non-covalently linked in a virtually limitless variety of sequences

C. are constructed to serve various functions in living cells

D. belong to 20 different types

4. **Choose an appropriate word or expression from the list below and write it down in the underline before its corresponding definition.**

> neurotransmitter, evolution, hydrogen bond, amino acid, polysaccharide, adenosine triphosphate, intermediate, enzyme, catabolism, chromosome

(1) _____The set of metabolic pathways that breaks down molecules into smaller units

(2) _____Monomeric subunits of proteins

(3) _____Carbohydrate molecule composed of long chains of monosaccharide units bound together by glycosidic linkages and on hydrolysis give the constituent monosaccharides or oligosaccharides

(4) _____A nucleoside triphosphate used in cells as a coenzyme often called the "molecular unit of currency" of intracellular energy transfer

(5) _____A packaged and organized structure containing most of the DNA of a living organism

(6) _____Proteins that act as biological catalysts

(7) _____Electrostatic attraction between polar molecules that occurs when a hydrogen (H) atom bound to a highly electronegative atom such as nitrogen, oxygen or fluorine

(8) _____A short-lived, unstable molecule in a chemical reaction

(9) _____Endogenous chemicals that transmit signals across a synapse or junction from one neuron (nerve cell) to another "target" neuron, muscle cell or gland cell

(10) _____Change in the heritable traits of biological populations over successive generations

5. **Translate the following sentences and paragraphs into Chinese.**

(1) Biochemistry determine how the collections of inanimate molecules that constitute living organisms interact with each other to maintain and perpetuate life.

(2) Enzymes are catalysts that accelerate the rates of biological reactions. Each enzyme is very specific in its function and acts only in a particular metabolic reaction.

(3) One of the most fruitful approaches to understand biological phenomena has been to purify an individual chemical component, such as a protein, from a living organism and to characterize its chemical structure or catalytic activity.

(4) The chemical principles that govern the properties of biological molecules include the covalent

笔记

bonding of carbon with itself and with other elements as well as the functional groups that appear in common biological molecules.

(5) The basic unit of DNA is a linear polymer of four different monomeric subunits arranged in a precise linear sequence.

(6) Biochemistry is an intrinsically beautiful and fascinating body of knowledge. We now know the essence and many of the details of the most fundamental processes in biochemistry, such as how a single molecule of DNA replicates to generate two identical copies of itself and how the sequences of bases in a DNA molecule determines the sequence of amino acid in an encoded protein. Our ability to describe these processes in detailed, mechanistic terms places a firm chemical foundation under other biological science.

(7) Proteins are the agents of biological function. Virtually every cellular activity is dependent on one or more particular proteins. Thus, a convenient way to classify the enormous number of proteins is by the biological roles they fill. By far the largest class of proteins is enzyme. A number of proteins do not perform any obvious chemical transformation but nevertheless regulate the ability of other proteins to carry out their physiological functions. Such proteins are referred to as regulatory proteins. Transport proteins, storage proteins and structural proteins are proteins carry out respective functions.

Text B
Discovery of Insulin, and the Making of a Medical Miracle

Background

Insulin is a hormone that regulates the amount of glucose (sugar) in the blood and is required for the body to function normally. Insulin is produced by β-cells in the pancreas, also called the islets of Langerhans. These cells continuously release a small amount of insulin into the body, but release surges of the hormone in response to a rise in the blood glucose level.

Certain cells in the body change the food ingested into energy, or blood glucose, that cells can use. Every time a person eats, the blood glucose rises. Raised blood glucose triggers the cells in the islets of Langerhans to release the necessary amount of insulin. Insulin allows the blood glucose to be transported from the blood into the cells. Cells have an outer wall, called a membrane, which controls what enters and exits the cell. Researchers do not yet know exactly how insulin works, but they do know insulin binds to receptors on the cell membrane. This activates a set of transport molecules so that glucose and proteins can enter the cell. The cells can then use the glucose as energy to carry out its functions. Once transported into the cell, the blood glucose level is returned to normal within hours.

Without insulin, the blood glucose builds up in the blood and the cells are starved of their energy source. Some of the symptoms that may occur include fatigue, constant infections, blurred eye sight, numbness, tingling in the hands or legs, increased thirst, and slowed healing of bruises or cuts. The cells will begin to use fat, the energy source stored for emergencies. When this lasts for too long a time the body produces ketones, chemicals produced by the liver. Ketones can poison and kill cells if they build up in the body over an extended period of time. This can lead to serious illness and coma.

People who do not produce the necessary amount of insulin have diabetes. There are two general

笔记

types of diabetes. The most severe type, known as Type I or juvenile-onset diabetes, is when the body does not produce any insulin. Type I diabetics usually inject themselves with different types of insulin three to four times daily. Dosage is taken based on the person's blood glucose reading, taken from a glucose meter. Type II diabetics produce some insulin, but it is either not enough or their cells do not respond normally to insulin. This usually occurs in obese or middle aged and older people. Type II diabetics do not necessarily need to take insulin, but they may inject insulin once or twice a day.

How Insulin Almost Wasn't Discovered

Before the discovery of insulin, diabetes was a feared disease that most certainly led to death. Patients wasted away, grew weak, and suffered indescribably before their inevitable death. They had insatiable thirst and hunger, but trying to satisfy their hunger only made things worse, and they continued to lose weight. Doctors knew that sugar worsened the condition of diabetic patients and that the most effective treatment was to put the patients on very strict diets where sugar intake was kept to a minimum. At best, this treatment could buy patients a few extra years, but it never saved them. In some cases, the harsh diets even caused patients to die of starvation.

During the nineteenth century, observations of patients who died of diabetes often showed that the pancreas was damaged. In 1869, a German medical student, Paul Langerhans, found that within the pancreatic tissue that produces digestive juices there were clusters of cells whose function was unknown. Some of these cells were eventually shown to be the insulin-producing beta cells. Later, in honor of the person who discovered them, the cell clusters were named the islets of Langerhans.

In 1889 in Germany, physiologist Oskar Minkowski and physician Joseph von Mering, showed that if the pancreas was removed from a dog, the animal got diabetes. But if the duct through which the pancreatic juices flow to the intestine was ligated - surgically tied off so the juices couldn't reach the intestine - the dog developed minor digestive problems but no diabetes. So it seemed that the pancreas must have at least two functions:

- To produce digestive juices
- To produce a substance that regulates the sugar glucose

This hypothetical internal secretion was the key. If a substance could actually be isolated, the mystery of diabetes would be solved. Progress, however, was slow.

In 1920, an unknown Canadian surgeon named Frederick Banting approached Professor John Macleod, the head of the University of Toronto's physiology department, with an idea about finding that secret. He theorized that the pancreatic digestive juices could be harmful to the secretion of the pancreas produced by the islets of Langerhans. He therefore wanted to ligate the pancreatic ducts in order to stop the flow of nourishment to the pancreas. This would cause the pancreas to degenerate, making it shrink and lose its ability to secrete the digestive juices. The cells thought to produce an antidiabetic secretion could then be extracted from the pancreas without being harmed. Unfortunately, Macleod, a leading figure in the study of diabetes in Canada, didn't think much of Banting's theories and rebuffed his suggestion. Despite this, Banting managed to convince Macleod that his idea was worth trying. Macleod gave Banting a laboratory with a minimum of equipment and ten dogs. Banting also got an assistant, a medical student by the name of Charles Best. The experiment was set to start in the summer of 1921.

Banting and Best began their experiments by removing the pancreas from a dog. This resulted in

笔记

the following:

- It's blood sugar rose.
- It became thirsty, drank lots of water, and urinated more often.
- It became weaker and weaker.

The dog had developed diabetes.

Experimenting on another dog, Banting and Best surgically ligated the pancreas, stopping the flow of nourishment, so that the pancreas degenerated. After a while, they removed the pancreas, sliced it up, and froze the pieces in a mixture of water and salts. When the pieces were half frozen, they were ground up and filtered. The isolated substance was named "isletin."

The extract was injected into the diabetic dog. Its blood glucose level dropped, and it seemed healthier and stronger. By giving the diabetic dog a few injections a day, Banting and Best could keep it healthy and free of symptoms. Banting and Best showed their result to Macleod, who was impressed, but he wanted more tests to prove that their pancreatic extract really worked. For the increased testing, Banting and Best realized that they required a larger supply of organs than their dogs could provide, and they started using pancreases from cattle. With this new source, they managed to produce enough extract to keep several diabetic dogs alive. The new results convinced Macleod that they were onto something big. He gave them more funds and moved them to a better laboratory with proper working conditions. He also suggested that they should call their extract "insulin." Now, the work proceeded rapidly. In late 1921, a third person, biochemist Bertram Collip, joined the team. Collip was given the task of trying to purify the insulin so that it would be clean enough for testing on humans. During the intensified testing, the team also realized that the process of shrinking the pancreases had been unnecessary. Using whole fresh pancreases from adult animals worked just as well.

In 1922 the insulin was tested on Leonard Thompson, a 14-year-old diabetes patient who lay dying at the Toronto General Hospital. He was given an insulin injection. At first he suffered a severe allergic reaction and further injections were cancelled. The scientists worked hard on improving the extract and then a second dose of injections were administered on Thompson. The results were spectacular. The scientists went to the other wards with diabetic children, most of them comatose and dying from diabetic keto-acidosis. They reacted just as positively as Leonard to the insulin extract.

Banting and Macleod were awarded the Nobel Prize in 1923 for the practical extraction of insulin. They were incensed that the other members of their team were not included, and they immediately shared their prize money with Best and Collip. They sold the original patent to the University of Toronto for one half-dollar. They were not looking for fame or fortune; they wanted to keep sick children from dying. They did eventually benefit financially, but that was the last thing on their minds.

Very soon after the discovery of insulin, the medical firm Eli Lilly started large-scale production of the extract. As early as in 1923, the firm was producing enough insulin to supply the entire North American continent. Although insulin doesn't cure diabetes, it's one of the biggest discoveries in medicine. When it came, it was like a miracle. People with severe diabetes and only days left to live were saved. And as long as they kept getting their insulin, they could live an almost normal life.

Working with human insulin

In 1982, the Eli Lilly Corporation produced a human insulin (Humulin®) that became the first

笔记

approved genetically engineered pharmaceutical product. This important achievement was the result of a vast network of basic and applied scientific advances that began in the 1950s with the classic structural studies on DNA by Watson and Crick and on insulin by Sanger.[1] Without needing to depend on animals, researchers could produce genetically engineered insulin in unlimited supplies. It also did not contain any of the animal contaminants. Using human insulin also took away any concerns about transferring any potential animal diseases into the insulin. While companies still sell a small amount of insulin produced from animals—mostly porcine—from the 1980s onwards, insulin users increasingly moved to a form of human insulin created through recombinant DNA technology.

Insulin is a protein consisting of two separate chains of amino acids, an A above a B chain, that are held together with disulfide bonds. The insulin A chain consists of 21 amino acids and the B chain has 30. Before becoming an active insulin protein, insulin is first produced as preproinsulin. This is one single long protein chain with the A and B chains not yet separated, a section in the middle linking the chains together and a signal sequence at one end telling the protein when to start secreting outside the cell. After preproinsulin, the chain evolves into proinsulin, still a single chain but without the signaling sequence. Then comes the active protein insulin, the protein without the section linking the A and B chains. At each step, the protein needs specific enzymes to produce the next form of insulin.

Lilly has prepared human insulin by two different means—initially, by a chain combination procedure and, since 1986, by transforming human proinsulin into human insulin. In the first method, the two insulin chains are produced separately. Manufacturers need the two mini-genes: one that produces the A chain and one for the B chain. Since the exact DNA sequence of each chain is known, they synthesize each mini-gene's DNA and insert them into plasmids. The recombinant, newly formed, plasmids are then transformed into bacterial cells. During a fermentation process, the millions of bacteria harboring the recombinant plasmid replicate roughly every 20 minutes through cell division, and each expresses the insulin gene.[2] After multiplying, the cells are taken out of the fermentation tanks and broken open to extract the protein chains. The two chains are then mixed together and joined by disulfide bonds through the reduction-reoxidation reaction. Although the chain combination procedure worked quite well, the proinsulin approach required fewer processing steps and, consequently, superseded the chain method in 1986. The sequence that codes for proinsulin is inserted into the non-pathogenic *E. coli* bacteria. The bacteria go through the fermentation process where they reproduce and produce proinsulin. Then the connecting sequence between the A and B chains is spliced away with an enzyme and the resulting insulin is purified.

The Future

The future of insulin holds many possibilities. Since insulin was first synthesized, diabetics needed to regularly inject the liquid insulin with a syringe directly into their bloodstream. This allows the insulin to enter the blood immediately. For many years it was the only way known to move the intact insulin protein into the body. In the 1990s, researchers began to make inroads in synthesizing various devices and forms of insulin that diabetics can use in an alternate drug delivery system.

Manufacturers are currently producing several relatively new drug delivery devices. Insulin pens look like a writing pen. A cartridge holds the insulin and the tip is the needle. The user set a dose, inserts the needle into the skin, and presses a button to inject the insulin. With pens there is no need to use a vial of insulin. However, pens require inserting separate tips before each injection. Another downside is that the pen does not allow users to mix insulin types, and not all insulin is available.

The insulin pump allows a controlled release in the body. This is a computerized pump, about the size of a beeper, that diabetics can wear on their belt or in their pocket. The pump has a small flexible tube that is inserted just under the surface of the diabetic's skin. The diabetic sets the pump to deliver a steady, measured dose of insulin throughout the day, increasing the amount right before eating. This mimics the body's normal release of insulin. Manufacturers have produced insulin pumps since the 1980s but advances in the late 1990s and early twenty-first century have made them increasingly easier to use and more popular. Researchers are exploring the possibility of implantable insulin pumps. Diabetics would control these devices through an external remote control.

Researchers are exploring other drug-delivery options. Ingesting insulin through pills is one possibility. The challenge with edible insulin is that the stomach's high acidic environment destroys the protein before it can move into the blood. Researchers are working on coating insulin with special materials that would protect the drugs from the stomach's acid.

In 2001 promising tests are occurring on inhaled insulin devices and manufacturers could begin producing the products within the next few years. Since insulin is a relatively large protein, it does not permeate into the lungs. Researchers of inhaled insulin are working to create insulin particles that are small enough to reach the deep lung. The particles can then pass into the bloodstream. Researchers are testing several inhalation devices much like that of an asthma inhaler.

Insulin patches are another drug delivery system in development. Patches would release insulin continuously into the bloodstream. The challenge is finding a way to have insulin pass through the skin. Ultrasound is one method researchers are investigating. These low frequency sound waves could change the skin's permeability and allow insulin to pass.

Other research has the potential to discontinue the need for manufacturers to synthesize insulin. Researchers are working on creating the cells that produce insulin in the laboratory. The thought is that physicians can someday replace the non-working pancreatic cells with insulin-producing cells. Another hope for diabetics is gene therapy. Scientists are working on correcting the insulin gene's mutation so that diabetics would be able to produce insulin on their own.

Word Study

1. allergic [əˈləːdʒik] *adj.* 过敏的
2. blur [bləː] *v.* 弄脏，使…模糊
3. bruise [bruːz] *n.* 淤青，擦伤；*v.* 碰伤、擦伤、挫伤
4. cartridge [ˈkɑːtridʒ] *n.* 弹药筒，笔芯，墨盒
5. code [kəud] *n.* 密码，法规，准则；*v.* 把…编码
6. comatose [ˈkəumətəus] *adj.* 昏睡状态的，昏迷的
7. cure [kjuə] *n.* 治疗，治愈，疗法；*v.* 治愈
8. degenerate [diˈdʒenəreit] *v.* 退化
9. diabetes [ˌdaiəˈbiːtiːz] *n.* 糖尿病
10. digestion [daiˈdʒestʃ ən] *n.* 消化
11. digestive [daiˈdʒestiv] *adj.* 消化的；*n.* 消化药

笔记

12. extract ['ekstrækt] *n.* 榨出物, 浓缩物, 提取物; ['ikstrækt], *v.* 拔出, 榨出, 提取

13. fatigue [fə'ti:g] *n.* 疲劳, 疲乏

14. filter ['filtə] *v.* 过滤, 渗透; *n.* 过滤器

15. harsh [hɑ:ʃ] *adj.* 粗糙的, 严厉的, 严酷的, 刺耳的

16. implantable [im'plɑ:ntəbl] *adj.* 可移植的, 可植入的

17. insatiable [in'seiʃəbl] *adj.* 不知足的, 贪得无厌的

18. islet ['ailət] *n.* 小岛

19. islets of Langerhans 兰格汉斯岛, 胰岛

20. isolate ['aisəleit] *v.* 使孤立, 隔离, 分离; *adj.* 孤立的, 单独的

21. keto-acidosis ['ketəuæsid'əusis] *n.* 酮酸中毒

22. ketone ['ki:təun] *n.* 酮

23. ligate [lai'geit] *v.* 绑, 扎

24. nourishment ['nə:riʃmənt] *n.* 营养

25. numbness [nʌmnəs] *n.* 麻木

26. obese [əu'bi:s] *adj.* 肥胖的

27. obesity [əu'bi:səti] *n.* 肥胖

28. pancreas ['pæŋkriəs] *n.* 胰脏

29. patch [pætʃ] *n.* 小片, 补丁, 贴剂

30. patent ['pætnt] *n.* 专利, 特许; *v.* 给予专利权; *adj.* 专利的

31. pathogenic ['pæθə'dʒenik] *adj.* 致病的

32. permeability [,pəmiə'biliti] *n.* 弥漫, 渗透

33. permeate ['pə:mieit] *v.* 弥漫, 渗透

34. physiology [,fizi'ɔ:lədʒi] *n.* 生理学

35. plasmid ['plæzmid] *n.* 质粒

36. porcine ['pɔ:sain] *adj.* 猪的

37. preproinsulin [pri:prəu'insjulin] *n.* 前胰岛素原

38. proinsulin [prəu'insəlin] *n.* 胰岛素原

39. recombinant [ri:'kɔmbənənt] *n.* 重组体, 重组子; *adj.* (基因) 重组的

40. splice [splais] *n.* 接合, 衔接; *v.* 拼接, 剪接

41. symptom ['simptəm] *n.* 症状

42. syringe [si'rindʒ] *n.* 注射器

43. tingling [tiŋgliŋ] *n.* 刺痛感

44. ultrasound ['ʌltrəsaund] *n.* 超声

Notes

1. This important achievement was the result of a vast network of basic and applied scientific advances that began in the 1950s with the classic structural studies on DNA by Watson and Crick and on insulin by Sanger. 译为: 这一重要成就归功于 20 世纪 50 年代以来在基础和应用科学领域取得的一系列研究成果, 其中包括沃森和克里克对 DNA 的结构研究和桑格对胰岛素结构的研究。"that began in the 1950s" 为修饰 "advances" 的定语从句。"classic structural studies on…by…and on…by…" 包含两个并列的结构。

2. During a fermentation process, the millions of bacteria harboring the recombinant plasmid replicate roughly every 20 minutes through cell division, and each expresses the insulin gene. 译

笔记

为：在发酵过程中，数百万计的携带重组质粒的细菌几乎每20分钟就会增殖一代，每一个细菌细胞都会表达胰岛素基因。"harboring the recombinant plasmid"为"bacteria"的后置定语。"each expresses…"中的each指的是前面提到的"millions of bacteria"。

Supplementary Parts

1. Medical and Pharmaceutical Terms Made Easier (3): Common Morphemes in English Terms for Biology and Biochemistry

Morpheme	Meaning	Example
acet	醋酸，乙酸，醋	acetone 丙酮
aden	腺	adenosine 腺苷
allo-	异	allopurinol 别嘌醇
andr	雄	androgen 雄性激素
angul	角	triangular 三角（形的）
anthrop	人	anthropometry 人体测量学
arachid	花生	arachidonic acid 花生四烯酸
aspar	天冬	asparagine 天冬酰胺
bio	生物，生命	biology 生物学
chol	胆	cholecalciferol 胆钙化醇
cinchon	金鸡纳	cinchona 金鸡纳树（皮）
clon	克隆	monoclonal 单克隆的，单细胞系的
corn	角	cornification 角（质）化
cyt	细胞	cytochromes 细胞色素
de-	脱，使…失去	denaturation 变性
dem	人	demography 人口学，人口统计学
endo-	内	endopeptidase 内肽酶
estr	雌	estrogen 雌激素
exo-	外	exopeptidase 外肽酶
fem	雌	female 女性的，雌性的
gamet	配子	gametocide 杀配子剂
gen	基因	genome 染色体基因，基因组
gluc	甘，葡萄糖	glucokinase 葡萄糖激酶
glyc	甘，甜	glycolysis 糖酵解
gon	角	goniometer 角度计
heter	异	heteroduplex 杂化双链
hydro	水	hydrolase 水解酶类
iso-	异构	isomerase 异构酶类
kerat	角	keratin 角蛋白
ket	酮	ketogenic amino acid 生酮氨基酸
kin	动	kinase 激酶
lact	乳	lactate 乳酸盐
lino	亚麻	linolenate 亚麻酸
lipo	脂肪	lipoprotein 脂蛋白
mal	苹果	malate 苹果酸
malt	麦芽	maltase 麦芽糖酶
mono	单	monooxygenase 单加氧酶
mort	死	mortality 死亡率
necr	死	necrology 死亡统计学，死亡通知
ped	儿童	pediatrics 儿科学
pent	戊	pentose 戊糖
pept	肽	peptidyl site 肽基位，P位

笔记

续表

Morpheme	Meaning	Example
phosph	磷	phospholipase 磷脂酶
phyll	叶	chlorophyll 叶绿素
phyt	植物	phytosterol 植物固醇
poly	多	polypeptide 多肽
pyridox	吡哆	pyridoxamine 吡哆胺
pyruv	丙酮酸	pyruvate kinase 丙酮酸激酶
rib	核	riboflavin 核黄素（维生素 B$_2$）
spor	孢子	sporicide 杀孢子剂
tel	末端	telomerase 端粒酶
term	终端	terminator 终止子
thym	胸腺	thymine (T) 胸腺嘧啶
trans	转	transaldolase 转醛缩酶
ur	尿	uracil (U) 尿嘧啶
vit	生命	vital 生命的，生机的
vivi	生命	vivisect 活体解剖
zyg	合子	zygote 合子
zym	酶	zymogen 酶原

(1)　Decompose the following words and translate them into Chinese.

1)　aminopeptidase _____

2)　amyloid _____

3)　argininemia _____

4)　fructokinase _____

5)　gelatinous _____

6)　glutamine _____

7)　histidinuria _____

8)　mannitol _____

9)　nucleoprotein _____

10)　proteinuria _____

11)　steatosis _____

12)　tyrosinosis _____

(2)　Fill in the blanks with the missing word root, prefix or suffix.

1)　_____ometry 人体测量学

2)　_____purinol 别嘌醇

3)　mono_____al 单克隆的，单细胞系的

4)　_____ogen 雌激素

5)　_____lysis 糖酵解

6)　_____merase 异构酶类

7)　_____protein 脂蛋白

8)　_____iatrics 儿科学

9)　chloro_____ 叶绿素

10)　_____peptide 多肽

11)　_____aldolase 转醛缩酶

12)　_____gen 酶原

笔记

2.　English-Chinese Translation Skills: 药学英语语篇特点与翻译

药学英语语篇是关于药学以及相关学科的文献,这就决定了药学英语语篇区别于其他类型的语篇,具有不同的语言功能、语言特点和表达方式,以及在传播中构建的作者与读者之间的人际关系。根据系统功能语言学的情景语境理论,药学英语语篇有三个变量,即:语场(field)、语旨(tenor)和语式(mode)。简单来说,语场是指语篇话题(subject matter)、内容以及场地(setting)等情境因素;语旨是指交际双方的社会角色;语式是指语言活动所采用的媒介(medium)或渠道(channel)。这三个变量相互影响,构成一个整体。翻译药学英语语篇时,要首先了解语篇作者是如何在讨论某个具体内容时,选择语言表达方式,构建何种读者和作者人际关系。这样才能够准确判断原文的交际意图、正式程度、交际对象和交际重点等,做到翻译得体。如:

例: **The Structure of DNA Allows for Its Repair and Replication with Near-Perfect Fidelity**

The capacity of living cells to preserve their genetic material and to duplicate it for the next generation results from the structural complementarity between the two halves of the DNA molecule. The basic unit of DNA is a linear polymer of four different monomeric subunits, deoxyribonucleotides, arranged in a precise linear sequence. It is this linear sequence that encodes the genetic information. Two of these polymeric strands are twisted with each other to form the DNA double helix, where each monomeric subunit in one strand pairs specifically with the complementary subunit in the opposite strand. In the enzymatic replication or repair of DNA, one of the two strands serves as a template for the assembly of another, structurally complementary DNA strand. Before a cell divides, the two DNA strands separate and each serves as a template for the synthesis of a complementary strand, generating two identical double-helical molecules, one for each daughter cell. If one strand is damaged, continuity of information is assured by the information present on the other strand.

翻译前仔细分析该语篇,可以发现该段是关于 DNA 结构的自身修复和复制。从语篇的语场来看,该段文字语言规范,结构严谨,专业性词汇密度高,属于专业性较强的学术文献;从语篇的语旨来看,该段文字作者以客观、科学的方式介绍研究信息或主要观点,属于同行之间的学术交流,本着尊重科学的严谨态度,没有刻意构建轻松愉快的作者 - 读者关系,从语篇的语式来看,该段文字采用书面语的形式,句式规范,逻辑性强,在实际应用的过程中应该还配有其他模态,比如图片、模型、PPT 等。翻译前对语篇进行分析可以为正确翻译原文,确定翻译风格具有重要意义。

参考译文: **DNA 的结构允许其以几近完美精准度的方式进行自身修复和复制**

活细胞保持其遗传物质和为下一代复制的能力来源于 DNA 分子两条单链之间的结构互补性。DNA 的基本单位是由四种不同脱氧核糖核苷酸单体亚单位精密排列成的线性序列。正是这种线性序列能够编码遗传信息。两条聚合 DNA 单链互相缠绕而形成 DNA 双螺旋结构,在这里一条链上每一个单体亚基都能在另一条链中找到其特定的互补的亚基。在 DNA 的酶复制或修复过程中,两条链中一条充当另一条的装配模板,即结构互补 DNA 链。在细胞分裂前,两条 DNA 链分离,每个 DNA 分子作为模板用以合成另一条互补链,生成两个相同的双螺旋分子,一个子细胞含有一个双螺旋分子。如果一条链被破坏了,遗传信息的连续性可以确保由另一条链得以呈现。

从参考译文可以看出,译文真实反映了原文作者传递的信息内容,译文语言规范,结构严谨,专业词汇使用正确。阅读译文可以感受到原文作者与读者的沟通是建立在具有共同学科知识基础上,作者在介绍专业信息的同时希望读者能够理解并作出相应回应,体现出学术交流平等直接关系。从译文语言媒介来看,语言简洁,句式短小精悍,没有主观性形容词,书面语特征明显,语言风格与原文基本吻合。

就语篇体裁而言,药学英语语篇也有多种语篇形式,如医药科普文章、医药广告、药典、药品说明书、医药实验报告、质量标准等,不同的语篇体裁具有不同的语篇特点和语境意义,正确分析并理解不同语篇体裁是做好药学英语翻译的重要前提之一。

Unit Four Pharmacology

Pharmacology is concerned with all facets of the interaction of chemicals with biological systems. When such interactions are applied to the cure or amelioration of disease, the chemicals are usually called drugs.

Most drugs produce effects by combining with biological receptors. The chemical bonds that form between drug molecule and receptor are usually reversible. The ease with which drug and receptor interact is influenced by the degree of complementarity of their respective three-dimensional structures. For this reason, minor chemical modification of a drug may produce profound changes in its pharmacological activity.

Pharmacology is a hybrid science. It freely draws upon the intellectual resources of all the basic medical sciences and contributes to every aspect of clinical medicine. Today receptor theory serves as a unifying concept for the explanation of the effects of chemicals on biological systems, whether these chemicals be of exogenous (pharmacological) or endogenous (physiological) origin. In general, a drug produces a particular effect by combining chemically with some specific molecular constituent (receptor) of the biological system upon which it acts. The function of the receptor molecule in the biological system is thereby modified to produce a measurable effect.

药理学是全面研究化学物质与生物系统之间相互作用的一门学科。当这种相互作用被用于治疗或改善疾病时，这些化学物质即称为药物。

大多数药物通过与生物受体相结合而产生药效。药物分子与受体之间的化学偶联作用往往是可逆的。药物与受体相互作用易受它们各自的三维结构的互补程度影响。因此，即使是细微的化学修饰也可能引起药物药理学活性的重大改变。

药理学是一门交叉科学，它最大限度地综合了各个基础医学科学的知识资源，并且有助于临床医学的每一方面。当今，受体理论作为一个共识的概念，用于解释化学物质对生物系统的作用，无论这些化学物质是外源性的（药理学的）还是内源性的（生理学的）。总之，药物通过与其作用（影响）的生物系统的某些特定分子成分（受体）的化学结合而产生特定的作用，从而使生物系统中受体分子的功能改变而产生明显的作用。

笔记

53

Text A
The Scope of Pharmacology

In its entirety, pharmacology embraces the knowledge of the history, source, physical and chemical properties, compounding, biochemical and physiological effects, mechanisms of action, absorption, distribution, biotransformation and excretion, and therapeutic and other uses of drugs. Since a drug is broadly defined as any chemical agent that affects living processes, the subject of pharmacology is obviously quite extensive.

For the physician and the medical student, however, the scope of pharmacology is less expansive than indicated by the above definitions. The clinician is interested primarily in drugs that are useful in the prevention, diagnosis, and treatment of human disease, or in the prevention of pregnancy. His study of the pharmacology of these drugs can be reasonably limited to those aspects that provide the basis for their rational clinical use. Secondarily, the physician is also concerned with chemical agents that are not used in therapy but are commonly responsible for household and industrial poisoning as well as environmental pollution. His study of these substances is justifiably restricted to the general principles of prevention, recognition, and treatment of such toxicity or pollution. Finally, all physicians share in the responsibility to help resolve the continuing sociological problem of the abuse of drugs.

A brief consideration of its major subject areas will further clarify how the study of pharmacology is best approached from the standpoint of the specific requirements and interests of the medical students and practitioners. At one time, it was essential for the physician to have a broad botanical knowledge, since he had to select the proper plants from which to prepare his own crude medicinal preparations. However, fewer drugs are now obtained from natural sources, and, more importantly, most of these are highly purified or standardized and differ little from synthetic chemicals. Hence, the interests of the clinician in pharmacognosy are correspondingly limited. Nevertheless, scientific curiosity should stimulate the physician to learn something of the sources of drugs, and this knowledge often proves practically useful as well as interesting. He will find the history of drugs of similar value.

The preparing, compounding, and dispensing of medicines at one time lay within the province of the physician, but this work is now delegated almost completely to the pharmacist.[1] However, to write intelligent prescription orders, the physician must have some knowledge of the physical and chemical properties of drugs and their available dosage forms, and he must have a basic familiarity with the practice of pharmacy. When the physician shirks his responsibility in this regard, he invariably fails to translate his knowledge of pharmacology and medicine into prescription orders and medication best suited for the individual patient.

Pharmacokinetics deals with the absorption, distribution, biotransformation, and excretion of drugs. These factors, coupled with dosage, determine the concentration of a drug at its sites of action and, hence, the intensity of its effects as a function of time. Many basic principles of biochemistry and enzymology and the physical and chemical principles that govern the active and passive transfer and the distribution of substances across biological membranes are readily applied to the understanding of this important aspect of pharmacology.[2]

The study of the biochemical and physiological effects of drugs and their mechanisms of action is termed as pharmacodynamics. It is an experimental medical science that dates back only to the later half of the nineteenth century. As a border science, pharmacodynamics borrows freely from both the subject matter and the experimental techniques of physiology, biochemistry, microbiology, immunology, genetics, and pathology. It is unique mainly in that attention is focused on the characteristics of drugs. As the name implies, the subject is a dynamic one. The student who attempts merely to memorize the pharmacodynamic properties of drugs is foregoing one of the best opportunities for correlating the entire field of preclinical medicine. For example, the actions and effects of the saluretic agents can be fully understood only in terms of the basic principles of renal physiology and of the pathogenesis of edema. Conversely, no greater insight into normal and abnormal renal physiology can be gained than by the study of the pharmacodynamics of the saluretic agents.

Another ramification of pharmacodynamics is the correlation of the actions and effects of drugs with their chemical structures. Such structure-activity relationships are an integral link in the analysis of drug action, and exploitation of these relationships among established therapeutic agents has often led to the development of better drugs. However, the correlation of biological activity with chemical structure is usually of interest to the physician only when it provides the basis for summarizing other pharmacological information.

The physician is understandably interested mainly in the effects of drugs in man. This emphasis on clinical pharmacology is justified, since the effects of drugs are often characterized by significant interspecies variation, and since they may be further modified by disease. In addition, some drug effects, such as those on mood and behavior, can be adequately studied only in man. However, the pharmacological evaluation of drugs in man may be limited for technical, legal, and ethical reasons, and the choice of drugs must be based in part on their pharmacological evaluation in animals. Consequently, some knowledge of animal pharmacology and comparative pharmacology is helpful in deciding the extent to which claims for a drug based upon studies in animals can be reasonably extrapolated to man.[3]

Pharmacotherapeutics deals with the use of drugs in the prevention and treatment of disease. Many drugs stimulate or depress biochemical or physiological function in man in a sufficiently reproducible manner to provide relief of symptoms or, ideally, to alter favorably the course of disease. Conversely, chemotherapeutic agents are useful in therapy because they have only minimal effects on man but can destroy or eliminate parasites. Whether a drug is useful for therapy is crucially dependent upon its ability to produce its desired effects with only tolerable undesired effects. Thus, from the standpoint of the physician interested in the therapeutic uses of a drug, the selectivity of its effects is one of its most important characteristics. Drug therapy is rationally based upon the correlation of the actions and effects of drugs with the physiological, biochemical, microbiological, immunological, and behavioral aspects of disease. Pharmacodynamics provides one of the best opportunities for this correlation during the study of both the preclinical and the clinical medical sciences.

Toxicology is the aspect of pharmacology that deals with the adverse effects of drugs. It is concerned not only with drugs used in therapy but also with the many other chemicals that may be responsible for household, environmental, or industrial intoxication. The adverse effects of the pharmacological agents employed in therapy are properly considered an integral part of their total pharmacology. The toxic effects of other chemicals are such an extensive subject that the physician must usually confine his attention to the general principles applicable to the prevention, recognition, and treatment of drug poisonings of any cause.

笔记

Word Study

1. approach [əˈprəutʃ] *vt.* (着手)探讨/处理，(开始)对付

2. behavioral [biˈheivjərəl] *adj.* 关于行为的，关于态度的

3. biotransformation [baiətrænsfəˈmeiʃ(ə)n] *n.* 生物转化

4. botanical [bəˈtænik(ə)l] *adj.* 植物的，植物学的；*n.* 植物性药材

5. chemotherapeutic(al) [ˌkeməuˌθerəˈpju:tik(l)] *adj.* 化学治疗的；*n.* 化学治疗剂

6. clinician [kliˈniʃ(ə)n] *n.* 临床医生

7. converse [kənˈvə:s] *adj.* 相反的，逆的，颠倒的

8. delegate [ˈdeləgeit] *v.* 授权，把…委托给；*n.* 代表

9. diagnosis [ˌdaiəgˈnəusis] *n.* 诊断(法)

10. edema [iˈdi:mə] *n.* 浮肿，水肿

11. embrace [imˈbreis] *vt.* 包含，包括

12. entirety [inˈtaiərəti] *n.* 全部，整体

13. ethical [ˈeθik(ə)l] *adj.* 伦理的，道德的，(药品)合乎规格的，凭处方出售的

14. excretion [ikˈskri:ʃ(ə)n] *n.* 排泄(物)，分泌(物)

15. exploitation [ˌeksplɔiˈteiʃ(ə)n] *n.* 利用，开发，剥削

16. extrapolate [ikˈstræpəleit] *v.* 推断，推知；extrapolate to 推广到……

17. for(e)go [fɔ:ˈgəu] *v.* 放弃，摒弃，拒绝

18. genetics [dʒəˈnetiks] *n.* 遗传学

19. immunological [ˌimjunəˈlɔdʒikl] *adj.* 免疫的，免疫学的

20. integral [inˈtegrəl] *adj.* 完整的，整体的，组成的

21. interspecies [intrəˈspi:ʃi:z] *n.* 种类之间，种间

22. intoxication [inˌtɔksiˈkeiʃ(ə)n] *n.* 中毒，醉酒

23. invariably [inˈvɔəriəb(ə)li] *adv.* 不变地，永恒地；总是

24. justifiably [dʒʌstiˈfaiəbli] *adv.* 正当地，有理地，情有可原地

25. parasite [ˈpærəsait] *n.* 寄生生物

26. pathology [pəˈθɔlədʒi] *n.* 病理学，病理，病状

27. pharmacognosy [fɑ:məˈkɔgnəsi] *n.* 生药学，药材学

28. pharmacotherapeutics [fɑ:məkʌθerəpˈju:tiks] *n.* 药物治疗学，药物疗法

29. practitioner [prækˈtiʃ(ə)nə] *n.* 从业者(尤指医生、律师等)，职业医生，专业人才，开业者

30. preclinical [priˈklinikəl] *adj.* 临床用以前的，临床前的

31. pregnancy [ˈpregnənsi] *n.* 怀孕，怀胎，怀孕期

32. province [ˈprɔvins] *n.* 范围，领域，分科

33. ramification [ˌræmifiˈkeiʃn] *n.* 分枝，细节，分歧

34. renal [ˈri:n(ə)l] *adj.* 肾(脏)的

35. reproducible [ri:prəˈdju:səbl] *adj.* 能再现的，能再复制的，能再生产的，能繁殖的

36. saluretic [səˌlu:ˈretik] *adj.* (促)尿食盐排泄的；*n.* (促)尿食盐排泄剂

37. selectivity [səˌlekˈtiviti] *n.* 选择，精选，选择性

38. shirk [ʃə:k] *v.* 逃避(义务、责任等)，推掉

Notes

笔记

1. The preparing, compounding, and dispensing of medicines at one time lay within the province of

the physician, but this work is now delegated almost completely to the pharmacist. 英英注释：
The preparing, compounding, and dispensing of medicines was once included in the work of the
physician, but it is now done completely by the pharmacist.

2. Many basic principles of biochemistry and enzymology and the physical and chemical principles that
govern the active and passive transfer and the distribution of substances across biological membranes
are readily applied to the understanding of this important aspect of pharmacology. 译为：在对药理学
这一重要方面的理解过程中常常运用到许多有关生物化学和酶学方面的基本原理和物理化学
方面的一些基本法则，而这些原理和法则决定着物质在生物膜之间主动和被动转运及分布。

3. Consequently, some knowledge of animal pharmacology and comparative pharmacology is
helpful in deciding the extent to which claims for a drug based upon studies in animals can be
reasonably extrapolated to man. 译为：因此，动物药理学和比较药理学方面的知识有助于确定
以动物实验为基础研制的某种新药有多大可能用于人体。

Exercises

1. **Decide whether each of the following statements is true (T) or false (F) according to the
passage.**

(1) Pharmacodynamics, which is concerned with the study of the biochemical and physiological
effects of drugs and their mechanisms of action, is an experimental medical science.

(2) It's unreasonable for a physician to be interested mainly in the effects of drugs on human beings,
for the pharmacological evaluation of drugs in them may be limited due to technical, legal, and
ethical reasons.

(3) As the effects of drugs are often characterized by significant interspecies variation and may be
further modified by disease, clinical pharmacology has never been emphasized.

(4) The physician is not interested in drugs that are useful in the prevention, diagnosis, and treatment
of human disease, but in chemical agents that are commonly responsible for household and
industrial poisoning as well as environmental pollution.

(5) A drug is said to be useful in therapy if it has the ability to produce its desired effects with only
tolerable undesired effects.

(6) Toxicology deals not only with drugs used in therapy but also with many other chemicals that
may be responsible for household, environmental, or industrial intoxication.

2. **Questions for oral discussion.**

(1) How do you understand pharmacology in broad sense or less expansive sense?

(2) What are the traditional major subject areas in the study of pharmacology from the viewpoint of
the specific requirements and interests of medical students and practitioners?

(3) How is pharmacodynamics defined in this passage?

(4) Why is it understandable that the physician is interested mainly in the effects of drugs on human
beings?

3. **Choose the best answer to each of the following questions.**

(1) Which of the following parts of knowledge of drugs should be included in pharmacology?

　　A. The effects of drugs on man.

　　B. The correlation of biological activity with chemical structure.

　　C. The history, source, physical and chemical properties, compounding, biochemical and physiological
effects, mechanisms of action, absorption, distribution, biotransformation and excretion.

D. The prevention, recognition, and treatment of drug poisonings.

(2) Which of the following is what a clinician is primarily interested in according to the text?

A. Drugs which can be reasonably limited to those aspects that provide the basis for their rational clinical use.

B. Chemical agents that are not used in therapy but are commonly responsible for household and industrial poisoning as well as environmental pollution.

C. Drugs which are useful in the prevention, diagnosis and treatment of human disease, or in the prevention of pregnancy.

D. Drugs which help resolve the continuing abuse of drug.

(3) Why was the physician not interested in pharmacognosy?

A. He didn't have to select the proper plants for his prescription.

B. He had a broad botanical knowledge.

C. Fewer drugs were obtained from natural sources.

D. Natural drugs had little difference with synthetic ones.

(4) Which of the following is the best way of studying pharmacology for medical students and practitioners?

A. to have a broad botanical knowledge

B. to select a plant and its preparation

C. to have the ability to purify natural plants

D. to have curiosity that stimulates them to learn about sources of drugs

(5) What are the tasks related to medicines almost completely delegated to the pharmacists now?

A. the physical and chemical properties of medicines

B. the preparing, compounding, and dispensing of medicines

C. dosage forms of medicines available

D. the therapeutic and other uses of medicines

(6) What is a main unique aspect of pharmacodynamics?

A. Pharmacodynamics is an experimental medical science.

B. Pharmacodynamics is focused on the characteristics of drugs.

C. Pharmacodynamics borrows freely from both the subject matter and the experimental techniques of physiology, biochemistry, microbiology, genetics and pathology.

D. Pharmacodynamics correlates the entire field of preclinical medicine.

(7) What time of history does pharmacodynamics date back to?

A. the second half of the seventeenth century

B. the second half of the eighteenth century

C. the second half of the nineteenth century

D. the second half of the twentieth century

(8) What does the research on pharmacodynamics focus on?

A. study of clinical effect of drugs

B. study of the process of drugs in the body

C. study of the effect and the mechanism of drugs on the body

D. study of the correlation of the actions and effects of drugs with their chemical structure

笔记

(9) Which of the following is true when drugs are selected?

A. It has to be based in part on legal reasons.

B. It has to be based in part on ethical reasons.

C. It has to be based in part on the pharmacological evaluation in man.

D. It has to be based in part on the pharmacological evaluation in animals.

(10) Why are chemotherapeutic agents useful in therapy?

A. They stimulate or depress biochemical or physiological function in man in a sufficiently reproducible manner to provide relief of symptoms or, ideally, to alter favorably the course of disease.

B. They can produce desired effects with only tolerable undesired effects.

C. They have only minimal effects on man but can destroy or eliminate parasites.

D. The selectivity of their effects is one of their most important characteristics.

4. Fill in each of the following blanks with an appropriate word or expression according to the meaning of the sentence(s).

(1) The clinician is interested primarily in drugs that are useful in the prevention, _____ and treatment of human disease, or in the prevention of pregnancy.

(2) A brief consideration of its major subject areas will further clarify how the study of pharmacology is best approached from the standpoint of the specific requirements and interests of the medical students and _____.

(3) _____ deals with the absorption, distribution, biotransformation, and excretion of drugs.

(4) _____ is an experimental medical science that dates back only to the second half of the nineteenth century.

(5) Pharmacodynamics borrows freely from both the subject matter and the experimental techniques of physiology, biochemistry, _____, immunology, genetics and pathology.

(6) Another _____ of pharmacodynamics is the correlation of the actions and effects of drugs with their chemical structures.

(7) _____ deals with the use of drugs in the prevention and treatment of disease.

(8) Drug therapy is rationally based upon the correlation of the actions and effects of drugs with the physiological, biochemical, microbiological, _____, and behavioral aspects of disease.

(9) It is concerned not only with drugs used in therapy but also with many other chemicals that may be responsible for household, environmental, or industrial _____.

(10) Chemotherapeutic agents are useful in therapy because they have only minimal effects on man but can destroy or eliminate _____.

5. Translate the following sentences and paragraphs into Chinese.

(1) Such structure-activity relationships are an integral link in the analysis of drug action, and exploitation of these relationships among established therapeutic agents has often led to the development of better drugs.

(2) The student who attempts merely to memorize the pharmacodynamic properties of drugs is foregoing one of the best opportunities for correlating the entire field of preclinical medicine.

(3) However, the pharmacological evaluation of drugs in man may be limited for technical, legal, and ethical reasons, and the choice of drugs must be based in part on their pharmacological evaluation in animals.

(4) At one time, it was essential for the physician to have a broad botanical knowledge, since he had to select the proper plants from which to prepare his own crude medicinal preparations.

(5) Since a drug is broadly defined as any chemical agent that affects living processes, the subject of

笔记

pharmacology is obviously quite extensive.

(6) Pharmacokinetics deals with the absorption, distribution, biotransformation, and excretion of drugs. These factors, coupled with dosage, determine the concentration of a drug at its sites of action and, hence, the intensity of its effects as a function of time. Many basic principles of biochemistry and enzymology and the physical and chemical principles that govern the active and passive transfer and the distribution of substances across biological membranes are readily applied to the understanding of this important aspect of pharmacology.

(7) The study of the biochemical and physiological effects of drugs and their mechanisms of action is termed as pharmacodynamics. It is an experimental medical science that dates back only to the later half of the nineteenth century. As a border science, pharmacodynamics borrows freely from both the subject matter and the experimental techniques of physiology, biochemistry, microbiology, immunology, genetics, and pathology. It is unique mainly in that attention is focused on the characteristics of drugs. As the name implies, the subject is a dynamic one. The student who attempts merely to memorize the pharmacodynamic properties of drugs is foregoing one of the best opportunities for correlating the entire field of preclinical medicine. For example, the actions and effects of the saluretic agents can be fully understood only in terms of the basic principles of renal physiology and of the pathogenesis of edema. Conversely, no greater insight into normal and abnormal renal physiology can be gained than by the study of the pharmacodynamics of the saluretic agents.

Text B
Adverse Drug Reactions

Adverse drug reactions are unwanted effects caused by normal therapeutic doses. Drugs are great mimics of diseases, and adverse drug reactions present with diverse clinical signs and symptoms. The classification proposed by Rawlins and Thompson divides reactions into type A and type B.

Type A reactions, which constitute the great majority of adverse drug reactions, are usually a consequence of the drug's main pharmacological effect (e.g. bleeding from warfarin) or a low therapeutic index (e.g. nausea from digoxin), and they are therefore predictable. They are dose-related and usually mild, although they may be serious or even fatal (e.g. intracranial bleeding from warfarin). Such reactions are usually due to incorrect dosage (too much or too long), for the individual patient or to disordered pharmacokinetics, usually impaired drug elimination. The term "side-effects" is often applied to minor type A reactions.

Type B (idiosyncratic) reactions are not predictable from the drug's main pharmacological action, are not dose-related and are severe, with a considerable mortality. The underlying pathophysiology of type B reactions is poorly if at all understood, and often has a genetic or immunological basis. Type B reactions occur infrequently (1:1000-1:10 000 treated subjects being typical).

Three further minor categories of adverse drug reactions have been proposed.

1. Type C—continuous reactions due to long-term drug use (e.g. neuroleptic-related tardive dyskinesia or analgesic nephropathy);

2. Type D—delayed reactions (e.g. alkylating agents leading to carcinogenesis, or retinoid-associated teratogenesis);

3. Type E—end-of-use reactions such as adrenocortical insufficiency following withdrawal of

笔记

corticosteroids, or withdrawal syndromes following discontinuation of treatment with clonidine, benzodiazepines, tricyclic antidepressants or beta-adrenoreceptor antagonists.

There are between 30 000 and 40 000 medicinal products available directly or on prescription in the UK. A recent survey suggested that approximately 80% of adults take some kind of medication during any 2-week period. Exposure to drugs in the population is thus substantial, and the incidence of adverse reactions must be viewed in this context.[1] Type A reactions are believed to be responsible for up to 3% of acute hospital admissions and 2%-3% of consultations in general practice.[2] In hospital, clinically significant adverse reactions are estimated to complicate 10%-20% of all admissions, prolonging hospital stay and causing suffering and an appreciable number of fatalities, as well as wasting resources. They are the most frequent and severe in neonates, the elderly, women, patients with hepatic or renal disease, and individuals with a history of previous adverse drug reactions. Adverse drug reactions often occur early in therapy (during the first 1-10 days). The drugs most commonly implicated are digoxin, antimicrobials, diuretics, potassium salt replacements, analgesics, sedatives and major tranquillizers, insulin, aspirin, glucocorticosteroids, antihypertensives and warfarin.

Factors involved in the etiology of adverse drug reactions can be classified as follows:

1. **patient factors**

   Intrinsic:

   Age- neonate, infant and elderly

   Sex- hormonal environment

   Genetic abnormalities (e.g. enzyme or receptor polymorphisms)

   Previous adverse drug reactions, allergy, atopy

   Presence of organ dysfunction- disease

   Personality and habits–alcoholic, drug addict, nicotine, compliance

   Extrinsic:

   Environment–sun

   Xenobiotics (e.g. drugs, herbicides)

   Malnutrition

2. **Prescriber factors**

   Incorrect drug or drug combination

   Incorrect route of administration

   Incorrect dose

   Incorrect duration of therapy

3. **Drug factors**

   Drug-drug interactions

   Pharmaceutical–batch problems, shelf-life, incorrect dispensing

Adverse Drug Reaction Monitoring/Surveillance Pharmacovigilance

The evaluation of drug safety is complex, and there are many methods for monitoring adverse drug reactions. Each of these has its own advantages and shortcomings, and no single system can offer the absolute security that public opinion expects. The ideal method would identify adverse drug reactions with a high degree of sensitivity and specificity and respond rapidly. It would detect rare but severe adverse drug reactions, but would not be overwhelmed by common ones, the incidence of

笔记

which would quantify together with predisposing factors.[3] Continued surveillance is mandatory after a new drug has been marketed, as it is inevitable that the preliminary testing of medicines in humans during drug development, although excluding many ill effects, cannot identify uncommon adverse effects. A variety of early detection methods have been introduced to identify adverse drug reactions as swiftly as possible.

Phase I / II / III Trials

Early (phase I / II) trials are important for assessing the tolerability and dose-response relationship of new therapeutic agents. However, these studies are very insensitive at detecting adverse reactions because they are performed on relatively few subjects (perhaps 200-300). This is illustrated by the failure to detect the serious toxicity of several drugs (e.g. practolol, benoxaprofen, temafloxacin, felbamate, dexfenfluramine and fenfluramine, troglitazone) before marketing. However, phase III clinical trials can establish the incidence of common adverse reactions and relate this to therapeutic benefit. Analysis of the reasons given for dropping out of phase III trials is particularly valuable in establishing whether common events such as headache, constipation, lethargy or male sexual dysfunction are truly drug related. The Medical Research Council Mild Hypertension Study unexpectedly identified impotence as being more commonly associated with thiazide diuretics than with placebo or beta-adrenoreceptor antagonist therapy in this way.

The problem of adverse drug reaction recognition is much greater if the reaction resembles spontaneous disease in the population, such that physicians are unlikely to attribute the reaction to drug exposure.[4] The numbers of patients that must be exposed to enable such reactions to be detected are probably greater than those quoted by more than one or two orders of magnitude.

Word Study

1. addict ['ædikt] *n.* 沉溺，成瘾（者）
2. admission [əd'miʃn] *n.* 住院，入院
3. adrenocortical [ə,dri:nəu'kɔ:təkəl] *adj.* 肾上腺皮质的
4. alkylate ['ælkə,leit] *v.* 使烷基化
5. allergy ['ælədʒi] *n.* 过敏
6. analgesic [,ænəl'dʒi:zik] *n.* 止痛剂，镇痛剂
7. antagonist [æn'tægənist] *n.* 拮抗剂
8. antidepressant [ænti:dip'resənt] *n.* 抗抑郁药
9. antihypertensive ['ænti,haipə'tensiv] *n.* 抗高血压药
10. appreciable [ə'pri:ʃəbl] *adj.* 可感知的，很可观的
11. atopy ['ætəpi] *n.* 特异反应性；特应性
12. benoxaprofen [benɔk'sæprəfn] *n.* 苯噁洛芬
13. benzodiazepines [,benzɔdai'æzə,pin] *n.* 苯二氮䓬类药物
14. batch [bætʃ] *n.* 一批，批处理，批次
15. carcinogenesis [,kɑ:sinəu'dʒenisis] *n.* 癌变
16. clonidine ['klɔni,di:n] *n.* 可乐定（一种降压药）
17. compliance [kəm'plaiəns] *n.* 依从性
18. constipation [,kɔnstə'peiʃən] *n.* 便秘

19. consultation [ˌkɑːnslˈteiʃn] *n.* 咨询，会诊

20. corticosteroids [ˌkɔːtikəusˈtirɔidz] *n.* 皮质甾类，皮质类固醇类

21. dexfenfluramine [deksfenˈfluərəmiːn] *n.* 右芬氟拉明

22. digoxin [daiˈgɔksin] *n.* 地高辛

23. dispense [disˈpens] *v.* 配药，发药

24. diuretic [ˌdaijuˈretik] *n.* 利尿剂

25. dyskinesia [ˌdiskiˈniːʒə] *n.* 运动障碍

26. extrinsic [eksˈtrinsik] *adj.* 外在的

27. fatality [fəˈtæləti] *n.* 死亡，病死

28. felbamate [ˈfelbəmeit] *n.* 苯丙氨酯

29. fenfluramine [fenˈfluərəmiːn] *n.* （减肥用，食欲抑制药）芬氟拉明

30. glucocorticosteroids [gˈluːkəukɔːtikɔstirɔidz] *n.* 皮质类固醇类，糖皮质激素类

31. hepatic [hiˈpætik] *adj.* 肝的

32. herbicide [ˈhəːbisaid] *n.* 除草剂

33. hormonal [hɔːˈməunl] *adj.* 激素的

34. idiosyncratic [ˌidiəsiŋˈkrætik] *adj.* 特质的，特殊的，异质的

35. implicate [ˈimplikeit] *vt.* 牵涉，意味着，暗示

36. impotence [ˈimpətəns] *n.* 阳痿

37. infant [ˈinfənt] *n.* 婴儿，幼儿

38. intracranial [intrəˈkreiniəl] *adj.* 头盖内的，颅内的

39. intrinsic [inˈtrinsik] *adj.* 内在的

40. lethargy [ˈleθədʒi] *n.* 嗜睡，倦怠

41. magnitude [ˈmægnituːd] *n.* 大小，量级

42. malnutrition [ˌmælnuˈtriʃn] *n.* 营养不良

43. mandatory [ˈmændətəri] *adj.* 命令的，强制性的，法定的

44. monitor [ˈmɔnitə] *v.* 监控，监测，监视

45. neonate [ˈniːəneit] *n.* 新生儿

46. nephropathy [niˈfrɔpəθi] *n.* 肾病

47. neuroleptic [njuərəˈleptik] *n.* 精神抑制药，安定药

48. nicotine [ˈnikətiːn] *n.* 尼古丁

49. pathophysiology [ˈpæθəuˌfiziˈɔlədʒi] *n.* 病理生理，病理生理学

50. pharmacovigilance [fɑːməkʌˈvidʒiləns] *n.* 药物警戒

51. placebo [pləˈsiːbəu] *n.* 安慰剂

52. polymorphism [pɔliˈmɔːfizəm] *n.* 多态性，多形性

53. practolol [ˈpræktəlɔl] *n.* 普拉洛尔（心得宁）

54. predispose [ˌpriːdiˈspəuz] *v.* 预先处理

55. surveillance [səˈveiləns] *n.* 监视，监督

56. tardive [ˈtɑːdiv] *adj.* 迟缓的，迟发的

57. temafloxacin [ˌtiməflɔkˈsʌsin] *n.* 替马沙星

58. teratogenesis [ˌterətəuˈdʒenisis] *n.* 畸形生长，[胚]畸形发生

59. thiazide [ˈθaiəˌzaid] *n.* [药]噻嗪化物；噻嗪类（利尿药）

60. tolerability [ˈtɔːlərəbl] *adj.* 可容忍的；容忍度

61. tranquillizer [ˈtræŋkwilaizə] *n.* 安定剂，镇定剂

笔记

62. tricyclic [traiˈsaiklik] *adj.* 三环的

63. troglitazone [trəugliˈteizəu] *n.* 曲格列酮

64. replacement [ripˈleismənt] *n.* 补充

65. retinoid [ˈretinɔid] *n.* 维 A 酸，视黄酸，类视色素，类维生素 A

66. sedative [ˈsedətiv] *n.* 镇静剂

67. spontaneous [spɔnˈteiniəs] *adj.* 自发的，本能的，自然产生的

68. syndrome [ˈsindrəum] *n.* 症候群，综合征

69. warfarin [ˈwɔːfərin] *n.* 华法林，双香豆素（抗凝剂）

70. withdrawal [wiðˈdrɔːəl] *n.* 撤退，退回，取消

71. xenobiotics [zenəbaiˈɔtiks] *n.* 外源性物质

Notes

1. Exposure to drugs in the population is thus substantial, and the incidence of adverse reactions must be viewed in this context. 译为：可见人群中暴露药物是多见的，因此在这种情况下必须注意不良反应的发生。"exposure to…"意思是"暴露于……"，"in this context"意思是"在这种情况下"。

2. consultations in general practice 会诊，全科医疗。

3. It would detect rare but severe adverse drug reactions, but would not be overwhelmed by common ones, the incidence of which would quantify together with predisposing factors. 译为：它（这种方法）能够检测罕见且严重的药物不良反应，而不是只是顾及一般的不良反应，并且可以对这些罕见且严重的反应的发生率及易感因素进行量化。"the incidence of which…"为非限制性定语从句。

4. The problem of adverse drug reaction recognition is much greater if the reaction resembles spontaneous disease in the population, such that physicians are unlikely to attribute the reaction to drug exposure. 译为：如果药物不良反应与人群的自发性疾病相似，以至于医生不大可能将其归因于药物暴露，那么对不良反应的认识问题就更加重要。在这句话中，"such that"相当于"to such an extent that"（到……程度以至于）。

Supplementary Parts

1. Medical and Pharmaceutical Terms Made Easier (4): Common Morphemes in Terms of English for Pharmacology

Morpheme	Meaning	Example
adreno	肾上腺	adrenoceptor 肾上腺受体 adrenergic（药物或其作用）类似肾上腺素的
alg	痛	analgesia 镇痛
alges/i	对痛的感受性	hyperalgesia 痛觉过敏
anti	抗	antianemic drugs 抗贫血药 antitussive 止咳药
carcino	癌	carcinogenicity 致癌性；致癌力
chem/o	化学，药	chemotherapy 化学疗法
chrono	时间	chronopharmacology 时辰药理学
contra	对抗	contraceptives 避孕药
dynam	动力	pharmacodynamics 药（物）效（应）动力学，药效学
erg/o	工作，能力	adrenergic 肾上腺素能的

笔记

续表

Morpheme	Meaning	Example
esthesi/o	感受	anesthesia 麻醉
hist/o	组织	histology 组织学
hypn/o	睡眠	hypnotic 催眠剂
idi/o	自己，个人	idiosyncracy 特异反应性，特异性
-ia	症	insomnia 失眠症
		hypoglycemia 低血糖（症）
immuno	免疫	immunopharmacology 免疫药理学
mut	突变	mutagenicity 致突变性
narc/o	麻木	narcosis 麻醉，昏迷状态
neuro	神经	neuropharmacology 神经药理学
pharmac/o	药	pharmacognosy 生药学
-phylaxis	保卫，保护	anaphylactic 过敏性的
pyr/o	热，发热	pyrogenic 致热的
rhythm	规律，节律	antiarrhythmic drugs 抗心律失常药
somn/i	睡眠	insomnia 失眠
sopor/i	沉睡	soporific 催眠的
spasm/o	痉挛	spasmodic 痉挛的
terato	畸形	teratogenicity 致畸性
-therapy	治疗	thermotherapy 温热疗法
ton/o	紧张	atony 张力缺乏，弛缓
tox/o	毒	toxin 毒素
toxic/o	毒	toxicology 毒理学
tuss/i	咳嗽	antitussive 镇咳剂

Word-matching.

1) histology	A. 抗贫血药
2) antiarrhythmic drugs	B. 致突变性
3) anesthesia	C. 肾上腺素能的
4) anaphylactic	D. 特异反应性
5) spasmodic	E. 痉挛的
6) idiosyncracy	F. 抗心律失常药
7) antianemic drugs	G. 麻醉
8) mutagenicity	H. 异染色体
9) teratogenicity	I. 利胆剂
10) adrenergic	J. 组织学
11) allosome	K. 过敏性的
12) cholagogue	L. 致畸性

2. English-Chinese Translation Skills: 药学英语翻译中的直译与意译

直译（literal translation）和意译（free translation）是英汉翻译两种不同的方法。所谓"直译"，就是在不失原文语言形式和语篇风格，比较完整地按照原文意义翻译，直译不是"逐字翻译"也不是"词典翻译"，直译的重点在于译文的"准确"，但也要求译文通顺。所谓"意译"就是为了完整表达原文内容，抛弃原文语言形式，按照译入语的习惯重新造句，意译不是乱译或者漏译、错译，意译的重点在于"通顺"，但也不失意义正确。药学英语语篇属于科技文献，注重客观事实，在翻译时主要采用直译法。如：

笔记

例 1：Type B (idiosyncratic) reactions are not predictable from the drug's main pharmacological action, are not dose-related and are severe, with a considerable mortality.

参考译文：B 型不良反应（特异性反应）无法从药物的主要药理作用预测到，与药物剂量无关，且较严重，死亡率高。

药学英语原文结构复杂，加上英汉语言结构上的差异，翻译时要适当调整译文语言结构，使得译文通畅，这种译法还属于直译。如：

例 2：Several of the traditional diseases that were major causes of death before the antibiotic era, e.g. tuberculosis and diphtheria, are now re-emerging in resistant form, adding to the problems posed by infections in which antibiotic resistance has long been a problem, and those like West Nile virus and severe acute respiratory syndrome (SARS) that have been recognized in recent years. Not only has the development of resistance to established antibiotics become a challenge, so too has the ability of microorganisms to take advantage of changing practices and procedures in medicine and surgery.

参考译文：在抗生素时代之前一些曾经是主要死因的传统疾病，如肺结核和白喉，现在又以抗性形式出现，这加剧了由长期存在的抗生素耐药性带来的感染问题，以及那些类似于西尼罗河病毒和 SARS（严重急性呼吸综合征）等近年来人们才有所认识的疾病带来的问题。这不仅对已有抗生素耐药性的发展是一种挑战，而且对微生物在药物和手术方面利用不断改变的实践和操作能力也是一种挑战。

说明：例句原文由两个小句组成，专业词汇多，句子结构复杂。第一小句的主句是 Several of the traditional diseases are now re-emerging in resistant form. 主语 diseases 后面有 that 引导的定语从句，主句后面有非谓语动词 adding to… 作状语，而且在这个状语中又包含有两个定语从句。第二小句又是一个特殊英语句型 Not only…, so too…。译文很好地将原文复杂结构进行拆分，用短小句子将原文的意思一层层表述出来，既忠实原文，又符合汉语表达习惯。

另外，药学英语语篇中含有很多化学、医学、药学名称，这些词的处理肯定是直接翻译。一般来讲，医药名词的翻译具有单一性，基本属于词典翻译。如：

例 3：**Identification:**

A: *Infrared Absorption* <197K>

B: *Ultraviolet Absorption* <197U>

Solution: 5µg per ml.

Medium: 0.1N hydrochloric acid in methanol (1 in 100).

C: it responds to *Thin-layer Chromatographic Identification Test* <201>, a test solution in methanol containing about 1 mg per ml and a solvent system consisting of a mixture of methylene chloride and methanol (4:1) being used.

参考译文：

鉴别：

A. 红外吸收（附录 197K）

B. 紫外吸收（附录 197U）

溶液：5µg/ml

介质：0.1N 盐酸的甲醇溶液（1 → 10）

C. 薄层色谱法（附录 201）每 1 ml 中约含供试品 1 mg 的甲醇溶液作为供试品溶液，二氯甲烷 - 甲醇（4:1）为展开剂。

这种"词典翻译"法也不是完全照词典释义，也是要根据原文内容，对术语在词典中的释义进行选择，这类翻译大多出现在药典、药品说明书、医药实验报告中。

笔记

Early advances in medicinal chemistry were concerned principally with the estimation, isolation, structural determination, and synthesis of medicinal agents of natural origin. A second major area was the synthesis of simplified fragments of complex drug molecules. In this phase of its development medicinal chemistry was almost indistinguishable from organic chemistry. The golden age (1940－1960) in the discovery of medicinals by these empirical strategies came to an end concomitant with the thalidomide tragedy. An arid middle age marked by pessimism in drug synthesis in both industrial and academic quarters ensued because of the combined difficulties of toxicity, carcinogenicity, and teratogenicity, and the relatively low return from random synthesis. It is characteristic of historical trends, however, that transitions to a new era are obscured and difficult to identify. In medicinal chemistry the doldrums in new drug development are actually yesterday's news, even though the renaissance that has begun is still not widely recognized. Underlying this new age is a foundation that includes the explosive development of molecular biology since 1960, the advances in physical chemistry and physical organic chemistry made possible by high-speed computer and new, powerful analytic methods including various types of chromatography, radioimmunoassay, mass spectrometry, X-ray crystallography, and nuclear magnetic resonance spectroscopy.

药物化学早期的发展主要是关于具有药用价值的天然产物的判定、分离、结构鉴定以及合成。第二个主要的发展阶段是将复杂的药物分子进行结构简化并合成。药物化学发展的这一阶段几乎完全与有机化学区分不开。通过经验式策略发现药物的黄金时段（1940－1960）随着沙利度胺（又称反应停）悲剧的出现而结束。之后由于随机合成伴随着可能致毒、致癌、致畸以及其相对低的回报率等多重困难，无论是在工业界还是在学术界，人们的悲观态度使得药物合成走进了低产的中期。然而，历史发展的特征就是旧时代向新世纪的转化往往是模糊和难以分辨的。在药物化学里，新药开发延续着昨日的低迷，然而尽管当时很少有人意识到，新药研发的复兴之火已经被点燃了。新时期药物化学的发展是建立在20世纪60年代以来包括分子生物学爆炸性发展的基础上，高速计算机及新的有力的分析方法，包括各种类型的色谱分析，放射性免疫分析法，质谱，X射线晶体学，磁共振，使得物理化学和物理有机化学的发展成为可能。

笔记

Such newly refined techniques will bring to us an understanding of drug metabolism and its relationship to drug toxicity, carcinogenicity, teratogenicity, and mutagenicity that will make it possible to minimize or eliminate these hazards. We already know that untoward reactions often are caused by reactive metabolites, and we are gaining an understanding of the chemical and biological factors involved in the production of such substances. In the study of receptors, the combined power of physical chemistry, physical organic chemistry, bioorganic chemistry, and the techniques of quantitative drug design have given such results as the histamine-H_2 blockers, a sophisticated antimetabolite and enzyme inhibitor theory, and a detailed understanding of structure-activity relationships in hormones. Again, the elucidation of the opiate receptor and the finding of endogenous opiate-like substances promise to revolutionize the development of analgesic agents. Work on immuno-stimulatory and immuno-suppressive agents is dramatically altering our helplessness in the face of viral diseases and immune system disorders such as arthritis.

这些最新的尖端技术使我们认识了药物代谢及其与致毒、致癌、致畸和致突变之间的关系,从而使得将这些危害降低、消除成为可能。我们已经知道不良反应是由活性代谢物引起的,同时我们也获知影响着这些代谢物产生的化学和生物因素。在受体研究中,物理化学、物理有机化学、生物有机化学和药物定量设计技术的联合应用得出了如下这些结果:组胺 H_2 受体拮抗剂、复杂的抗代谢物和酶抑制剂理论,以及激素构效关系的详细理解。同时,对阿片受体的阐明与内源性阿片样物质的发现预示着止痛剂开发的变革。对免疫增强剂和免疫抑制剂的研究正显著地改变着我们以往对病毒疾病和免疫系统疾病(如关节炎等)束手无力的状况。

Text A
Combinatorial Chemistry and New Drugs

In a process called combinatorial chemistry, we generate a large number of related compounds and then screen the collection for the ones that could have medicinal value.

This approach differs from the most common way pharmaceutical makers discover new drugs. They typically begin by looking for signs of a desired activity in almost anything they can find, such as diverse collections of synthetic compounds or of chemicals derived from bacteria, plants or other natural sources. Once they identify a promising substance (known in the field as a lead compound), they laboriously make many one-at-a-time modifications to the structure, testing after each step to determine how the changes affected the compound's chemical and biological properties.

Often these procedures yield a compound having acceptable potency and safety. For every new drug that has been made to market in this way, however, researchers quite likely tinkered with and abandoned thousands of other compounds en route. The entire procedure is time-consuming and expensive: it takes many years and hundreds of millions of dollars to move from a lead compound in the laboratory to a bottle of medicine on the shelf of local pharmacy.

The classical approach has been improved by screening tests that work more rapidly and reliably than in the past and by burgeoning knowledge about how various modifications are likely to change a molecule's biological activity. But as medical science has advanced, demand for drugs that can intervene in disease processes has escalated. To find those drugs, researchers need many more compounds to screen as well as a way to find lead compounds that require less modification.

Drug-makers have two basic combinatorial techniques at their disposal. The first, known as parallel synthesis, was invented in the mid 1980s by H. Mario Geysen, now at Glaxo Wellcome[1]. He initially used parallel synthesis as a quick way to identify which small segment of any given large protein bound to an antibody. Geysen generated a variety of short protein fragments, or peptides, by combining multiple amino acids (the building blocks of peptides and proteins) in different permutations. By performing dozens or sometimes hundreds of reactions at the same time and then testing to see whether the resulting peptides would bind to the particular antibody of interest, he rapidly found the active peptides from a large universe of possible molecules.

In a parallel synthesis, all the products are assembled separately in their own reaction vessels. To carry out the procedure, chemists often use a so-called microtitre plate—a sheet of molded plastic that typically contains eight rows and 12 columns of tiny wells, each of which holds a few milliliters of the liquid in which the reactions will occur. The array of rows and columns enables workers to organize the building blocks they want to combine and provides a ready means to identify the compound in a particular well.

Chemists often start a combinatorial synthesis by attaching the first set of building blocks to inert, microscopic beads made of polystyrene (often referred to as solid support.) After each reaction, researchers wash away any unreacted material, leaving behind only the desired products, which are still tethered to the beads. Although the chemical reactions required to link compounds to the beads and later to detach them introduce complications to the synthesis process, the ease of purification can outweigh these problems.

In many laboratories today, robots assist with the routine work of parallel synthesis, such as delivering small amounts of reactive molecules into the appropriate wells. In this way, the process becomes more accurate and less tedious.

The second technique for generating a combinatorial library, known as a split-and-mix synthesis, was pioneered in the late 1980s by Arpad Furka, now at Advanced ChemTech in Louisville, KY. In contrast to parallel synthesis, in which each compound remains in its own container, a split-and-mix synthesis produces a mixture of related compounds in the same reaction vessel. This method substantially reduces the number of containers required and raises the number of compounds that can be made into the millions.[2] The trade-off, however, is that keeping track of such large numbers of compounds and then testing them for biological activity, can become quite complicated.

As we mentioned earlier, one of the problems with a split-and-mix synthesis is identifying the composition of a reactive compound within a large mixture. Kit Lam of the University of Arizona has developed a way to overcome this obstacle. He noted that at the end of a split-and-mix synthesis, all the molecules attached to a single bead are of the same structure. Scientists can pull out from the mixture the beads that bear biologically active molecules and then, using sensitive detection techniques, determine the molecular makeup of the compound attached. Unfortunately, this technique will work only for certain compounds, such as peptides or small segments of DNA.

Nevertheless, because of the difficulties of identifying compounds made in a split-and-mix synthesis, most pharmaceutical companies today continue to rely on parallel synthesis.

Word Study

1. array [əˈrei] *n.* 排列
2. bead [biːd] *n.* 珠子，滴，念珠
3. burgeon [ˈbəːdʒən] *v.* 迅速成长，迅速发展
4. combinatorial [kɔmbinəˈtɔːriəl] *adj.* 组合的，混合的
5. en route [ən ˈruːt] *adv.* 在途中，在路上
6. escalate [ˈeskəleit] *v.* 变得更严重，变得更糟糕
7. inert [iˈnəːt] *adj.* 惰性的
8. intervene [intəˈviːn] *v.* 干涉，干预
9. laboriously [ləˈbɔːriəsli] *adv.* 漫长而艰苦地，枯燥乏味地
10. microtitre [maikrəˈtaitə] *n.* 微量滴定
11. peptide [ˈpeptaid] *n.* 肽
12. permutation [pəːmjuˈteiʃn] *n.* 排列组合
13. polystyrene [ˌpɔliˈstairiːn] *n.* 聚苯乙烯
14. potency [ˈpəutənsi] *n.* (药品、毒品、化学品的) 效力，效能
15. segment [ˈsegment] *n.* 部分，片，断
16. tether [ˈteðə] *v.* 拴住，系住
17. tedious [ˈtiːdiəs] *adj.* 沉闷的，冗长乏味的
18. tinker [ˈtikə] *v.* 改进，修理

Notes

1. Glaxo Wellcome: 葛兰素威康 (Glaxo Wellcome) 公司是一家以研究和开发为基础的制药集团公司，和史克必成 (Smith Kline) 强强联合，于 2000 年 12 月成立英国葛兰素史克公司，总部在英国。

2. This method substantially reduces the number of containers required and raises the number of compounds that can be made into the millions. 译为：这种方法大量减少了所需容器的数量，并将可生成化合物的数量提高到几百万个。

Exercises

1. **Decide whether each of the following statements is true (T) or false (F) according to the passage.**

(1) With the more efficient screening tests and burgeoning knowledge about how a molecule's biological activities are likely to be changed, the traditional approach of discovering new drugs has been improved.

(2) With the parallel synthesis used to identify which small segment of any given large protein would bind to an antibody, Mario Geysen generated a variety of short protein fragments by combining multiple amino acids in different permutations.

(3) A parallel synthesis and a split-and-mix synthesis are different in that in a split-and-mix synthesis, all the products are assembled separately in their respective reaction vessels.

(4) In many laboratories, robots are used in the routine work of parallel synthesis to deliver small amounts of reactive molecules into appropriate wells, thus making the process more accurate and less tedious.

(5) In a parallel synthesis, each compound remains in its own container; while in a split-and-mix synthesis, the related compounds are mixed up in the same reaction vessel.

(6) In order to solve the difficulties of identifying the compounds made in a parallel synthesis, scientists pull out from the mixture the beads that bear biologically active molecules and determine the molecular makeup of the compound attached.

2. **Questions for oral discussion.**

(1) What are the two basic combinatorial techniques drug-makers have at their disposal?

(2) Which combinatorial technique is preferred by most pharmaceutical companies today? And why?

(3) What is the difference between combinatorial chemistry and the most common way drug makers discover new drugs?

(4) According to this passage, what role do robots play in laboratories today?

3. **Choose the best answer to each of the following questions.**

(1) H. Mario Geysen initially used parallel synthesis as a quick way to identify which small _____ of any given large protein bound to an antibody.

    A. division   B. pieces
    C. part   D. fragment

(2) Chemists often start a combinatorial synthesis by attaching the first set of building blocks to _____, microscopic beads made of polystyrene.

    A. solid   B. inert
    C. soft   D. active

(3) The chemical reactions required to link compounds to the beads and later to detach them _____ to the synthesis process.

    A. induce complications   B. make easy
    C. introduce complications   D. introduce easy

(4) In a parallel synthesis, all the products are _____ separately in their own reaction vessels.

笔记

A. combined   B. assembled

C. joined   D. assorted

(5) In many laboratories today, robots assist with the routine work of parallel synthesis, such as _____ small amounts of reactive molecules into the appropriate wells.

A. sending   B. transporting

C. delivering   D. giving

(6) Scientists can pull out from the mixture the beads that bear biologically active molecules and then, using sensitive detection techniques, _____ the molecular makeup of the compound attached.

A. determine   B. make sure

C. find   D. search

(7) Most pharmaceutical companies today continue to _____ parallel synthesis. Which of the following is not appropriate to be filled in the blank?

A. count in   B. count on

C. depend on   D. rely on

(8) Once they identify a promising substance, they _____ make many one-at-a-time modifications to the structure.

A. laboriously   B. hardly

C. easy   D. effectively

(9) Often these procedures yield a compound having acceptable _____ and safety.

A. strength   B. effect

C. potency   D. effort

(10) In many laboratories today, robots _____ the routine work of parallel synthesis.

A. help   B. assist with

C. assist in   D. assist to

4. **Fill in each of the following blanks with an appropriate word or expression according to the meaning of the sentences.**

(1) By looking for signs of a _____ activity in almost anything, combinatorial chemistry generates a large number of related compounds and then screen the collection for the ones with medicinal value.

(2) In a combinatorial synthesis, with the requirements that compounds are required to be linked to the beads and later to be _____ from them, the chemical reactions actually make the synthesis more complicated, whereas the purification easier.

(3) Once they identify a _____ substance (known in the field as a lead compound), they laboriously make many one-at-a-time modifications to the structure, etc.

(4) Nevertheless, because of the difficulties of identifying compounds made in a split-and-mix synthesis, most pharmaceutical companies today continue to rely on _____ synthesis.

(5) The split-and-mix synthesis produces a mixture of related compounds in the same reaction _____.

(6) In many laboratories today, robots _____ the routine work of parallel synthesis.

(7) The _____, however, is that keeping track of such large numbers of compounds can become quite complicated.

(8) Drug-makers have two basic _____ at their disposal, split-and-mix synthesis and parallel synthesis.

笔记

(9) As medical science has advanced, demand for drugs that can intervene in disease processes has _____.

(10) Although the chemical reactions required to link compounds to the beads and later to detach them introduce complications to the synthesis process, the ease of purification can _____ these problems.

5. **Translate the following sentences and paragraphs into Chinese.**

(1) In a process called combinatorial chemistry, the scientists generate a large number of related compounds and then screen the collection for the ones that could have medicinal value.

(2) In a parallel synthesis, chemists often use a so-called microtitre plate to carry out the procedure and all the products are assembled separately in their own reaction vessels.

(3) In contrast to parallel synthesis, in which each compound remains in its own container, a split-and-mix synthesis produces a mixture of related compounds in the same reaction vessel. This method substantially reduces the number of containers required.

(4) As we mentioned earlier, one of the problems with a split-and-mix synthesis is identifying the composition of a reactive compound within a large mixture.

(5) Early advances in medicinal chemistry were concerned principally with the estimation, isolation, structural determination, and synthesis of medicinal agents of natural origin.

(6) At the end of a split-and-mix synthesis, all the molecules attached to a single bead are of the same structure. Scientists can pull out from the mixture the beads that bear biologically active molecules and then, using sensitive detection techniques, determine the molecular makeup of the compound attached.

(7) For every new drug that has been made to market in this way, however, researchers quite likely tinkered with and abandoned thousands of other compounds en route. The entire procedure is time-consuming and expensive: it takes many years and hundreds of millions of dollars to move from a lead compound in the laboratory to a bottle of medicine on the shelf of local pharmacy.

Text B
Lead Compounds

Before any medicinal chemistry project can get underway, a lead compound is required. A lead compound will have some property considered therapeutically useful. The property sought will depend on the tests used to detect the lead compound, which in turn depends on the drug's target. The level of biological activity may not be particularly high, but that does not matter. The lead compound is not intended to be used as a clinical agent. It is the starting point from which a clinically useful compound can be developed. Similarly, it does not matter whether the lead compound is toxic or has undesirable side effects. Again, drug design aims to improve the desirable effects of the lead compound and to remove the undesirable effects.

Lead compounds can be obtained from a variety of different sources such as the flora and fauna of the natural world, or synthetic compounds made in the laboratory. There is also the potential of designing lead compounds using computer modeling or NMR spectroscopic studies.

In order to search for lead compounds, a suitable test is required. This could be a test that reveals a physiological effect in a tissue preparation, organ or test animal. Alternatively, it could be a cellular effect, resulting from the interaction of a lead compound with a particular target, such as a receptor or an enzyme; or a molecular effect, such as the binding of a compound with a receptor. In the last two situations, the molecular target is considered important to a particular disease state, and in such cases, the lead compound may not have the desired physiological activity at all! For example, there have been several examples where the natural agonist for a receptor was used as the lead compound in order to design a receptor antagonist. Here, the crucial property for the lead compound was that it should be recognized and bound to the binding site of the target receptor. The lead compound was then modified to bind as an antagonist rather than as an agonist. For example, the chemical messenger histamine was used as the lead compound in developing the anti-ulcer agent cimetidine. Histamine is an agonist that activates histamine receptors in the stomach wall to increase the release of gastric acid. Cimetidine acts as an antagonist at these receptors, thus reducing the levels of gastric acid released and allowing the body to heal the ulcer.

The natural world is particularly rich in potential lead compounds. For example, plants, trees, snakes, lizards, frogs, fungi, corals and fish have all yielded potent lead compounds which have either resulted in clinically useful drugs or have the potential to do so. There is a good reason why nature should be so rich in potential lead compounds. Years of evolution have resulted in the "selection" of biologically potent natural compounds that have proved useful to the natural host for a variety of reasons. For example, a fungus that produces a toxin can kill off its microbiological competitors and take advantage of available nutrients.

Large numbers of novel structures are synthesized in research laboratories across the world for a diverse range of synthetic projects. This is a potential source of lead compounds, and pharmaceutical companies will often enter into arguments with research teams in order to test their compounds. Many of these structures may have been synthesized in research topics unrelated to medicinal chemistry, but are still potential lead compounds. The history of medicinal chemistry has many examples of lead compounds that were discovered from synthetic projects that had no medicinal objective in mind.[1] For example, prontosil was manufactured as a dye, but was the lead compound for the development of the sulfonamides.

Strategies in the Search for New Lead Compounds

A retrospective analysis of the ways leading to discovery of new drugs suggests that there are four types of successful strategies leading to new lead compounds.

The first strategy consists of systematic screening of sets of compounds arbitrarily chosen for their diversity, by selected biological assays. This approach was useful in the past for the discovery of new antibiotics such as streptomycin and for the identification of compactin as an HMG-CoA reductase inhibitor. Presently, as high-throughput screening (HTS), it is applied in a very general manner to synthetic as well as to natural compounds. Experience gathered has confirmed that high-throughput screening allows for the rapid identification of numerous hits, and the literature is full of success stories obtained with that approach. Among them, one could mention the discovery of insulin mimetics, of ORL1 receptor agonists, of protein tyrosine phosphatase-1 B inhibitors, of selective neuropeptide Y5 receptor antagonists, of selective COX-2 inhibitors, of corticotropin releasing factor (CRF) receptor modulators, and of CXCR2 receptor antagonists. Yet the HTS strategy for drug discovery has several limitations. It suffers from inadequate diversity, has low hit rates, and often leads to compounds with poor bioavailability or toxicity profiles.

The second strategy is based on the modification and improvement of existing active molecules.

笔记

The objective is to start with known active principles and, by various chemical transformations, prepare new molecules (sometimes referred to as "me-too compounds") for which an increase in potency, a better specific activity profile, improved safety, and a formulation that is easier to handle by physicians and nurses or more acceptable to the patient are claimed. A typical illustration of this approach is found in the series of lovastatin analogues (lovastatin, simvastatin, pravastatin, fluvastatin, atorvastatin, rosuvastatin, etc.). In the pharmaceutical industry, motivations for this kind of research are often driven by competitive and economic factors. Indeed, if the sales of a given medicine are high and if a company is in a monopolistic situation protected by patents and trademarks, other companies will want to produce similar medicines, if possible with some therapeutic improvements. They will therefore use the already commercialized drug as a lead compound and search for ways to modify its structure and some of its physical and chemical properties while retain or improve its therapeutic properties.

The third approach resides in the retroactive exploitation of various pieces of biological information that sometimes results from new discoveries made in biology and medicine and sometimes is just the fruits of more or less serendipitous observations. Examples are the chance discovery of the vasodilating activity of nitroglycerol, the antibiotic activity of Penicillium notatum, and the clinical observation of the activity of sildenafil on erectile dysfunction. Research programs based on the exploitation of clinical observations of side effects are of great interest in the discovery of new tracks as they are based on information about activities observed directly in man and not in animals.[2] They can also detect new therapeutic activities even when no pharmacological models in animals exist.

Finally, the fourth route to new active compounds is a rational design based on the knowledge of the molecular cause of the pathological dysfunction. Examples are the design of captopril as a hypotensive drug or of cimetidine as a treatment for peptic ulcers. This approach depends heavily on the progress made in fundamental research, particularly in the identification and structural elucidation of a new receptor or enzyme subclass involved in a specific disease.

It would be imprudent to compare hastily the merits of each of these approaches. Indeed, "poor" research can end with a universally recognized medicine and, conversely, a brilliant rationale can remain sterile. It is therefore of the highest importance that decision makers in the pharmaceutical industry appeal to all four above-mentioned strategies and that they realize that the strategies are not mutually exclusive.

The present trend is mass screening of huge libraries containing several thousand molecules. This was made possible by the association of combinatorial chemistry with high-throughput screening (HTS). However, other alternatives leading to interesting hits exist.

Word Study

1. captopril ['kæptəpril] *n.* 卡托普利，甲巯丙脯酸
2. cimetidine [sai'metidi:n] *n.* 西咪替丁（抗消化性溃疡药）
3. compactin ['kɔmpaktin] *n.* 美伐他汀 (mevastatin) 的商品名
4. coral ['kɔrəl] *n.* 珊瑚；*adj.* 珊瑚（色）的
5. fauna ['fɔ:nə] *n.* 动物群
6. flora ['flɔ:rə] *n.* 植物群落
7. high-throughput screening (HTS) [həi' θru:put 'skriniŋ] *n.* 高通量筛选
8. lizard ['lizəd] *n.* 蜥蜴

笔记

9. nitroglycerol [naitrəuˈglisərəl] *n.* 硝酸甘油
10. prontosil [ˈprɔntəsil] *n.* 百浪多息(一种磺胺类药的商品名)
11. retroactive [retrəuˈæktiv] *adj.* 追溯的,有追溯力的
12. sildenafil [siˈdenəfil] *n.* 西地那非,万艾可,伟哥
13. tyrosine [ˈtairəsi:n] *n.* 酪氨酸

Notes

1. The history of medicinal chemistry has many examples of lead compounds that were discovered from synthetic projects that had no medicinal objective in mind. 译为:在药物化学的发展历史上有许多先导化合物的例子表明这些先导化合物是在一些并没有药物研究目的的合成项目中发现的。注意该句中在第一个大的定语从句中含有一个小的定语从句。

2. Research programs based on the exploitation of clinical observations of side effects are of great interest in the discovery of new tracks as they are based on information about activities observed directly in man and not in animals. 译为:由于这些信息是直接通过观察临床患者得来的,而不是来自动物实验的信息,因而,对药物副作用的临床观察是药物新的活性研究的有效方式。句中"are of great interest in…"意思是"对……很有用"。

Supplementary Parts

1. Medical and Pharmaceutical Terms Made Easier (5): Common Morphemes of Colors in Medical and Pharmaceutical English Terms

Morpheme	Meaning	Example
erythro-	红	erythrocyte 红细胞
rubro-		rubriblast 原红细胞
xantho-	黄	xanthoma 黄色瘤
cyano-	蓝	cyanosis 发绀;苍白病,黄萎病
chloro-	绿	chlorophyll 叶绿素
vio-	紫	viomycin 紫霉素
albo-	白	albumin 清蛋白,白蛋白
leuko-		leukocyte 白细胞
leuco-		leucocidin 杀白细胞素
melano-	黑	melanoma(恶性)黑素瘤,(良性)胎记瘤
nigro-		nigrometer 黑度计
polio-	灰,白灰	poliomyelitis 脊髓灰质炎(小儿麻痹症)
glauco-	绿灰	glaucoma 青光眼,绿内障
chrom-	色	chromosome 染色体

Word-matching.

1) chlorophyll	A. 红细胞
2) cyanosis	B. 染色体
3) xanthoma	C. 叶绿素
4) chromosome	D. 黑度计
5) nigrometer	E. 杀白细胞素
6) rubriblast	F. 紫霉素
7) leucocidin	G. 清蛋白,白蛋白
8) leukocyte	H. 青光眼,绿内障

笔记

续表

9) viomycin	I. 白细胞
10) erythrocyte	J. 黄色瘤
11) albumin	K. 发绀；苍白病，黄萎病
12) glaucoma	L. 原红细胞

2.　English-Chinese Translation Skills: 药学英语翻译技巧 (1)：词性转换

词性转换法是翻译中常用手段，这是由英汉两种语言表达差异造成的。词性转换几乎可以在所有词性间进行，例如把原文的名词译为汉语的动词，把原文的副词译为汉语的形容词，或把原文的形容词译为汉语的名词等。例如：

例 1：A second major area was the **synthesis** of simplified fragments of complex drug molecules.

参考译文：第二个主要的发展阶段是**合成**复杂的药物分子的简单片段。

例 2：The institute claimed that phosphate also stabilized penicillin **beyond** its buffer effect.

参考译文：该研究所声称磷酸盐也能稳定青霉素，其效果**超过**了它的缓冲作用。

说明：本句原文中的介词 beyond 在译文中用了动词"超过"来表达。若不将 beyond 转译，句子难以有效译出。在英语中的介词或介词短语在许多情况下可以译成汉语中的动词。

例 3：The objective is to start with known active principles and, by various chemical transformations, prepare new molecules (sometimes referred to as "me-too compounds") for which an increase in potency, a better specific activity profile, improved safety, and a formulation that is **easier** to handle by physicians and nurses or more **acceptable** to the patient are claimed.

参考译文：目的就是利用已知的活性物质，通过一系列的化学转化，制备药效更强，作用更专一，安全性更高的新的化合物分子（有时也称为"me-too 化合物"），并且形成**更容易**被医师和护士应用，为患者**接受**的新剂型。

说明：在上面例句中，easier 和 acceptable 在原文中都是形容词做表语，构成"形容词 + to + 动词"结构，而汉语中没有这样结构，翻译时就需要结构转换，用符合汉语的语言结构表达原义，译文将 easier 转换成了副词修饰"（被医师和护士）应用"，将 acceptable 转换成了动词"接受"，使得译文更加顺畅。

英汉翻译中词性转换也包括英语表达结构中常见的非谓语动词形式，汉语中没有这种词性，在英译汉时需要根据这些非谓语动词的意义和语法功能进行词性转换，译成准确、通顺的汉语，如：

例 4：By **preserving** energy metabolism in cell **exposed** to hypoxia or ischaemia, trimetazidine prevents a decrease in intracellular ATP level, thereby **ensuring** the proper functioning of ionic pumps and transmembrane sodium-potassium flow while **maintaining** cellular homeostasis.

参考译文：曲美他嗪通过保护细胞在缺氧或缺血情况下的能量代谢，阻止细胞内 ATP 水平的下降，从而保证了离子泵的正常功能和透膜钠 - 钾流的正常运转，同时维持细胞内环境的稳定。

说明：在上面例句中，原句有四个非谓语动词形式：preserving, exposed, ensuring 和 maintaining，起着不同语法功能。在翻译时，为了译文通顺就必须根据意义表达需要将这些非谓语动词形式翻译成对应的动词形式，以符合汉语的习惯传递信息。

笔记

Unit Six　Pharmaceutics

Pharmaceutics is the discipline of pharmacy that deals with the process of turning a new chemical entity (NCE) or old drugs into a medication to be safely and effectively administered by patients. Pharmaceutics aims to deliver drugs to the target sites, and maintain appropriate drug concentrations over time, which helps relate the formulation of drugs to their delivery and disposition in the body. Branches of pharmaceutics mainly include pharmaceutical formulation, pharmaceutical manufacturing, physical pharmacy, biopharmaceutics and pharmacokinetics. Pharmaceutical formulation involves the design, development and evaluation of dosage forms and drug delivery systems. Biopharmaceutics and pharmacokinetics study the absorption, distribution, metabolism and excretion of drugs and metabolites in humans, animals and tissue culture.

药剂学作为药学的分支学科，主要研究将新型化学药物或已知药物以适当的剂型安全有效地应用于患者。药剂学研究重点在于实现靶部位的定点释药，并维持有效的体内药物浓度，这有助于制定药物体内的传递和处置。其分支学科主要包括药物制剂、药品生产、物理药学、生物药剂学和药物代谢动力学等。药物制剂包括药物剂型和传递系统的设计、开发和评估。生物药剂学和药物代谢动力学研究药物在人体、动物以及组织培养中的吸收、分布、代谢和消除过程。

笔记

Text A
Biopharmaceutics

Bioavailability

The therapeutic response of a drug depends on the concentration of the drug being achieved and maintained at the target site. For systemically acting drugs, i.e. drugs that reach target sites via systemic circulation, a dynamic equilibrium exists between the concentration of drug at its site(s) of action and the concentration of drug in the blood plasma. As a result, the therapeutic concentration of a drug at its site(s) of action can be adjusted by its plasma concentration. The unbound drug concentration in plasma represents a more accurate therapeutic index than the drug concentration in whole plasma since a drug may often reversibly bind to plasma proteins. Only drugs that are unbound can permeate through the vascular endothelium and distribute to tissues and hence its site(s) of action. Drug concentrations in whole blood may not be an appropriate therapeutic index because drugs can bind to or enter blood cells. However, to determine the concentration of an unbound drug in plasma requires complex and sensitive analytical methods to differentiate unbound drugs from bound drugs. Based upon the assumption that the plasma drug concentration is directly proportional to the therapeutic effect of the drug, plasma drug concentration is thus regarded as an index to evaluate drug concentration at the site(s) of action and the therapeutic effects of the drug. However, one should not draw inferences about the therapeutic effects of a drug simply from its plasma concentration until it has been established that the two are consistently correlated.

The drug concentration in blood plasma depends on numerous factors including the dose that enters the systemic circulation, the rate at which this occurs, the rate and extent of drug distribution between the systemic circulation and tissues and other fluids, and the rate of elimination from the body.

Apart from the intravenous route of administration, where a drug is introduced directly into the blood circulation, all other routes of administration involve the absorption of drug from the site of administration into the blood circulation.[1] Drugs must be absorbed in a sufficient quantity and at a sufficient rate to achieve a certain blood plasma concentration which, in turn, will produce an appropriate concentration of drug at its site(s) of action to elicit the desired therapeutic response.

There are two aspects of drug absorption which are important in clinical practice, namely, the rate and the extent to which the administered dose is absorbed. Simply because a certain dose of a drug is administered to a patient, there is no guarantee (except for intravenous administration) that all of that dose will reach the systemic circulation. The fraction of an administered dose of drug that reaches the systemic circulation in unchanged form is known as the bioavailable dose. The relative amount of an administered dose of a particular drug which reaches the systemic circulation intact and the rate at which this occurs is known as the bioavailability of that drug. Bioavailability is thus concerned with the quantity and the rate at which the intact form of a particular drug appears in the systemic circulation following administration of that drug. The bioavailability exhibited by a drug is thus very important in determining whether a therapeutically effective concentration is achieved at the site(s) of action of the drug.

In defining bioavailability in these terms, it is assumed that intact drug is the therapeutically

笔记

active form of the drug. This definition of bioavailability would not be valid in the case of a prodrug, whose therapeutic action normally depends on it being converted into its therapeutically active form prior to or on reaching the systemic circulation. It should also be noted that in the context of bioavailability, the term systemic circulation refers primarily to venous blood (excluding the hepatic portal blood during the absorption phase) and arterial blood which carries the intact drug to the tissues.

According to the definition of bioavailability, an administered dose of a particular drug in an oral dosage form will be 100% bioavailable only if: ⅰ) the drug is completely released from the dosage form into solution in the gastrointestinal fluids[2]; ⅱ) the released drug must be completely stable in the gastrointestinal fluids and all of the drug must pass through the gastrointestinal barrier into the mesenteric circulation without being metabolized; ⅲ) all of the absorbed drug must enter the systemic circulation without being metabolized on passing through the liver. Any factor that adversely affects either the release of the drug from the dosage form, its dissolution in the gastrointestinal fluids, its stability in the gastrointestinal fluids, its permeation through and stability in the gastrointestinal barrier or its stability in the hepatic portal circulation will influence the bioavailability exhibited by that drug from the dosage form in which it was administered.

Biopharmaceutics

Many factors have been found to influence the time course of a drug in the plasma and hence at its site(s) of action. These include food taken by the patient, the disease state, the age of the patient, the site(s) of absorption of the administered drug, the coadministration of other drugs, the physical and chemical properties of the administered drug, the type of dosage form, the composition and method of manufacture of the dosage form and the size of dose and frequency of administration of the dosage form. Thus, a given drug may exhibit differences in its bioavailability if it is administered in the same type of dosage form by different routes of administration, e.g. an aqueous solution of a given drug administered by the oral and intramuscular routes of administration. A given drug may also show differences in its bioavailability from one type of dosage form to another when given by the same route, e.g. a tablet, a hard gelatin capsule and an aqueous suspension administered by the peroral route. A given drug may show different bioavailabilities from different formulations of the same dosage given by the same route of administration. Variability in the bioavailability exhibited by a given drug from different formulations of the same type of dosage form or from different types of dosage forms, can cause patients to be under- or overmedicated. The result may be therapeutic failure or serious adverse effects particularly in the case of drugs which have a narrow therapeutic range.

The entry of a drug into the systemic circulation following the administration of a drug product usually involves two processes: ⅰ) the release of the drug from its dosage form in the biological fluids at the absorption site; ⅱ) the transport of the dissolved drug across biological membranes into the systemic circulation.

Therefore, biopharmaceutics is the study of the relationships between physical and chemical properties, dosage, and administration of a drug and its activity in humans and animals.

Word Study

1. assumption [əˈsʌmpʃn] *n.* 假设

2. bioavailability [ˌbaiəuəˌveiləˈbiliti] *n.* 生物利用度

3. biopharmaceutics [baiɔfɑːməsˈjuːtiks] *n.* 生物药剂学

4. elimination [iˌlimiˈneiʃn] *n.* 消除

5. plasma [ˈplæzmə] *n.* 血浆

6. systemic circulation [siˈstemik ˌsəːkjuˈleiʃn] *n.* 体循环

7. therapeutic index [ˌθerəˈpjuːtik ˈindeks] *n.* 治疗指数

8. vascular endothelium [ˈvæskjələ ˌendəuˈθiːliəm] *n.* 血管内皮

Notes

1. Apart from the intravenous route of administration...all other routes of administration involve the absorption of drug from the site of administration into the blood circulation. 译为：除静脉注射途径药物可以直接进入血液循环，其他全身给药途径都涉及药物从给药部位吸收进入血液循环的过程。where 引导的非限定性定语从句修饰 the intravenous route of drug administration。

2. According to the definition of bioavailability ... into solution in the gastrointestinal fluids. 译为：因此，依据生物利用度的定义，只有当药物从其制剂中完全释放到溶液时，这种药物以口服形式服用的剂量才可以百分之百地被生物利用。

Exercises

1. **Decide whether each of the following statements is true (T) or false (F) according to the passage.**

(1) The concentration of a drug in whole plasma is the most accurate index of the drug concentration at the site(s) of action.

(2) It is difficult to measure the total concentration of both unbound and bound drug in total plasma.

(3) The clinical effect of a drug is assumed to be directly related to the plasma drug concentration.

(4) Systemically acting drugs administered by all routes involve the absorption of drug from the place of administration into the blood.

(5) Bioavailability of a drug indicates whether a therapeutically effective concentration is achieved at the site(s) of action of that drug.

(6) Prodrugs are not therapeutically effective unless they are changed into therapeutically active forms before or after reaching the systemic circulation.

2. **Questions for oral discussion.**

(1) In clinical practice, what is regarded as an index of drug concentration at site(s) of action of a particular drug?

(2) What are the two aspects of drug absorption that are important in clinical practice?

(3) What is the definition of a bioavailable dose? What is the bioavailability of a drug?

(4) What are the processes involved in the entry of a drug into the systemic circulation?

3. **Choose the best answer(s) to each of the following questions.**

(1) Pharmaceutics is an interdisciplinary subject involving _____.

   A. formulation, manufacturing, physical pharmacy, and biopharmaceutics

   B. manufacturing

   C. physical pharmacy

   D. biopharmaceutics

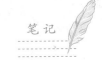
笔记

(2) Formulation is about the design, development and evaluation of dosage forms, _____.

    A. discovery of novel drugs

    B. analytical methods

    C. drug delivery systems and manufacturing process

    D. dosing regimen

(3) Biopharmaceutics mainly studies the *in vivo* process of drugs and metabolites in humans, animals and tissue culture, which specifically involves _____.

    A. absorption and distribution

    B. absorption, distribution, metabolism, and excretion

    C. metabolism and excretion

    D. absorption and excretion

(4) Regarding the definition of bioavailability (BA), BA is related to _____.

    A. total plasma drug concentration only

    B. unbound drug concentration in the plasma

    C. unbound drug concentration at the target site

    D. total plasma drug concentration, and the administered drug dose

(5) Plasma drug concentration is affected by following factors such as _____.

    A. rate of absorption

    B. rate and extent of distribution

    C. rate of elimination

    D. all of above

(6) Which of the following routes of administration will involve the absorption of drugs?

    A. i.v. injection

    B. i.v. infusion

    C. Subcutaneous injection, transdermal and oral

    D. None of above

(7) Which of the following factors may influence the time course of a drug in the plasma and hence at its site of action?

    A. Food   B. Disease state

    C. Route of administration   D. All of above

(8) Please identify the potential biological barriers for an orally administered tablet to be absorbed into the systemic circulation.

    A. Skin epidermis   B. Gastrointestinal epithelium

    C. Oral mucosal membrane   D. All of above

(9) Given the same administration dose, which of the following will likely result in varying bioavailabilities for the same drug administered to the same person?

    A. tablets (p.o.) vs. solutions (p.o.)

    B. solutions for injection (i.v.) vs. oral solutions (p.o.)

    C. coated tablets (p.o.) vs. hard gelatin capsules (p.o.)

    D. All of above

(10) Which of the following statements is true?

    A. Bioavailability is only related to the administered dose and the total drug concentration in the blood circulation.

笔记

B. Plasma protein binding does not affect the bioavailability of a specific drug.

C. A given drug in different dosage forms may show differences in bioavailability if given by the same route.

D. Biopharmaceutical studies do not involve animal experiment.

4. Complete the following vocabulary work.

(1) Fill in the blanks with appropriate letters.

1) ph ☐☐☐☐☐☐ tics

2) pharmacok ☐☐☐☐☐☐

3) ADME refers to a_____, d_____, m_____ and e_____.

4) sys ☐☐☐☐ circu ☐☐☐☐☐☐

5) intrav ☐☐☐☐ in ☐☐☐ ion

(2) Translate following words or expressions into Chinese

1) bioavailability:

2) dose:

3) dosage:

4) metabolism:

5) oral administration:

5. Translate the following sentences and paragraphs into Chinese.

(1) Absorption is the process of a drug entering systemic circulation from its site of administration. A drug must pass through one or more layers of cells to reach the general circulation.

(2) Many factors impact drug absorption, especially orally administered drugs, such as the physicochemical properties of the drug, dosage form, food, and patient age.

(3) After absorption, most drugs undergo extensive distribution to organs and tissues in the body, while the degree of drug accumulation depends on the lipophilicity and local blood flow within the organ or the tissue.

(4) Highly perfused organs receive most of the drugs. After entering the blood circulation, most drugs will more or less bind with plasma proteins. However, the binding is loose and reversible, and is always under equilibrium.

(5) Bioavailable dose is the fraction of an administered dose of unchanged drug that reaches the systemic circulation.

(6) Apart from the intravenous route of administration, where a drug is introduced directly into the blood circulation, all other routes of administration involve the absorption of drug from the site of administration into the blood circulation. Drugs must be absorbed in a sufficient quantity and at a sufficient rate to achieve a certain plasma concentration which, in turn, will produce an appropriate concentration of drug at its site(s) of action to elicit the desired therapeutic response.

(7) According to the definition of bioavailability, an administered dose of a particular drug in an oral dosage form will be 100% bioavailable only if: ⅰ) the drug is completely released from the dosage form into solution in the gastrointestinal fluids; ⅱ) the released drug must be completely stable in the gastrointestinal fluids and all of the drug must pass through the gastrointestinal barrier into the mesenteric circulation without being metabolized; ⅲ) all of the absorbed drug must enter the systemic circulation without being metabolized on passing through the liver.

笔记

Text B
Formulation and Advanced Drug Delivery Systems

(Adapted from *Drug Delivery and Targeting, Martin's Physical Pharmacy and Pharmaceutical Sciences*, 3rd Edition)

Drug Delivery Systems

"Drugs" taken by a patient exert a biological function by interacting with specific receptors at the site of action. The drug is intended to be delivered to the target site at a certain rate and concentration, which minimizes the side effects and maximizes the therapeutic effect. Human body presents great barriers against drug delivery and targeting which render an otherwise potent drug ineffective *in vivo*. Dosage forms thus serve many purposes including facilitating drug administration and improving drug delivery. Traditional and classical dosage forms mainly include injections, oral formulations (solutions, suspension, tablets, and capsules), topical creams and ointments. Unfortunately, most traditional dosage forms are unable to facilitate adequate drug absorption, gain access to the target site, prevent nonspecific drug distribution and premature metabolism and excretion, or match drug input with the dose requirement. Therefore, alternative routes of drug administration and advanced drug delivery systems are proposed to meet these delivery challenges and improve drug therapy.

Advanced drug delivery systems are defined as a formulation or device that delivers drug to a specific site in the body at a certain rate. Advanced drug delivery systems usually represent a more sophisticated system that incorporates advanced technologies such as controlled, pulsatile, targeted, or bioresponsive drug delivery. This chapter aims to introduce the currently available delivery systems and advanced drug delivery systems under development.

1. Controlled Drug Delivery

Controlled drug delivery is defined as the delivery of drug or active pharmaceutical ingredient (API) in the body at a predetermined rate. A controlled drug delivery system is therefore one that provides temporal or spatial control or both over drug delivery in the body.

Implant An implant is a single unit drug delivery system designed for delivering drug at predetermined rate over an extended period of time. For example, drugs can be mixed with either nondegradable or biodegradable polymers. The resulting polymeric matrix can be surgically implanted to achieve controlled drug release *in vivo*. Implants help eliminate the need for continuous intravenous infusion or repeated injections for maintaining therapeutic drug concentrations, which greatly improves patient compliance by reducing or eliminating the patient-involved dosing.[1]

Osmotic pump An osmotic pump is usually composed of a core tablet surrounded by a semipermeable membrane containing a laser-created hole. The core tablet contains two layers, one with drug and the other with the electrolyte. When the tablet is swallowed, the semipermeable membrane permits the entry of fluid from the stomach and intestines to the tablet, which dissolves/suspends the drug. As pressure increases due to the inward diffusion of water molecules, drug is pumped out of the tablet through the hole. Thus, drug delivery is controlled by the osmotic gradient between the contents of the core tablet and fluids in the gastrointenstinal (GI) tract.

笔记

2. Advanced Drug Delivery Systems

Representative examples of drug delivery systems designed for different routes of administration are described below.

Buccal Drug Delivery Systems The buccal and sublingual mucosa in the oral cavity provide an excellent alternative for the delivery of drugs. The buccal mucosa offers several advantages for controlled drug delivery: (ⅰ) the mucosa is well supplied with both vascular and lymphatic drainage; (ⅱ) "first-pass" intestinal/hepatic metabolism and presystemic degradation in the GI tract are avoided; (ⅲ) the area is well suited for a retentive device and is usually acceptable to the patient; and (ⅳ) with the right DDS design, the permeability and the local environment of the mucosa can be controlled and manipulated to accommodate drug permeation.

The most commonly used dosage form through this route is a small tablet, which is designed to dissolve rapidly and be absorbed readily into the systemic circulation. Other dosage forms include gels, adhesive patches for systemic or local mucosal delivery.

Pulmonary Drug Delivery Systems The respiratory tract including the nasal mucosa, pharynx, large and small airway structures (trachea, bronchi, bronchioles, alveoli), provides a large mucosal surface for drug absorption, which presents a more convenient way of administration compared with parenteral route. [2]Aerosols are widely used to deliver drugs in the respiratory tract. The deposition of the particles in the respiratory tract is driven by the inhalation regime, the particle size, shape, density, charge, and hygroscopicity.

Inhaled medications have been used for years for the treatment of lung diseases, and are widely accepted as the optimal route of administration of first-line therapy for asthma and chronic obstructive pulmonary diseases. Aerosols have already been developed to deliver peptide and protein drugs, e.g. gonadotrophin-releasing factor, vasopressin, and insulin. Peptides and proteins easily undergo hydrolysis and degradation in the GI tract due to the presence of various enzymes and stomach acid. Thus, peptide and protein delivery via pulmonary route offers an alternative to parenteral administration, which is considered a better way to deliver proteins and peptides than sticking people with needles.

Transdermal Drug Delivery Systems The skin has been used for centuries as the site for the topical administration of drugs, but only recently has it been used as a pathway for systemic drug delivery. The skin mainly functions as a barrier to prevent water loss and the entry of external agents. However, some drugs with proper physicochemical properties are proven to penetrate the skin in sufficient amounts to produce a systemic effect. The transdermal route is of particular interest for drugs that have a systemic short elimination half-life or undergo extensive first-pass metabolism, therefore, requiring frequent dosing.[3]

Regarding the fabrication transdermal patches, drugs are often mixed with a polymer matrix or encapsulated within a membrane. An adhesive layer is then impregnated with the drug-containing complex. Placing the patch on the skin allows the drug to diffuse through the skin and into the body. The most widely used so far are nitroglycerine-containing patches for angina, a transdermal product containing clonidine for hypertension as well as the product containing scopolamine for motion sickness. A transdermal device containing 17-β-estradiol for postmenopausal women protects that drug from degradation in the digestive tract.

Current systems can deliver only drugs of proper molecular size and solubility. But with iontophoresis, a drug is literally propelled across the skin by a positive electric charge. The use of this

笔记

system should expand the number of drugs that can be administered transdermally.

3. Targeted Drug Delivery

Drugs administered by routine parenteral routes are distributed throughout the body and reach nontarget organs/tissues thus leading to extensive adverse effects and low therapeutic efficacy. Most drugs undergo metabolism in the liver and excretion by kidney. As a result, only a small fraction of the administered drug dosage will reach the target (diseased) organ or tissues. The concept of targeted drug delivery was introduced by German chemist Paul Ehrlich more than a century ago. However, making drugs with high therapeutic selectivity or targetability has remained a great challenge for pharmaceutical scientists. The goal of targeted drug delivery is to deliver drugs specifically to diseased organs, tissues and cells while not exposing healthy organs or tissues. Additionally, targeted drug delivery should ensure minimal drug loss during the transit to the target site, protect the drug from metabolism and premature clearance, retain the drug at the target site for desired period of time, facilitate the drug transport into target cells and deliver drug to the appropriate intracellular organism.

Carrier-linked Prodrug Strategy This strategy aims to develop prodrugs by conjugating drug molecules to monoclonal antibodies (mAbs) or ligands for specific recognition and interaction with antigens or receptors expressed on target cell surface. The delivery systems consist of three components: drug, carrier, and the targeting moiety. Carrier-linked prodrugs are obtained by conjugating the drug molecules to low- to high-molecular-weight molecules such as sugars, growth factors, antibodies, peptides, natural and synthetic polymers that can transport the drugs to the target site and subsequently release drugs there.

Central Nervous System (CNS) Drug Delivery Drug delivery to brain remains a great challenge due to the presence of a blood-brain barrier (BBB) regulating the entry of molecules to the brain. The BBB makes the brain inaccessible to CNS-targeted drugs in the systemic circulation, more so for biotherapeutics such as peptides, proteins, and nucleic acids.[4] Transport mechanisms that could be utilized to develop CNS-targeted drug delivery systems include: passive diffusion, active transport, and receptor-mediated transport. The physicochemical properties of the drug molecules are critical to the brain drug delivery. Usually, increasing the hydrophobicity of a drug molecule is likely to increase its transport across the BBB. For low-molecular weight drugs in the range of 400–600 Da, highly lipid soluble molecules such as barbiturate drugs can rapidly cross the BBB into the brain. However, the presence of p-glycoprotein efflux pumps will present a major barrier for the passive diffusion of small molecules across the BBB, if those small molecule drugs were substrates for p-glycoprotein. Examples include vinblastine, vincristine, and cyclosporine. In addition, drugs that are highly charged or bind strongly to plasma proteins may show low transport efficiency across the BBB.

Over the years, different strategies have been developed to overcome the BBB and achieve brain targeted drug delivery. Polymeric implants, for example, Gliadel® (Guilford Pharmaceuticals, Baltimore, MD), have been developed as an adjunct to surgery for prolonging patient survival with brain tumor. Besides the invasive strategies for local drug delivery to CNS, extensive efforts have been contributed to developing systemic approaches for CNS drug delivery. One strategy to improve poor drug uptake in the brain is to administer compounds as prodrugs that can be shuttled by transporters specifically expressed at the blood-brain barrier. Using this approach, researchers have succeeded in designing drug-carrier conjugates that can specifically interact with glucose transporters

笔记

(GluT1), amino acid transporters (LAT1) and choline transporters, thereby targeting the drugs to the brain.

Word Study

1. alveoli [æl'viːəlai] *n.* 肺泡
2. angina [æn'dʒainə] *n.* 心绞痛
3. asthma ['æsmə] *n.* 哮喘
4. bronchi ['brɔŋkai] *n.* 支气管,（尤指肺两侧的）支气管
5. bronchiole [brɔŋtʃa'iəl] *n.* 细支气管
6. buccal ['bʌkəl] *adj.* 面颊的，口的，口腔的
7. choline ['kəuliːn] *n.* 胆碱
8. colloid ['kɔlɔid] *n.* 胶体
9. efflux pump ['eflʌks pʌmp] *n.* 外排泵
10. estradiol [estrə'daiəul] *n.* 雌二醇
11. glycoprotein [ˌglaikəu'prəutiːn] *n.* 糖蛋白
12. gonadotropin [ˌgɔnədəu'trɔpin] *n.* 促性腺激素
13. hygroscopicity [haigrəskɔ'pisiti] *n.* 收湿性
14. hypertension [ˌhaipə'tenʃn] *n.* 高血压
15. impregnate ['impregneit] *v.* 灌注，使饱和，使怀孕
16. iontophoresis [aiɔntəfə'riːsis] *n.* 离子导入
17. lymphatic drainage [lim'fætik 'dreinidʒ] *n.* 淋巴引流
18. nitroglycerine [ˌnaitrəu'glisəriːn] *n.* 硝酸甘油
19. osmotic pump [ɔz'mɔtik pʌmp] *n.* 渗透泵
20. pharynx ['færiŋks] *n.* 咽
21. postmenopausal ['pəustmenəu'pɔːzəl] *adj.* 绝经后的
22. premature ['primətʃə] *adj.* 过早的，提前的
23. pulsatile ['pʌlsətail] *adj.* 脉冲的，跳动的
24. respiratory tract [rə'spirətri trækt] *n.* 呼吸道
25. scopolamine [skəu'pɔləmiːn] *n.* 东莨菪碱
26. spatial ['speiʃl] *adj.* 空间的
27. sublingual [sʌb'liŋgwəl] *adj.* 舌下的
28. temporal ['tempərəl] *adj.* 时间的
29. thermodynamically [θəːməudai'næmikəli] *adv.* 热力学的
30. trachea [trə'kiːə] *n.* 气管

Notes

1. Implants help eliminate the need for continuous intravenous infusion or repeated injections for maintaining therapeutic drug concentrations, which greatly improves patient compliance by reducing or eliminating the patient-involved dosing. 译为：植入剂有助于减少患者对连续静脉输注或反复注射给药以维持治疗血药浓度的需求，并可以极大降低或减少患者参与的给药以提高患者顺应性。

2. The respiratory tract including the nasal mucosa, pharynx, large and small airway structures (trachea, bronchi, bronchioles, alveoli), provides a large mucosal surface for drug absorption,

笔记

which presents a more convenient way of administration compared with parenteral route. 译为：呼吸道由鼻黏膜、咽部、大小气道（气管、支气管、细支气管、肺泡）等结构组成，呼吸道黏膜上皮表面积巨大有助于药物吸收，药物经呼吸道黏膜给药相较经肠外方式给药更为方便。

3. The transdermal route is of particular interest for drugs that have a systemic short elimination half-life or undergo extensive first-pass metabolism, therefore, requiring frequent dosing. 译为：透皮给药途径尤其适用于消除半衰期短或易于受首过代谢影响而需要反复给药的药物。

4. The BBB makes the brain inaccessible to CNS-targeted drugs in the systemic circulation, more so for biotherapeutics such as peptides, proteins, and nucleic acids. BBB 是 blood brain barrier 的缩写。血脑屏障使通过全身给药的靶向中枢神经的药物难以进入大脑，对于生物治疗类药物如多肽、蛋白和核酸的屏障作用更为突出。"more so"后面引导的为省略句式，补充完整为"The BBB makes the brain more inaccessible to biotherapeutics such as peptides, proteins, and nucleic acids"。

Supplementary Parts

1. Medical and Pharmaceutical Terms Made Easier (6): Common Morphemes in English Terms for Pharmaceutics

Morpheme	Meaning	Example
aero	气体	aerosol 气溶胶，气雾剂，烟雾剂
amphi	二、两栖	amphiphilic agent 两亲剂
anti	抗	antioxidant 抗氧化剂
de	去、脱	defoamer 去泡剂
lip	脂肪	lipophilic 亲脂性的
lyo	液体	lyophilic 亲液性的
lyt	溶解	carcinolytic 溶癌的
morph	形态、形状	amorphous 无定形的，无组织的
oleo	油	oleophilic 亲油性的
philic	亲	amphiphilic agent 两亲剂
phobic	害怕、疏远	hydrophobic 狂犬病的，恐水病的，患恐水病的，疏水的
solv	溶解	dissolve 溶解
therm	热	thermostat 恒温器

(1) Write down different prefixes or suffixes according to the Chinese meanings, and then give one sample word using the same prefix or suffix.

Meaning	Prefix or suffix	Sample word	Meaning
剂，者	ant	coagulant	凝血剂

笔记

续表

Meaning	Prefix or suffix	Sample word	Meaning
反对,相反,抗			
霉菌素			
灌肠剂			

(2)　Fill in the blanks with the missing word root, prefix or suffix.

1)　pro_____普鲁卡因

2)　fungi_____ 杀真菌剂

3)　_____foamer 去泡剂

4)　vermi_____ 驱蠕虫药

5)　_____in 胰岛素

6)　_____philic 亲脂性的

7)　_____philic 亲液性的

8)　carcino_____ 溶癌的

9)　_____philic 亲油性的

10)　tuberculo_____ 结核菌抑制药

11)　dis_____ 溶解

12)　hydro_____ 狂犬病的

2.　English-Chinese Translation Skills: 药学英语翻译技巧 (2): 句子成分转换

英汉两种语言句子结构基本相同,有主语、谓语、宾语和定语、状语、补语等,但是不同的句子成分表达方式不完全相同,因此在翻译过程中,常常需要转换句子成分,才能使译文通顺、易懂。句子成分转换法是把英语句子某一成分(如主语)译成汉语句子另一成分(如宾语)等。在多数情况下,词性转换会导致句子成分的转换,句子成分转换法的目的是使译文通顺,更加符合汉语习惯。如:

例 1: The concentration of drug in blood plasma depends on **numerous factors**. **These** include the relative amount of an administered dose that enters the systemic circulation, the rate at which this occurs, the rate and extent of distribution of the drug between the systemic circulation and other tissues and fluids and the rate of elimination of the drug from the body.

参考译文: 很多因素决定着血浆中的药物浓度,包括所用药物进入体循环的相对的量,进入的速度,体循环、其他组织及体液之间的分布的速度和广度,以及药物从体内排出的速度。

说明: 例句原文有两个小句说明决定血浆药物浓度的因素,为了保持语篇结构平衡,numerous factors 作第一小句的宾语,第二句主语用 these,衔接上一小句。在翻译成汉语时,numerous 变成了主语,原句第二句主语 these 则省略了,这样的句子成分转换符合汉语言表达习惯。

例 2: Finally, all of the absorbed drug must pass into the systemic circulation **without being metabolized on passing through the liver**.

笔记

参考译文：最后，所有的药物都必须能够进入体循环而不在通过肝脏时被代谢掉。

说明：原例句有两个介词短语 without being metabolized 和 on passing through the liver，语法功能都是状语，在译成汉语时，第二个介词短语保持时间状语功能："在通过肝脏时"，而第一个介词短语则转换成了动词结构"不……被代谢掉"，符合汉语表达习惯。

例 3：Prolonged presence close to the site of the action, improved drug bioavailability, and easier administration of large drug doses **belong to** the benefits of pellets.

参考译文：微丸有助于延长药物在目标作用部位的作用时间，提高药物的生物利用度，且易于大剂量药物的服用。

说明：原句是一个倒装句结构，谓语动词是 belong to，在翻译成汉语时，为了符合汉语表达习惯，原句的宾语成分 the benefit of pellets 变成了主语，而且省略了谓语成分 belong to，将宾语成分中的名词 benefits 译成了动词"有助于"，避免了类似"微丸的好处包括……"这样生硬的译法。原句主语成分有三个名词词组：prolonged presence close to the site of the action，improved drug bioavailability 和 easier administration of large drug doses，其中，非谓语动词 prolonged 和 improved 作定语，翻译成汉语时都转换成了动词。

句子成分转换是英汉翻译过程中的一个技巧，属于直译策略。药学英语翻译首先还是要对原文句子结构，包括不同语法成分的功能准确理解，不要被句子表层结构限制，拘泥于句子的结构形式，而应把重点放在传达原文逻辑意义上，灵活使用句子成分转换法。

Unit Seven Pharmaceutical Analysis

Drug analysis has evolved from a special technique of the 20th century into an ever-maturing science-the science of pharmaceutical analysis. By utilizing the methodologies and techniques in physics, chemistry, biology and microbiology, pharmaceutical analysis focuses on qualitative and quantitative analysis of drugs, quality control and development of new drugs. This science relates to a wide range of studies, including quality control, clinical pharmacy, analysis of traditional Chinese medicine and natural drugs, drug metabolic analysis, forensic toxicological analysis, doping control and formulation analysis, etc. Pharmaceutical analysis assumes the most important task in drug quality control, which involves physical and chemical inspection of finished drugs, quality control in drug production, quality observation in storage, rapid analysis of preparations formulated in hospitals, establishment of quality standards in the R&D of novel drugs as well as the analysis of drugs *in vivo*. With the vigorous development of pharmaceutical science, the science of pharmaceutical analysis is facing increasing challenges from various related sciences. Instead of being only limited to static quality control of drugs, it has developed into a comprehensive and dynamic analytical study on drug manufacturing, *in-vivo* dynamics and metabolism.

药物分析从 20 世纪初的一种专门技术,逐步发展成为一门日臻成熟的科学——药物分析学。它运用物理学、化学、生物学和微生物学等方法和技术,研究药物的定性和定量分析,药物的质量控制和新药开发。该学科涉及的研究范围包括药品质量控制、临床药学、中药与天然药物分析、药物代谢分析、法医毒物分析、兴奋剂检测和药物制剂分析等。药物分析在药品的质量控制中担任着最主要的任务,包括药物成品的理化检验、药物生产过程中的质量控制、药物贮存过程中的质量考察、医院调配制剂的快速分析、新药研究开发中的质量标准制订以及体内药物分析等。随着药物科学的迅猛发展,各相关学科对药物分析学不断提出新的要求。它已不再仅仅局限于对药物进行静态的质量控制,而是发展到对制药过程、生物体内和代谢过程进行综合评价和动态分析研究。

笔记

91

Text A
What Do Analytical Chemists Do?

Analytical chemistry is concerned with the chemical characterization of matter and the answers to two important questions: what is it (qualitative) and how much is it (quantitative). Chemicals make up everything we use or consume, and knowledge of the chemical composition of many substances is important in our daily lives. Analytical chemistry plays an important role in nearly all aspects of chemistry, for example, agricultural, clinical, environmental, forensic, manufacturing, metallurgical, and pharmaceutical chemistry. The nitrogen content of a fertilizer determines its value. Foods must be analyzed for contaminants (e.g. pesticide residues) and for essential nutrients (e.g. vitamin content). The air in cities must be analyzed for carbon monoxide. Blood glucose must be monitored in diabetics (and, in fact, most diseases are diagnosed by chemical analysis). The presence of trace elements from gun powder on a murder defendant's hand will prove a gun was fired. The quality of manufactured products often depends on proper chemical proportions, and measurement of the constituents is a necessary part of quality control. The carbon content of steel will determine its quality. The purity of drugs will determine their efficacy.

What is Analytical Science?

The above description of analytical chemistry provides an overview of the discipline of analytical chemistry. There have been various attempts to define the discipline more specifically. The late Charles N. Reilley said: "Analytical chemistry is what analytical chemists do." The discipline has expanded beyond the bounds of just chemistry, and many have advocated using the name *analytical science* to describe the field. This term is used in a National Science Foundation report from workshops on "Curricular Developments in the Analytical Sciences." Even this term falls short of recognition of the role of instrumentation development and application. One suggestion is that we use the term analytical science and technology.

The Federation of European Chemical Societies held a contest to define analytical chemistry, and the following suggestion by K. Cammann was selected.

Analytical chemistry provides the methods and tools needed for insight into our material world ... for answering four basic questions about a material sample:

- What?
- Where?
- How much?
- What arrangement, structure or form?

The Division of Analytical Chemistry of the American Chemical Society provides a comprehensive definition of analytical chemistry, which may be found on their website. It is reproduced in most part here:

Analytical chemistry seeks ever improved means of measuring the chemical composition of natural and artificial materials. The techniques of this science are used to identify the substances which may be present in a material and to determine the exact amounts of the identified substance.

Analytical chemists work to improve the reliability of existing techniques to meet the demands for better chemical measurements which arise constantly in our society. They adopt proven

笔记

methodologies to new kinds of materials or to answer new questions about their composition and their reactivity mechanisms.[1] They carry out research to discover completely new principles of measurement and are at the forefront of the utilization of major discoveries, such as lasers and microchip devices for practical purposes. Their efforts serve the needs of many fields:

- In medicine, analytical chemistry is the basis for clinical laboratory tests which help physicians diagnose disease and chart progress in recovery.

- In industry, analytical chemistry provides the means of testing raw materials and for assuring the quality of finished products whose chemical composition is critical. Many household products, fuels, paints, pharmaceuticals, etc. are analyzed by the procedures developed by analytical chemists before being sold to the consumer.

- Environmental quality is often evaluated by testing for suspected contaminants using the techniques of analytical chemistry.

The nutritional value of food is determined by chemical analysis for major components such as protein and carbohydrates and trace components such as vitamins and minerals. Indeed, even the calories in a food are often calculated from its chemical analysis. Analytical chemists also make important contributions to fields as diverse as forensics, archaeology, and space science.[2]

Qualitative and Quantitative Analyses: What Does Each Tell Us?

The discipline of analytical chemistry consists of qualitative analysis and quantitative analysis. The former deals with the identification of elements, ions, or compounds present in a sample (we may be interested in whether only a given substance is present), while the latter deals with the determination of how much of one or more constituents is present. The sample may be solid, liquid, gas, or a mixture. The presence of gunpowder residue on a hand generally requires only qualitative knowledge, not of how much is there, but the price of coal will be determined by the percentage of sulfur impurity present.

Qualitative tests may be performed by selective chemical reactions or with the use of instrumentation. The formation of a white precipitate when adding a solution of silver nitrate to a dissolved sample indicates the presence of chloride. Certain chemical reactions will produce colors to indicate the presence of classes of organic compounds, for example, ketones. Infrared spectra will give "fingerprints" of organic compounds or their functional groups.

A clear distinction should be made between the terms selective and specific:

- A selective reaction or test is one that can occur with other substances but exhibits a degree of preference for the substance of interest.[3]

- A specific reaction or test is one that occurs only with the substance of interest.

Unfortunately, few reactions are specific but many exhibit selectivity. Selectivity may be achieved by a number of strategies. Some examples are:

- Sample preparation (e.g., extractions, precipitation)
- Instrumentation (selective detectors)
- Target analyte derivatization (e.g., derivatize specific functional groups with detecting reagents)
- Chromatography, which provides powerful separation

For quantitative analysis, a history of the sample composition will often be known (it is known that blood contains glucose), or else the analyst will have performed a qualitative test prior

 笔记

to performing the more difficult quantitative analysis. Modern chemical measurement systems often exhibit sufficient selectivity that a quantitative measurement can also serve as a qualitative measurement. However, simple qualitative tests are usually more rapid than quantitative procedures. Qualitative analysis is composed of two fields: inorganic and organic. The former is usually covered in introductory chemistry courses, whereas the latter is best left until after the student has had a course in organic chemistry.[4]

In comparing qualitative versus quantitative analysis, consider, for example, the sequence of analytical procedures followed in testing for banned substances at the Olympic Games. The list of prohibited substances includes about 500 different active constituents: stimulants, steroids, beta-blockers, diuretics, narcotics, analgesics, local anesthetics, and sedatives. Some are detectable only as their metabolites. Many athletes must be tested rapidly, and it is not practical to perform a detailed quantitative analysis on each. There are three phases in the analysis: the fast-screening phase, the identification phase, and possible quantification phase. In the fast-screening phase, urine samples are rapidly tested for the presence of classes of compounds that will differentiate them from "normal" samples, using various techniques including immunoassays, gas chromatography, and liquid chromatography. About 5% of the samples may indicate the presence of unknown compounds that may or may not be prohibited but need to be identified. Samples showing a suspicious profile during the screening undergo a new preparation cycle (possible hydrolysis, extraction, derivatization), depending on the nature of the compounds that have been detected. The compounds are then identified using the highly selective combination of gas chromatography/mass spectrometry (GC/MS). In this technique, complex mixtures are separated by gas chromatography, and they are then detected by mass spectrometry, which provides molecular structural data on the compounds. The MS data, combined with the time of elution from the gas chromatograph, provide a high probability of the presence of a given detected compound. GC/MS is expensive and time-consuming, and so it is used only when necessary. Following the identification phase, some compounds must be precisely quantified since they may normally be present at low levels, for example, from food, pharmaceutical preparations, or endogenous steroids, and elevated levels must be confirmed. This is done using quantitative techniques such as spectrophotometry or gas chromatography.

Word Study

1. analyte ['ænəlait] *n.* 分析物，待测物
2. chromatography [,krəumə'tɔgrəfi] *n.* 色谱法；色谱；层析；层析法
3. elution [i'lju:ʃən] *n.* 洗脱
4. extraction [iks'trækʃən] *n.* 萃取
5. forensic [fə'rensik] *adj.* 法医的
6. hydrolysis [hai'drɔlisis] *n.* 水解（作用）
7. immunoassay [imjunəu'æsei] *n.* 免疫测定
8. impurity [im'pjurəti] *n.* 不纯，杂质
9. late [leit] *adj.* 已故的
10. metallurgical [metə'lə:dʒikəl] *adj.* 冶金的，冶金学的
11. precipitation [prisipi'teiʃən] *n.* 沉淀
12. spectrophotometry [spektrəufəu'tɔmitri] *n.* 分光光度测定法

笔记

Notes

1. They adopt proven methodologies to new kinds of materials or to answer new questions about their composition and their reactivity mechanisms. 译为：他们将已证实的方法应用于新型材料，或回答关于其组成及反应机制的新问题。句中"adopt...to..."意思是"使用……来……"。

2. Analytical chemists also make important contributions to fields as diverse as forensics, archaeology, and space science. 译为：分析化学家在法医学、考古学和太空科学等多个领域也做出了重要贡献。句中，"as diverse as…"强调"范围很广，覆盖……"。

3. A selective reaction or test is one that can occur with other substances but exhibits a degree of preference for the substance of interest. 译为：选择性反应或检测是指可以和其他物质发生反应但对感兴趣物质显示一定程度的偏好的反应。句中，"one"指的是"a reaction or test"。

4. The former is usually covered in introductory chemistry courses, whereas the latter is best left until after the student has had a course in organic chemistry. 译为：前者通常涵盖于介绍性的化学课程中，而后者只有在学生学完一门有机化学课程后再去涉猎为好。注意句中的"The former…, whereas the latter…"是指"前者……，而后者……"。

Exercises

1. **Decide whether each of the following statements is true (T) or false (F) according to the passage.**

(1) Analytical chemistry is concerned with two important questions: what is it (qualitative) and how much is it (quantitative).

(2) Measurement of chemical constituents from manufactured products is unnecessary for quality control.

(3) Analytical chemistry seeks ever improved means of measuring the chemical composition of natural and artificial materials.

(4) Infrared spectra will give "fingerprints" of inorganic compounds or their functional groups.

(5) Modern chemical measurement systems often exhibit sufficient selectivity that a quantitative measurement can also serve as a qualitative measurement.

(6) Gas chromatography/mass spectrometry (GC/MS) is a highly selective technique.

2. **Questions for oral discussion.**

(1) What is analytical chemistry concerned with?

(2) What is analytical science?

(3) What is the difference between "selective" and "specific"?

(4) What are the three phases in testing for banned substances at the Olympic Games?

3. **Choose the best answer to each of the following questions.**

(1) Blood _____ must be monitored in diabetics (and, in fact, most diseases are diagnosed by chemical analysis).

　　A. protein　　　　　　　　　　　B. pH

　　C. glucose　　　　　　　　　　　D. hemoglobin

(2) In medicine, analytical chemistry is the basis for _____ laboratory tests which help physicians diagnose disease and chart progress in recovery.

　　A. clinical　　　　　　　　　　　B. polymer

笔记

C. agricultural   D. fuel

(3) In industry, analytical chemistry provides the means of testing raw materials and for assuring the quality of finished products whose chemical _____ is critical.

A. composition   B. compound

C. concentration   D. class

(4) _____ quality is often evaluated by testing suspected contaminants using the techniques of analytical chemistry.

A. Agricultural   B. Environmental

C. Nutritional   D. Engineering

(5) The formation of a white precipitate when adding a solution of silver nitrate to a dissolved sample indicates the presence of _____.

A. nitrate   B. sulfide

C. chloride   D. sulfate

(6) _____ spectra will give "fingerprints" of organic compounds or their functional groups.

A. Infrared   B. Ultraviolet

C. Visible   D. Mass

(7) Chromatography provides powerful _____.

A. instrumentation   B. precipitation

C. extraction   D. separation

(8) The list of prohibited substances at the Olympic Games includes about 500 different active constituents, such as _____.

A. stimulants   B. steroids

C. beta-blockers   D. all of the above

(9) Doped compounds are identified using the highly selective combination of gas _____ -mass spectrometry (GC-MS).

A. phase   B. concentration

C. flow   D. chromatography

(10) _____ spectrometry provides molecular structural data on the compounds.

A. Infrared   B. Mass

C. Visible   D. Ultraviolet

4. Choose an appropriate word from the list below and write it down in the underline before its corresponding definition.

qualitative, quantitative, mass spectrometry, infrared spectroscopy, ultraviolet spectroscopy, chromatography, pharmaceutical, contaminant, structure, nutrition

(1) _____ data are collected through participant observation and interviews, and analyzed by themes from description by informants.

(2) _____ data are collected through measuring things, and analyzed through numerical comparisons and statistical inferences.

(3) Torn muscles retract, and lose strength, _____, and tightness.

(4) _____ is the spectroscopy that deals with the infrared region of the electromagnetic spectrum, that is light with a longer wavelength and lower frequency than visible light.

(5) _____ refers to absorption spectroscopy or reflectance spectroscopy in the ultraviolet spectral region.

笔记

(6) _____ is the collective term for a set of laboratory techniques for the separation of mixtures.

(7) _____ is an analytical technique that sorts ions based on their mass (or "weight").

(8) _____ is the science that interprets the substances in food in relation to maintenance, growth, reproduction, health and disease of an organism.

(9) The _____ industry develops, produces, and markets drugs for use as medications.

(10) In environmental chemistry, _____ is in some cases virtually equivalent to pollution.

5. Translate the following sentences and paragraphs into Chinese.

(1) Qualitative analysis is to identify the elements, ions and compounds contained in a sample while quantitative analysis is to determine the exact quantity.

(2) Analytical chemistry has expanded beyond the bounds of just chemistry, and many have advocated using the name analytical science to describe the field. Even this term falls short of recognition of the role of instrumentation development and application.

(3) Analytical chemists work to improve the reliability of existing techniques to meet the demands for better chemical measurements which arise constantly in our society.

(4) Many household products, fuels, paints, pharmaceuticals, etc. are analyzed by the procedures developed by analytical chemists before being sold to the consumer.

(5) For quantitative analysis, a history of the sample composition will often be known (it is known that blood contains glucose), or else the analyst will have performed a qualitative test prior to performing the more difficult quantitative analysis.

(6) Qualitative tests may be performed by selective chemical reactions or with the use of instrumentation. For example, the formation of a white precipitate when adding a solution of silver nitrate to a dissolved sample indicates the presence of chloride. Infrared spectra will give "fingerprints" of organic compounds or their functional groups.

(7) The first phase in the testing of banned substances is called fast-screening phase, in which qualitative analysis such as GC or LC is adopted to test suspicious samples. In the second phase, GC-MS is employed for further testing of those suspicious samples. Finally, spectrophotometry or GC is applied for accurate quantification.

Text B
Analytical Techniques

Separation Techniques

Nearly all the samples presented to the pharmaceutical analyst are mixtures, sometimes very complex ones. The determination of the amount of each isolated component is usually a simple matter. The analysis of these same components in each other's presence may, however, be difficult or even impossible because of interference by one substance in the assay of another.[1] Interference can take several forms. The interfering substance can respond quantitatively to the analytical method for the desired component. An example is the interference caused by acetic acid in the assay of hydrochloric acid by titration with alkali. This is not an entirely hopeless situation, for the analysis will at least yield the sum of the amounts of the desired component and the interfering component. Another common example is the interference observed in absorption spectroscopy when two solutes have overlapping absorption bands. Sometimes the interference is a partial, non-quantitative response to the assay. For example, the nonaqueous titration of weakly acidic drugs in tablets containing stearic acid may be unsuccessful because of consumption of titrant by the stearic acid; this is not a reproducible effect, probably because of incomplete dissolution of stearic acid in the titration medium. It is very difficult to compensate for interferences of this type. Another commonly encountered form of interference is an impairment of the analytical method for the desired component, leading to non-quantitative results even for this component. A trace of copper in a sample of magnesium can vitiate a visual complexometric titration of the magnesium by poisoning the indicator. Another instance is the quenching of quinine fluorescence by hydrochloric acid.

When an analytical method cannot be applied directly to a mixture because of possible interference, a separation of the mixture into its components may be necessary.

Physical and Instrumental Methods

Physical and instrumental methods are analytical methods based upon measurements of physical properties and measurements with instruments. Separation of the properties of matter into physical and chemical properties is arbitrary but often convenient. A physical property can be defined as a quality of matter that is manifested without the occurrence of chemical reactions. The arbitrariness enters when we define chemical reactions. Solubility, for example, can be thought of as either a chemical or a physical property.

Part of the analyst's task is to describe the characteristics of ("to characterize") materials. Such physical properties as melting point, boiling point, density, refractive index, and spectral properties can help to accomplish this. Some of these properties also form the basis of quantitative analytical methods. These include some old, classical subjects (such as density and refractive index) and some modern ones (such as nuclear magnetic resonance and mass spectrometry). Both the old and the new methods are useful in current analytical practice. It is an interesting development that an old technique sometimes achieves new importance when it is modified with the incorporation of modern advances in instrumentation.[2]

Titrimetric Analysis

The basic experimental operation in titrimetric analysis is called titration. In titration, a solution of one reactant of accurately known concentration (the titrant, or standard solution) is added to a second solution of sample whose amount or concentration is to be determined. Titrant is added to the sample until the amount of titrant added is chemically equivalent to the amount of sample. The stage at which this equivalence occurs is called the equivalence point of the titration, and its experimental estimate is called the titration end point. From the amount of titrant used to reach the end point, from its concentration, and from the known stoichiometry of the substance, the concentration of the solution can be calculated. Usually the volume of titrant is measured, and then titrimetric analysis is also called volumetric analysis.

Titrimetry is a classical method of analysis, but even in modern analytical practice it is very important, as can be seen by browsing through the United States Pharmacopoeia/Nation Formulary (the legal compendium of specifications and the standards for drug purity and quality).[3]

In many assay procedures, a titration serves as the final step, being preceded by other chemical reactions, separation techniques, or other manipulations. It may be noted here that titrimetry is a widely applicable approach for quantitative analysis, and is often coupled with other methods.

One of the advantages of titrimetry as an analytical approach is that it is an absolute method of analysis. The meaning of this statement will not be fully clear until we have studied methods lacking this attribute, but it simply means that, by titrimetric analysis, the purity of a sample compound can be determined without reference to a separate specimen of that same compound (whose purity might itself be in doubt). For example, a sodium hydroxide solution can be standardized against primary standard grade potassium biphthalate, and then the purity of a sample of acetic acid can be determined by titration with the NaOH solution. Thus the purity of the acetic acid has been obtained without making any assumptions about acetic acid (that is, without using acetic acid as a primary standard). Such assumptions were, of course, made about the potassium biphthalate, and independent evidence must be available to support them.

A titration is feasible when ① the titration reaction is rapid compared with the speed of titration; ② its equilibrium constant is large enough to give a sharp "break" at the end point; ③ a method of end point detection is available. Whether or not the titration should be used for a particular analysis will depend upon many factors, including the sensitivity required, possible interfering substances that would also be titrated and alternative methods of analysis.

Gas Chromatography

Gas chromatography is a separation technique whereby a vaporized sample is carried by a flowing stream of (usually) inert gas through a tube which is either filled with fine particles or is wall-coated with a low-volatility liquid. The tube is termed the column. If the column is filled with dry particles, the technique is called gas-solid chromatography. In gas-liquid chromatography, the particles or the inside walls are coated with a low-volatility liquid. Gas chromatography can be used for the analysis of gas, liquid, and solid samples, providing that the latter two can be thermally vaporized without significant decomposition.

The practical aspects of gas chromatography can best be described by a general instrument diagram, in which the carrier gas module is simply a pressurized source of the inert carrier gas, usually a compressed gas cylinder. The sample introduction module encompasses the sample injection system, which is usually a heated block and may include associated sampling valves for gas samples. The vaporized sample then proceeds to the column module where it is separated into its various components. The components then emerge individually into the detection module, where their presence is sensed by the appropriate detector. The detector signal is then fed into a data acquisition module, which can be a simple recorder, an integrator, a computer, or some combination of the three.

The graphic presentation of a gas chromatogram is relative detector response plotted on the y-axis versus time plotted on the x-axis. The relative position of the individual peaks along the time axis is determined by the separating capability of the column for that mixture, and the size of the peaks (height or area) is a measure of the amount of component present in the mixture.[4]

Word Study

1. absorption [əbˈsɔːpʃən] *n.* 吸收
2. acquisition [ækwiˈziʃən] *n.* 采集
3. compensate [ˈkɔmpənseit] *v.* 补偿

笔记

4. complexometric [kɔmpleksi'metrik] *adj.* 络合滴定的
5. constant ['kɔnstənt] *n.* 常数
6. consumption [kən'sʌmpʃən] *n.* 消耗
7. decomposition [diːkɔmpə'ziʃən] *n.* 分解
8. density ['densiti] *n.* 密度
9. graphic ['græfik] *adj.* 图形的
10. impairment [im'pɛəmənt] *n.* 损害
11. instrument ['instrumənt, 'instrəmənt] *n.* 仪器
12. integrator ['intigreitə] *n.* 积分仪
13. interference [intə'fiərəns] *n.* 干扰
14. nonaqueous ['nɔn'eikwiəs] *adj.* 非水的
15. overlap ['əuvəlæp] *v.* 重叠
16. quantitative['kwɔntitətiv] *adj.* 定量的
17. quenching ['kwentʃiŋ] *n.* 淬灭，熄灭，抑制
18. quinine ['kwainain] *n.* 奎宁
19. reactant [ri'æktənt] *n.* 反应物
20. refractive [ri'fræktiv] *adj.* 折射的
21. sensitivity [sensi'tiviti] *n.* 灵敏度
22. solubility [sɔlju'biliti] *n.* 溶解性
23. spectrometry [spek'trɔmitri] *n.* 光谱测定法, 频谱测定法, 能谱测定, 度谱术
24. spectroscopy [spek'trɔskəpi] *n.* 光谱法
25. standardize ['stændədaiz] *v.* 标定
26. stoichiometry [stɔiki'ɔmitri] *n.* 化学计量学
27. titrant ['taitrənt] *n.* 滴定剂
28. titration [tai'treiʃən] *n.* 滴定
29. titrimetric [taitri'metrik] *adj.* 滴定分析的
30. titrimetry [tai'trimitri] *n.* 滴定分析法
31. vitiate ['viʃieit] *v.* 污染
32. volatility [vɔlə'tiliti] *n.* 挥发性
33. volumetric [vɔlju'metrik] *adj.* 容量的，测定体积的

Notes

1. The analysis of these same components in each other's presence may, however, be difficult or even impossible because of interference by one substance in the assay of another. 译为：然而，对其中各个组分进行分析却是困难的，甚至几乎不可能进行，因为在对某组分进行分析时，其他组分对其测定有干扰。其中"in each other's presence"指"在彼此共同存在的情况下"。

2. It is an interesting development that an old technique sometimes achieves new importance when it is modified with the incorporation of modern advances in instrumentation. 译为：有意思的是，随着现代仪器分析方法的进步，当改进的老方法与其相结合时，可以使老方法重新受到重视。

3. Titrimetry is a classical method of analysis, but even in modern analytical practice it is very important, as can be seen by browsing through the United States Pharmacopoeia/Nation Formulary (the legal compendium of specifications and the standards for drug purity and quality).

笔记

译为：滴定分析虽然是一种经典的分析化学方法，但是在现代分析技术中它也占有重要的地位，这一点可以通过浏览美国药典 / 国家处方集（关于药物纯度和质量的法定规范和标准集）看出来。其中"as"引导非限制性定语从句。

4. The relative position of the individual peaks along the time axis is determined by the separating capability of the column for that mixture, and the size of the peaks (height or area) is a measure of the amount of component present in the mixture. 译为：坐标轴上各组分峰的相对位置取决于色谱柱对混合体系的分离效能，峰的大小（峰高或峰面积）是衡量各组分在混合体系中含量的指标。

Supplementary Parts

1. Medical and Pharmaceutical Terms Made Easier (7): Common Morphemes in English Terms for Pharmaceutical Analysis

Morpheme	Meaning	Example
a-	无，非	aprotic solvent 无质子溶剂
alkal	碱	alkaloid 生物碱
amino	氨基	aminoglycoside 氨基糖苷
amper	安培，电流	amperometric 电流测定的
aque	水	nonaqueous titration 非水滴定法
argent	银	argentometry 银量法
auto	自动	autoprotolysis constant 质子自递常数
aux	辅助	auxochrome 助色团
brom	溴	bromimetry 溴量法
calor	热	calorimetry 量热法
chem	化学	chemometrics 化学计量学
chromato	颜色，色谱	chromatography 色谱法
coul	库仑	coulometric titration 库仑滴定法
electr	电	electrophoresis 电泳
fluor	荧光	fluorometry 荧光分析法
grav	重	electrogravimetry 电重量法
holo	全	holographic grating 全息光栅
homo	相同，均等	homolytic cleavage 均裂
iod	碘	iodimetry 碘量法
iso	相等	isoelectric focusing 等电聚焦
magnet	磁	electromagnetic spectrum 电磁波谱
photo	光	photodiode 光二极管
spectr	看，光	spectroscopy 光谱法
therm	热	thermospray 热喷雾
titri	滴定	titrimetric analysis 滴定分析法
volum	容量	volumetric analysis 容量分析法

(1) Decompose the following words and translate them into Chinese.

1) alkaloid　　　　　　　_____

2) amperometric　　　　_____

3) argentometry　　　　_____

4) auxochrome　　　　　_____

笔记

5) bromimetry _____
6) chromatography _____
7) electrophoresis _____
8) fluorometry _____
9) iodimetry _____
10) electromagnetic spectrum _____
11) spectroscopy _____
12) photodiode _____

(2)   Word-matching.

1) calorimetry	A. 氨基糖苷
2) volumetric analysis	B. 非水滴定法
3) titrimetric analysis	C. 电重量法
4) chemometrics	D. 热喷雾
5) thermospray	E. 容量分析法
6) nonaqueous titration	F. 库仑滴定法
7) electrogravimetry	G. 全息光栅
8) isoelectric focusing	H. 等电聚焦
9) aminoglycoside	I. 化学计量学
10) homolytic cleavage	J. 量热法
11) holographic grating	K. 均裂
12) coulometric titration	L. 滴定分析法

2.   English-Chinese Translation Skills: 药学英语翻译技巧 (3)：增、减词法

翻译时，为了对原文忠实，译文不能够对原文意思进行任意增加或者减少，但这并不是说译文必须完全对等于原文，在文字上也不能有任何增减。实际上，由于英汉两种语言表达习惯存在差异，为了确切、充分地表达译文原义，或者使译文表达更加顺畅且符合汉语习惯，往往需要对译文进行文字增补或者省略。增词法主要指增加原文中无其词但有其意的一些词，绝不是无中生有地随意增词；减词法主要指原文中有些词在译文中可以省略，不必翻译出来。有些原文中因结构需要必不可少的词语，如冠词、代词、介词等，如果原原本本地译成汉语就会成为不必要的冗词，译文就会显得十分累赘，不符合汉语表达习惯。

例 1：**The nutritional value of food** is determined by chemical analysis for major components **such as** protein and carbohydrates and trace components **such as** vitamins and minerals. Indeed, even **the calories in a food** **are often calculated from its chemical analysis**.

参考译文：食品的营养价值是通过对其中蛋白质、碳水化合物等主要成分以及维生素、矿物质等微量成分的化学分析而得以确定。实际上，甚至食物的热量也经常通过化学分析的方法来计算。

说明：在上面例句中，the nutritional value of food 和 the calories in a food 两个词组的结构不同，但是翻译中介词 in 省略了，没有机械地译成"……中的"。原文中的两个 such as 也根据汉语表达需要省略了，没有直译出来。另外在翻译 are often calculated from its chemical analysis 时，原文在"化学分析"后增加了"……的方法"，使得译文表达更加具体。

例 2：Do not take aluminum-containing antacids at all **while you are taking sucralfate**. This combination increases aluminum absorption into the bloodstream.

参考译文：服用硫糖铝时禁用含铝抗酸药，二者联用会增加铝在血液中的吸收。

笔记

说明：这个例句来自药品说明书，在翻译 while you are taking sucralfate 时，考虑到主语 you 没有明确意义，要省略。

例 3: However, there are limited examples of success in **developing** biotherapeutic modalities for central nervous system (CNS) diseases in the drug **development** pipeline.

参考译文：然而，在药物研发过程中，鲜有生物治疗模式用于中枢神经系统疾病的成功案例。

说明：上面例句有两个 develop，意思都是"研发、开发"等，从整个句子的翻译来讲，省略 in developing biotherapeutic modalities 中的 develop，避免了重复也不妨碍整句意思。

翻译中增、减词没有固定规律可言，主要还是出于译文表达需要，有时候在英文句子中没有什么省略，但是直接翻译成汉语，译文就不是很清楚，此时就必须根据汉语表达习惯适当增、减词。

例 4: The basic experimental operation in titrimetric analysis is called titration. **In titration**, a solution of one reactant of accurately known concentration (the titrant, or standard solution) is added to a second solution of sample whose amount or concentration is to be determined. Titrant is added to the sample until the amount of titrant added is chemically equivalent to the amount of sample.

参考译文：滴定分析中基本的实验操作就是滴定。在滴定过程中，将已知准确浓度的反应物溶液（滴定剂或标准溶液）加入到另外一种反应物溶液中，也就是样品量或浓度待测定的样品溶液中。滴定剂不断地加入到样品溶液中，直到加入滴定剂的量与样品中待测物的量达到化学平衡。

说明：原文有三个小句。第二个小句中 in titration 被译成"在滴定过程中"，增加了"过程中"，其中"is added to a second solution of sample whose amount or concentration…"译文增加了"也就是"；第三小句中 Titrant is added to the sample until…，译文增加了"不断地"，与原文中的"until（直到）"呼应，以及在翻译 to the amount of sample 时，译文增加了"待测物的"，与前文"titrant added（加入滴定剂的）"相呼应。原文句子结构完整，意思明确，没有缺少什么词，但是汉语译文增加了一些词，这些增词都没有改变原文意义，也不显得啰嗦，使译文表达更加通畅。

当然，这个例句中的第二句也涉及定语从句的翻译技巧，这在后面章节中另有讲解。

笔记

Unit Eight Natural Products

A natural product is a chemical compound or substance produced by a living organism - found in nature that usually has a pharmacological or biological activity for use in pharmaceutical drug discovery and drug design. A natural product can be considered as such even if it can be prepared by total synthesis.

Natural products may be extracted from tissues of terrestrial plants, marine organisms or microorganism fermentation broths. A crude (untreated) extract from any one of these sources typically contains novel, structurally diverse chemical compounds, which the natural environment is a rich source of.

Chemical diversity in nature is based on biological and geographical diversity, so researchers travel around the world obtaining samples to analyze and evaluate in drug discovery screens or bioassays. This effort to search for natural products is known as bioprospecting.

Pharmacognosy provides the tools to identify, select and process natural products destined for medicinal use. Usually, the natural product compound has some form of biological activity and that compound is known as the active principle - such a structure can act as a lead compound. Many of today's medicines are obtained directly from a natural source.

On the other hand, some medicines are developed from a lead compound originally obtained from a natural source. This means the lead compound can be produced by total synthesis, or can be a starting point (precursor) for a semisynthetic compound, or can act as a template for a structurally different total synthetic compound. This is because most biologically active natural product compounds are secondary metabolites with very complex structures. This has an advantage in that they are extremely novel compounds but this complexity also makes many lead compounds' synthesis difficult and the compound usually has to be extracted from its natural source - a slow, expensive and inefficient process. As a result, there is usually an advantage in designing simpler analogues.

天然产物是指由自然界的生物体产生的化合物或其他物质，通常具有一定的药理作用或生物活性，可用于药物发现和药物设计。尽管天然产物可以通过全合成来制备，上述定义仍然适用。

天然产物可提取自陆生植物、海洋生物或是微生物发酵液。来自上述任一来源的粗提取物通常含有新的、结构各异的化合物，自然界是这些化合物的丰富来源。

在自然界中，化学多样性实质上取决于生物多样性和地理多样性，因此研究者们会在世界各地获取样本并在药物发现筛选或生物鉴定中加以分析和评价。这项寻找天然产物的工作称为生物勘探。

生药学为药用天然产物的鉴别、筛选和加工提供了工具。通常，天然产物化合物具有一定的生物活性，被人们称作活性成分，这种结构可用作先导化合物。目前许多药物可直接从自然资源获取。

另一方面，有一些药物是以天然来源的先导化合物为基础研发而得。这意味着先导化合物可以通过全合成制备，可以作为半合成化合物的前体，或者作为模板来合成结构截然不同的全合成化合物。这是因为大多数具有生物活性的天然产物化合物是次级代谢产物，具有非常复杂的结构。它们的优势在于结构新颖；但结构的复杂性增加了合成难度，所以这些化合物通常是从其自然资源中提取 —— 耗时、昂贵又低效。因此，设计结构更简单的类似物通常会具有优势。

笔记

104

Text A
Drug Discovery and Natural Products

It may be argued that drug discovery is a recent concept that evolved from modern science during the 20th century, but this concept in reality dates back many centuries, and has its origins in nature. On many occasions, humans have turned to Mother Nature for cures, and discovered unique drug molecules. Thus, the term natural product has become almost synonymous with the concept of drug discovery. In modern drug discovery and development processes, natural products play an important role at the early stage of "lead" discovery, i.e. discovery of the active (determined by various bioassays) natural molecule, which itself or its structural analogues could be an ideal drug candidate.

Natural products have been enormous source of drugs and drug leads. It is estimated that 61 percent of the 877 small-molecular new chemical entities introduced as drugs worldwide during 1981–2002 can be traced back to or were developed from natural products. These include natural products (6 percent), natural product derivatives (27 percent), and synthetic compounds with natural-product- derived pharmacophores (5 percent) and synthetic compounds designed on the basis of knowledge gained from a natural product, i.e. a natural product mimic (23 percent). In some therapeutic areas, the contribution of natural products is even greater, e.g. about 78 per cent of antibacterials and 74 percent of anticancer drug candidates are natural products or structural analogues of natural products. In 2000, approximately 60 percent of all drugs in clinical trials for the multiplicity of cancers were of natural origins. In 2001, eight (simvastatin, pravastatin, amoxycillin, clavulanic acid, clarithromycin, azithromycin, ceftriaxone, cyclosporin and paclitaxel) of 30 top selling medicines were natural products or derived from natural products, and despite being neglected by the pharmaceutical companies, these eight drugs together totaled $16 billion in sales.

Despite the impressive record and statistics regarding the success of natural products in drug discovery, "natural product drug discovery" has been neglected by many big pharmaceutical companies in the recent past. The declining popularity of natural products as a source of new drugs began in the 1990s, because of some practical factors, e.g. the apparent lack of compatibility of natural products with the modern high throughput screening (HTS) programs, where significant degrees of automation, robotics and computers are used, the complexity in the isolation and identification of natural products and the cost and time involved in the natural product "lead" discovery process. Complexity in the chemistry of natural products, especially in the case of novel structural types, also became the rate-determining step in drug discovery programs. Attempts to discover new drug "leads" from natural sources has never stopped, despite being neglected by the pharmaceutical companies, but continued in academia and some semi-academic research organizations, where more traditional approaches to natural product drug discovery have been applied.

Neglected for years, natural product drug discovery appears to be drawing attention and immense interest again, and is on the verge of a comeback in the mainstream of drug discovery ventures. In recent years, a significant revival of interests in natural products as a potential source for new medicines has been observed among academics as well as several pharmaceutical companies. This extraordinary comeback of natural products in drug discovery research is mainly due to the following factors: combinatorial chemistry's promise to fill drug development pipelines with de novo synthetic small-molecular drug candidates is somewhat unsuccessful; the practical difficulties

笔记

of natural product drug discovery are being overcome by advances in separation and identification technologies and in the speed and sensitivity of structure elucidation and, finally, the unique and incomparable chemical diversity that natural products have to offer. Moreover, only a small fraction of the world's biodiversity has ever been investigated for bioactivity to date. For example, there are at least 250,000 species of higher plants that exist on this planet, but merely five to ten percent of these terrestrial plants have been investigated so far. In addition, re-investigation of previously investigated plants has continued to produce new bioactive compounds that have the potential for being developed as drugs. While several biologically active compounds have been found in marine organisms, e.g. antimicrobial compound cephalosporin C from marine organisms (*Cephalosporium acremonium* and *Streptomyces* spp.) and antiviral compounds such as avarol and avarone from marine sponges, e.g. *Dysidea avara*, research in this area is still at the starting point. The following notes are the summary of the traditional as well as the modern drug discovery processes involving natural products.

Natural Product Drug Discovery: the Traditional Way

In the traditional, rather more academic, method of drug discovery from natural products, drug targets are exposed to crude extracts, and in the case of a hit[1], i.e. any evidence of activity, the extract is fractionated and the active compound is isolated and identified. Every step of fractionation and isolation is usually guided by bioassays, and the process is called bioassay-guided isolation. The following scheme presents an overview of a bioassay-guided traditional natural product drug discovery process.

Sometimes, a straightforward natural product isolation route, irrespective of bioactivity, is also applied, which results in the isolation of a number of natural compounds (small compound library) suitable for undergoing any bioactivity screening. However, the process can be slow, ineffectual and labour intensive, and it does not guarantee that a "lead" from screening would be chemically workable or even patentable.

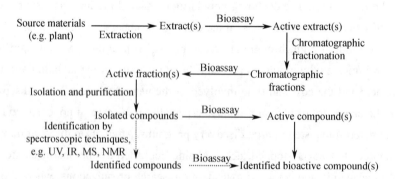

Natural Product Drug Discovery: the Modern Processes

Modern drug discovery approaches involve HTS[2], where, applying full automation and robotics, hundreds of molecules can be screened using several assays within a short time, and with very little amount of compounds. In order to incorporate natural products in the modern HTS programs, a natural product library (a collection of dereplicated natural products) needs to be built. Dereplication is the process by which one can eliminate recurrence or re-isolation of same or similar compounds from various extracts. A number of hyphenated techniques are used for dereplication, e.g. LC-PDA (liquid chromatography–photo-diode-array detector), LC-MS (liquid chromatography–mass detector) and LC-NMR (liquid chromatography–nuclear magnetic resonance spectroscopy).

While in the recent past it was extremely difficult, time consuming and labour intensive to build such a library from purified natural products, the situation has improved greatly with the advent of newer and improved technologies related to separation, isolation and identification of natural products. Now, it is possible to build a "high quality" and "chemically diverse" natural product library that can be suitable for any modern HTS programs. Natural product libraries can also be of crude extracts, chromatographic fractions or semi-purified compounds. However, the best result can be obtained from a fully identified pure natural product library as it provides scientists with the opportunity to handle the "lead" rapidly for further developmental work, e.g. total or partial synthesis, dealing with formulation factors, *in vivo* assays and clinical trials.

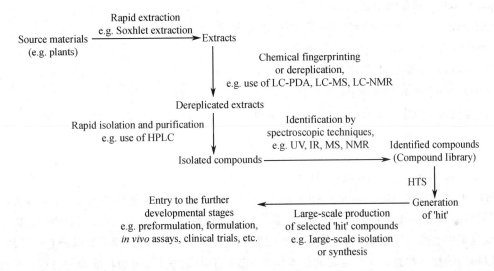

To continue to exploit natural sources for drug candidates, the focus must be on exploiting newer approaches for natural product drug discovery. These approaches include the application of genomic tools, seeking novel sources of organisms from the environment, new screening technologies and improved processes of sample preparation for screening samples. In addition, the recent focus on the synthesis of diversity-oriented combinatorial libraries based on natural-product-like compounds is an attempt to enhance the productivity of synthetic chemical libraries.

Word Study

1. amoxycillin [əmɔksə'silin] *n.* 阿莫西林
2. avarol [ə'værɔl] *n.* 阿瓦醇
3. avarone [əvə'rʌn] *n.* 阿瓦醌
4. azithromycin [eiziθrə'maisin] *n.* 阿奇霉素
5. bioassay [ˌbaiəu'æsei]   *n.* 生物检定，生物学鉴定法
6. candidate ['kændidit] *n.* 候选人，候补者，应试者
7. ceftriaxone [seftrai'æksn] *n.* 头孢曲松
8. cephalosporin [sefələu'spɔːrin]   *n.* 头孢菌素
9. cephalosporium acremonium *n.* 顶头孢菌
10. chromatographic [krəuˌmætə'græfik] *adj.* 色谱的

笔记

11. clarithromycin [klæriθrə'maisin] *n.* 克拉霉素

12. clavulanic acid [klaːviu'lænik'æsid] *n.* 克拉维酸

13. cyclosporin [ˌsaikləu'spɔːrin] *n.* 环孢霉素

14. dereplication [diˌrepli'keiʃən] *n.* 去重复化

15. *Dysidea avara n.* 贪婪倜海绵

16. entity ['entiti] *n.* 实体，存在，本质

17. hyphenated ['haifəneitid] *adj.* 带有连字符号的

18. LC-MS (liquid chromatography–mass spectrometry) *n.* 液相色谱质谱联用

19. LC-NMR (liquid chromatography–nuclear magnetic resonance) *n.* 液相色谱磁共振联用

20. LC-PDA (liquid chromatography–photo-diode-array) *n.* 二极管阵列液相色谱

21. marine [mə'riːn] *adj.* 海产的，海底的

22. mimic ['mimik] *n.* 模仿，临摹，仿制品

23. paclitaxel [ˌpækli'tæksəl] *n.* 紫杉醇

24. pharmacophore ['fɑːməkəfɔː] *n.* 药效团，药效基团，药效结构

25. pipeline ['paipˌlain] *n.* 导管，流水线

26. pravastatin ['prɑːvəstətin] *n.* 普伐他汀

27. simvastatin ['simvəstətin] *n.* 辛伐他汀

28. sponge [spʌndʒ] *n.* 海绵，海绵球，海绵动物

Notes

1. in the case of a hit: 一旦发现任何活性。

2. HTS 高通量筛选（High throughput screening）技术是指以分子水平和细胞水平的实验方法为基础，以微板形式作为实验工具载体，以自动化操作系统执行试验过程，以灵敏快速的检测仪器采集实验结果数据，以计算机分析处理实验数据，在同一时间检测数以千万的样品，并以得到的相应数据库支持运转的技术体系，它具有微量、快速、灵敏和准确等特点。简言之就是可以通过一次实验获得大量的信息，并从中找到有价值的信息。

Exercises

1. Decide whether each of the following statements is true (T) or false (F) according to the passage.

(1) 90% to 95 % of plants on this planet have not been investigated so far.

(2) To incorporate natural products in the modern HTS programmes, a natural product library is not useful.

(3) Natural products have been a source of drugs and drug leads.

(4) The traditional way of discovering drug from natural product is bioassay-guided.

(5) Academia and some semi-academic research organizations usually apply modern approaches to natural product drug discovery.

(6) Cephalosporin C is an antiviral compound.

2. Questions for oral discussion.

(1) What were some of the practical factors responsible for the declining popularity of natural products as a source of new drugs in the 1990s?

(2) Is the recent revival of interests in natural products as a potential source for new medicines timely? Give reasons for your answer.

笔记

(3) Compare the recent-past to the present. What do you think has changed in building a natural product library?

(4) Name two areas where natural products have contributed significantly. Give statistical evidence from this article to support your answer.

3. Choose the best answer to each of the following questions.

(1) What is the meaning of "drug candidate"?

   A. purified isolate   B. total extract

   C. a new drug on market   D. a compound with some bioactivity

(2) In the following solvents, whose polarity is the weakest?

   A. alcohol   B. ethyl acetate

   C. chloroform   D. acetone

(3) In order to extract most lipophilic ingredients from plants, which of the following solvents will you select?

   A. alcohol   B. butanol

   C. ethyl acctate   D. benzene

(4) In normal phase partition chromatography, the stationary phase commonly used is _____.

   A. chloroform   B. water

   C. n-butanol   D. ethyl acetate

(5) In glycosidic linkage hydrolysis, which of the following is the easiest in different glycosidic atoms?

   A. alcohol glycoside   B. N

   C. phenol glycosides   D. S

(6) Generally, free alkaloids can easily dissolve in _____.

   A. methanol   B. alcohol

   C. diethyl ether   D. chloroform

(7) What is the meaning of HTS?

   A. High Temperature Superconducting   B. Heat Transfer Salts

   C. High Throughput Screening   D. Heat-Treated Steel

(8) What category does simvastatin belong to?

   A. lipid regulating agents   B. antineoplastic agents

   C. antibiotics of aminoglycosides   D. analgesics

(9) What category does paclitaxel belong to?

   A. lipid regulating agents   B. antineoplastic agents

   C. antibiotics of aminoglycosides   D. analgesics

(10) What category does azithromycin belong to?

   A. lipid regulating agents   B. antineoplastic agents

   C. antibiotics of macrolides   D. analgesics

4. Match the words with the prefixes or suffixes according to the meaning(s).

1) angio-	A. pain
2) dermato-	B. heart
3) -algia	C. skin
4) -phobia	D. blood
5) cardio-	E. vessel

笔记

续表

6) hemato-	F. inflammation
7) tachy-	G. fast
8) -itis	H. slow
9) brady-	I. fear
10) -cyte	J. cell

5. Translate the following sentences and paragraphs into Chinese.

(1) Plant natural products have had, and continue to have, an important role as medicinal and pharmaceutical agents, not only as purified isolates and extractives, but also as lead compounds for synthetic optimization

(2) Plant secondary metabolites also show promise for cancer chemoprevention, which has been defined as "the use of non-cytotoxic nutrients or pharmacological agents to enhance intrinsic physiological mechanisms that protect the organism against mutant clones of malignant cells."

(3) Nevertheless, the vast majority of the world's quarter of a million plant species have not been evaluated in pharmaceutical screens, and the small percentage that has been tested has generally been screened for activity against only a few therapeutic targets

(4) Although many sampling programs designed to generate large numbers of samples for high-throughput screening programs have been characterized as random, it has been shown that they are not truly random nor haphazard, but that sampling occurs without preconceived selection of species

(5) Three main research approaches are used in my drug discovery and development process: ① bioactivity- or mechanism of action-directed isolation and characterization of active compounds, ② rational drug design-based modification and analog synthesis, and ③ mechanism of action studies

(6) Flavonoids are mainly water-soluble compounds. They can be extracted with 70% ethanol and remain in the aqueous layer, following partition of this extract with petroleum ether. Flavonoids are phenolic and hence change in colour when treated with base or with ammonia; thus they are easily detected on chromatograms or in solution. Flavonoids contain conjugated aromatic systems and thus show intense absorption bands in the UV and visible regions of the spectrum. Finally flavonoids are generally present in plants bound to sugar as glycosides and any one flavonoid aglycone may occur in a single plant in several glycosidic combinations. For this reason, when analysing flavonoids, it is usually better to examine the aglycones present in hydrolysed plant extracts before considering the complexity of glycosides that may be present in the original extract.

(7) While in the recent past it was extremely difficult, time consuming and labour intensive to build such a library from purified natural products, with the advent of newer and improved technologies related to separation, isolation and identification of natural products the situation has improved remarkably. However, the best result can be obtained from a fully identified pure natural product library as it provides scientists with the opportunity to handle the "lead" rapidly for further developmental work, e.g. total or partial synthesis, dealing with formulation factors, *in vivo* assays and clinical trials.

笔记

Text B
How to Approach the Isolation of a Natural Product?

Introduction

It may seem a dreadful task, faced with a liter of fermentation broth a dark, viscous sludge - knowing that in there is one group of molecules that has to be separated from all the rest. Those molecules possibly represent only about 0.0001% or 1 ppm of the total biomass and are dispersed throughout the organism, possibly intimately bound up with other molecules. Like the proverbial needle in a haystack, you have to remove lot of hay to be left with just the needle, without knowing what the needle looks like or where in the haystack it is.

1. What Are Natural Products?

The term "natural product" is perhaps quite misleading term. Strictly speaking, any biological molecule is a natural product, but the term is usually reserved for secondary metabolites, small molecules (mol wt < 1500 amu approx) produced by an organism but that are not strictly necessary for the survival of the organism, unlike the more prevalent macromolecules such as proteins, nucleic acids, and polysaccharides that make up the basic machinery for the more fundamental processes of life.

Secondary metabolites are a very broad group of metabolites, with no distinct boundaries, and grouped under no single unifying definition. Concepts of secondary metabolism include products of overflow metabolism as a result of nutrient limitation, or shunt metabolites produced during idiophase, defense mechanisms, regulator molecules, and so on. Perhaps the most cogent theory of secondary metabolism has been put forward by Zahner, who described secondary metabolism as evolutionary "elbow room". If a secondary metabolite has no adverse effect on the producing organism at any levels of differentiation, morphogenesis, transport, regulation, or intermediary metabolism, it may be conserved for a relatively long period during which time it may come to confer a selective advantage. Secondary metabolism therefore provides a kind of testing ground where new metabolites have the opportunity, as it were, to exist without being eliminated, during which time they may find a role that will give an advantage to the producing organism. This is supported by the fact that secondary metabolites are often unique to a particular species or group of organisms and, while many act as antifeedants, sex attractants, or antibiotic agents, many have no apparent biological role. It is likely that all these concepts can play some part in understanding the production of the broad group of compounds that come under the heading of secondary metabolite.

Isolation of natural products differs from that of the more commonly occurring biological macromolecules because natural products are smaller and chemically more diverse than the relatively consistent proteins, nucleic acids and carbohydrates, and isolation methods must take this into account.[1]

2. The Aim of the Extraction

The two most fundamental questions that should be asked at the onset of an extraction are:

(1) *What am I trying to isolate?*

There are a number of possible targets of isolation:

a. An unknown compound responsible for a particular biological activity.

b. A certain compound known to be produced by a particular organism.

c. A group of compounds within an organism that are all related in some way, such as by a common structural feature.

d. All of the metabolites produced by one natural product source that are not produced by a different "control" source, e.g., two species of the same genus, or the same organism grown under different conditions.

e. A chemical "dissection" of an organism, in order to characterize all of its interesting metabolites, usually those secondary metabolites, confined to that organism, or group of organisms, and not universal in all living systems, such an inventory might be useful for chemical, ecological, or chemotaxonomic reasons, among others.

(2) *Why am I trying to isolate it?*

The second fundamental question concerns what one is trying ultimately to achieve, for defining the aims can minimize the work required. Reasons for the extraction might be:

a. To purify sufficient amount of a compound to characterize it partially or fully.

b. More specifically, to provide sufficient material to allow for confirmation or denial of a proposed structure. As in many cases this does not require mapping out a complete structure from scratch but perhaps simply comparison with a standard of known structure; it may require less material or only partially pure material. There is no point in removing minor impurities if they do not get in the way of ascertaining whether the compound is, or is not, compound X.

c. The generation/production of the maximum amount of a known compound so that it can be used for further work, such as more extensive biological testing. (Alternatively, it may be more efficient to chemically synthesize the compound; any natural product that is of serious interest, i.e., is required in large amounts, will be considered as a target for synthetic chemistry.)

3. Purity

With a clear idea of what one is trying to achieve, one can then question the required level of purity. This in turn might give some indication of the approach to be taken and the purification methods to be employed.

For example, if you are attempting to characterize fully a complex natural product that is present at a low concentration in an extract, you will probably want to produce a compound that is suitable for NMR. The purity needed is dependent on the nature of the compound and of the impurities, but to assign fully a complex structure, material of 95%-100% purity is generally required. If the compound is present at high concentration in the starting material and there already exists a standard against which to compare it, structure confirmation can be carried out with less pure material and the purification will probably require fewer steps.

The importance of purity in natural products isolation has been highlighted by Ghisalberti, who described two papers that appeared at about the same time, both reporting the isolation from plants of ent-kauran-3-oxo-16, 17-diol. In one paper, the compound has a melting point of 173-174℃ and $[\alpha]_D$ -39.2° (CHCl$_3$); in the other, no melting point is reported, but the compound has an $[\alpha]_D$ -73.1° (CHCl$_3$). Either the compounds are different or one is significantly less pure than the other.

If a natural product is required for biological testing, it is crucial to know at least the degree of purity and, preferably, the nature of the impurities. It is always possible that the impurities are giving rise to all or part of the biological activities in question. If a compound is to be used to generate pharmacological or pharmacokinetic data, it is usually important that the material be very pure (generally >99% pure), particularly if the impurities are analogs of the main compound and may themselves be biologically active.

In some cases, a sample need only be partially purified prior to obtaining sufficient structural information. For example, it may be possible to detect the absence of a certain structural feature in crude mixture–perhaps by absence of a particular ultraviolet (UV) maximum–and conclude that the mixture does not contain compound A. In other cases, such as X-ray crystallography studies, material will almost be certainly required in an extremely pure state, generally >99.9% pure.

It is worth bearing in mind that the relationship between the degrees of purity achieved in a natural product extraction, and the amount of work required to achieve this, is very approximately exponential. It is often relatively easy to start with a crude, complex mixture and eliminate more than half of what is not wanted, but it can be a painstaking chore to remove the minor impurities that will turn a 99.5% pure sample into one that is 99.9% pure. It is also probably true to say that this exponential relationship also often holds for the degree of purity achieved versus the yield of natural product. In the same way that no chemical reaction results in 100% yield, no extraction step results in 100% recovery of the natural product. Compound will be lost at every stage; in many cases it may be that, to achieve very high levels of purity, it is necessary to sacrifice much of the desired material. In order to remove all the impurities it may be necessary to take only the cleanest "cuts" from a separation, thus losing much of the target material in the process (though these side fractions can often be reprocessed).

These factors may, of course, have some bearing on the level of purity deemed satisfactory, and it is useful to ask at each stage of the extraction, whether the natural product is sufficiently pure without any controversy.

At present, there are two main reasons why scientists extract natural products: to find out what they are and/or to carry out further experimental work using the purified compound. In the future, it may be easy to determine structures of compounds in complex mixtures; indeed, it is already possible to do this under some circumstances. Presently, most cases of structural determination of an unknown compound require that it be essentially pure. Likewise, to obtain valid biological or chemical data on a natural product usually requires that it be free from the other experimental variables present in the surrounding biological matrix.

Word Study

1. antifeedant [ˌænti'fiːdənt] *n.* 拒食素
2. broth [brɔːθ] *n.* 发酵液
3. chemotaxonomy ['keməutæk'sɔːnəmi] *n.* 化学分类学
4. chore [tʃɔː] *n.* 家庭杂务，讨厌的或累人的工作
5. cogent ['kəudʒənt] *adj.* 强有力的，使人信服的
6. ent-kauran [ent 'kaurən] *n.* 对映贝壳杉烷
7. haystack ['heistæk] *n.* 草堆
8. idiophase ['idiəfeiz] *n.* 繁殖期，生殖期，分化期
9. morphogenesis [ˌmɔːfə'dʒenisis] *n.* [胚] 形态发生，形态形成
10. shunt [ʃʌnt] *n.*, *v.* 分流，转轨
11. sludge [slʌdʒ] *n.* 泥泞，淤泥，沉淀物

笔记

Notes

1. Isolation of natural products differs from that of the more commonly occurring biological macromolecules because natural products are smaller and chemically more diverse than the relatively consistent proteins, nucleic acids and carbohydrates, and isolation methods must take this into account. 译为：天然产物的分离不同于通常出现的生物大分子，因为天然产物与常见的组成成分蛋白质、核酸和碳水化合物相比，分子量小且更具化学多样性，所以分离方法也要将这些因素考虑在内。

Supplementary Parts

1.　Medical and Pharmaceutical Terms Made Easier (8): Common Prefixes in Medical English Terms

Prefixes	Meaning	Example
a-,an-	无，没有	amorphous 无定形的
ab-	从，离开	abarticular 非关节的，关节外的
ad-	向，靠近，到……上	adrenal 肾上腺的
allo-	异	allosome 异染色体
ana-	向上，重回到	anabolism 合成代谢
ante-	在前	anteflexion [医学] 前屈（尤指子宫前屈）
anti-	反抗	antidote 解毒剂
auto-	自己	autotrophic 自造营养物质的，自给营养的
bi(n,s)-	两，加倍，二	biceps [解剖] 二头肌，强健的筋肉
brady-	慢	bradycardia [医学] 心动过缓
circum-	环行，围绕	circumduction 环行运动
co(n)-	与……在一起	cocarcinogenesis 助致癌作用
contra-	反，对抗	contraceptive 节育，避孕的
de-	从	deoxidation 脱氧
di-	二倍，加倍	diarthric 两关节的
dia-	通过	diathermy 透热疗法
dis	离开，分开	dislocation 脱位，脱臼
dys-	坏，痛的，困难	dysentery 痢疾
ecto-	外面，在外	ectoderm 外胚层
en-	内，在内	encephalic 脑的
endo-	内部	endocrine 内分泌
epi-	外面，上面，在上	epigastrium 上腹部
eu-	好，正常	euphoria 欣快，精神愉快
ex-	在之外，离开	excision 切除
extra-	在外面，超过	extracorporeal 体外的
hemi-	半	hemiparalysis 偏瘫
hetero-	异	heterogenous 异源的，异种的
homo-	同，等	homosexual 同性恋的
hyper-	超过，过多	hyperglycemia 高血糖
hypo-	低，少于正常	hypoglycemia 低血糖
in-	在内，进入	ingestion 摄入
in-	否定，不	incoagulability 不凝性

笔记

续表

Prefixes	Meaning	Example
infra-	在下，低于	infracostal 肋下的
inter-	在……之间	interventricular[解剖]（心脏）室间的
intra-	在内	intravenous 静脉内的
iso-	同	isotope 同位素，放射性核素
macro-,megalo-	巨大	macroglossia 巨舌
micro-	微小	microscope 显微镜
multi-	多	multipara 经产妇
oligo-	少	oliguria 少尿
para-	旁，附着，异常	paranephric 肾旁的，肾上腺的
per-	通过	peroral 经过口的，口周围的
peri-	周围	perihepatitis 肝周炎
pluri-	多	plurimenorrhea[医学] 多次行经
poly-	多	polyuria 多尿症
post-	在后，在……后方	postnasal 鼻后的
pre-	在前，在……前方	premolar 前磨牙
pro-	在前，在……后方	prognosis 预后
pros-	到，靠近，动上	prosthetics 修复学，装补学
pseudo-	假	pseudomembrane 假膜
semi-	半	semisynthetic 半合成的
sub-	在下	subcutaneous 皮下的
super-	高于，超过	superlactation 泌乳过多
supra-	高于，超过	supracranial 颅上的
syn-	与，在一起，合成	synapse *n.* 突触
tachy-	快	tachycardia 心动过速
trans-	穿过，越	transabdominal 通过腹部的

2. English-Chinese Translation Skills: 药学英语翻译技巧 (4)：解包袱法

解包袱（unpacking）法一词最初由美国翻译理论家、语言学家尤金·奈达（Eugene Nida）提出。他建议译者在使用各种翻译技巧前，必须先将纠缠在一起的语义逻辑关系像解包袱一样解开，然后理顺。解包袱法是针对修饰语和被修饰语之间的语义关系不明而提出的一种策略性翻译方法，旨在挣脱形式上的修饰关系，根据语境去理解语义，它是理解乃至翻译的一个法宝。英汉两种语言词组性质基本相似，如名词性词组、动词性词组、形容词词性词组等，但词组构成结构却不尽相同。如汉语中"食品商店"是卖食品的商店，"鞋帽商店"是卖鞋帽的商店，但是"儿童商店"是卖什么的商店呢？这些词组就像一个包袱，理解和翻译这些词组中词与词的关系就要一层层解开这个包袱。

在药学英语翻译中，正确"解包袱"还要了解药学英语语言特点以及药学基础知识。如：prepared sliced of Chinese crude drugs，根据正确的解包袱法，应该译成"中药饮片"，而不是"中药备好的切片"。

例 1：**The declining popularity of natural products** as a source of new drugs began in the 1990s, because of some practical factors, e.g. the apparent lack of compatibility of natural products with the modern high **throughput** screening (HTS) programs, where significant degrees of automation, robotics and computers are used, the complexity in the isolation and identification of natural products and the cost and time involved in the natural product "**lead**" discovery process.

笔记

　　参考译文：从20世纪90年代开始，因为一些实际原因，天然产物作为药物主要来源这一趋势明显开始下降，天然产物与现代高通量筛选（HTS）方法存在明显不兼容性，高通量筛选自动化程度高，大量使用机器人及计算机技术；在从天然产物发现"先导化合物"的过程中存在复杂的分离与鉴定以及经费和时间投入等方面的问题。

　　说明：翻译这段文章采用了"解包袱"法。原文中 the declining popularity of natural products 中的 popularity 就需要认真理解，这里的 popularity 不应该理解和翻译成"普及、流行"或者"通俗性、大众性"等，根据语境这里应该翻译成"趋势"。再如原文中 high throughput screening，从词组结构上看，throughput 修饰 screening，其基本意思是"吞吐量、吞吐率、生产量、生产能力"，但是对于专业技术名词词组翻译，解包袱时需要学科背景，随意解释和翻译会出现错译。high-throughput screening (HTS) 是近年来发展起来的药物筛选技术，具有微量、快速、灵敏和准确等特点，能在短时间内测试大量化合物的生物活性。根据专业性知识，high throughput screening 这个"包袱"可以成功解开，译成"高流通筛选"。另外，原文中 in the natural product "lead" discovery process，在理解和翻译时需要对 "lead" 进行仔细分析。这里的 lead 不是动词"领导、引导"等意思，而是形容词"领头的"，可以理解为"前期的"，药物化学中翻译成"先导的"，与文章涉及的"先导化合物"相呼应，具有隐喻意义。

　　例2：A primary reason for the lack of application of biotheorapeutics to neuroscience **targets**, is that the blood-brain barrier (BBB) isolates and protects central nervous system (CNS) structures creating a unique **biochemically and immunologically** privileged environment.

　　参考译文：生物治疗药物较少应用在神经科学领域的首要原因是由于血脑屏障创造了一个独特的具有生化活性和免疫活性的特殊环境，隔离并保护了中枢神经系统。

　　说明：在上面例句中，理解和翻译 neuroscience targets 时，要对 target 进行分析。在医药英语中，target 意思是"靶"，如 targeted delivery drugs system（靶向给药系统），target cell of immunologic reaction（免疫学反应靶细胞）等，neuroscience targets 中 target 采用了单词的基本意思，译成"靶向"。另外，a unique biochemically and immunologically privileged environment 中的两个副词 biochemically 和 immunologically，在理解和翻译时也需要解包袱，不能照字面翻译成"在生化和免疫方面"，而应该根据语言环境，进行词性转译，译成"具有生化活性和免疫活性的"，符合语义和汉语表达习惯。

笔记

Unit Nine　Biopharmaceuticals

The term biopharmaceuticals is most commonly used to refer to all therapeutic, prophylactic, and *in vivo* diagnostic agents produced using live organisms or their functional components. At least in the U.S., biopharmaceuticals are often considered to include products manufactured using both "new" technologies (recombinant DNA and monoclonal antibody/hybridoma) and "old" technologies (fermentation, non-recombinant cell culture-derived proteins, vaccines, and other products from live organisms including blood/plasma products). Thus, a biopharmaceutical results from bio-processing and can, therefore, be defined as the intersection of pharmaceutical technology and biotechnology. It is thus synonymous with biotechnology pharmaceuticals and pharmaceutical biotechnology products. Some 160 biopharmaceuticals have now gained medical approval and several hundreds are in the pipeline. Most biopharmaceuticals are protein-based, although two nucleic acid-based products are now on the US/European market. Development of biopharmaceutical products is a broad and multidisciplinary field. Science and technology are combined with new manufacturing, regulatory and commercial challenges. Effective formulation development and appropriate delivery strategies for biopharmaceuticals are critical and timely issues. From DNA-based products to antibodies, vaccines to therapeutics, administered by every route known to medicine, formulation and delivery system play a critical role in the ultimate success of biopharmaceutical products.

生物药物这一术语通常是指所有使用活体生物或它们的功能组分而生产的治疗、预防和体内诊断制剂。至少在美国，生物药物往往被认为是利用"新"技术（重组 DNA 和单克隆抗体 / 杂交瘤细胞）和"旧"技术（发酵，非重组细胞来源的蛋白、疫苗以及其他来自活生物体的产品例如血液 / 血浆制品）生产的药物。因此，由生物工艺得到的生物药物可以被看作是药学技术和生物技术交叉作用的结果。所以，它与生物技术药物和药物生物技术产品是同义词。目前大约有 160 种生物药物获批，还有数百个在研品种。虽然有两个核酸类生物药物在美国 / 欧洲上市，但大部分生物药物以蛋白质为基础。生物药物的开发涉及多个多学科领域。新的科学技术与生产、管理和营销环节中的挑战并存。对于生物药物而言，有效的剂型开发和合适的药物递送策略是急需解决的关键问题。从核酸类药物到抗体，从疫苗到治疗性药物，生物药物可以通过各种已知的途径给药，而剂型和递药系统对生物药物的最终成功应用起着决定性的作用。

笔记

Text A
Nonclinical Development of Biopharmaceuticals

Modern biologics are biotechnology-derived pharmaceuticals (also designated as "biopharmaceuticals", "biotech drugs" or "biotherapeutics") comprising different compound classes. Chemically, biologics are mainly represented by glycoproteins comprising L-amino acids and specific sugar molecules. They are mostly used for the diagnosis, prevention and treatment of serious and chronic diseases.

Therapeutic Biologics–Compound Classes

（i）Monoclonal antibodies (mAbs); （ii）recombinant protein therapeutics (rDNA products), such as replacement molecules for endogenous compounds (e.g. coagulation factors and insulin), and therapeutic cytokines (e.g. interferons and interleukins); （iii）hybrid and modified molecules [such as protein–synthetic constructs (pegylated, glycoengineered proteins)], fusion proteins (such as antibody fusion constructs), antibody fragments and biological conjugates (such as conjugated antibodies); （iv）nucleic acid molecules (such as antisense oligodeoxynucleotides; （v）vaccines directed against noninfectious disease targets); （vi）gene therapy products and therapeutically used viruses; and （vii）cell therapy products.

mAbs and rDNA-derived products make up the majority of marketed and close-to-market biologics. mAbs are becoming more prominent and now represent the majority of biologics with more than 150 compounds (30%-50% of all biologics in development) in company-sponsored clinical studies. Antibody fragments and fusion proteins have great potential as innovative therapeutic agents with their targeted therapy approach versus functional approaches.

Both biologics and small molecules have to be proven to be pure, safe and potent within their development. Nonclinical development comprises nonclinical drug safety (toxicology and safety pharmacology); nonclinical pharmacokinetics, or PK and bioanalytics for preclinical and clinical sample analysis, including immunogenicity evaluation. All these activities are prerequisites for moving into clinical development and must assess potential safety risks. As is the case for small molecules, some toxicology studies do not necessarily have to be performed before first use in humans but can be performed at later stages. The nonclinical testing strategy for biologics has to be adapted and refined from experience with small molecules. Differences in the physicochemical properties and resulting differences in PK, toxicity, immunogenicity[1] and bioactivities of biologics compared with small molecules are substantial. Risks other than those known from our extensive experience with small-molecule pharmaceuticals determine the development program of biologics. Binding specificity and affinity often limit species cross-reactivity and selection of adequate animal species. Immunogenicity as an inherent property of large molecules, like biologics, complicates the nonclinical testing strategy and needs an adapted experimental, as well as bioanalytical, testing strategy.

Bioanalytics of Biologics in Nonclinical and Clinical Development

Small molecules generally need a PK assay for quantification of the unchanged compound and its (major) metabolite(s). High-performance liquid chromatography (HPLC) and mass spectrometry (MS) have been highly developed as standard technologies in that field. By contrast, biologics require

笔记

several types of assay for quantification of the protein itself, its biological activity and the detection and characterization of binding antidrug antibodies (ADAs), neutralizing ADAs and, if necessary (especially for clinical sample analysis), assays to monitor antibodies that might have been generated in response to host cell proteins and/or other (high molecular) impurities or compound constituents (e.g. PEG moieties). This requires not only different technologies and a wider variety of assay types but also more capacity, time and logistical effort.

Assay Types Used in Nonclinical Development of Biologics

When developing a PK assay strategy, the needs of the nonclinical and clinical development program have to be considered, such as sensitivity of the assay based on nonclinical and estimated clinical dose, planed combination treatments, estimated target levels, pharmacokinetics/pharmacodynamics (PK/PD) modeling approaches and so on. Looking beyond assay technologies, sample-clean procedures routinely used for small molecules (e.g. solvent extraction and affinity chromatography) can usually not be used for biologics. Biologics are mostly analyzed without extraction or only with a crude protein precipitation step. Therefore, extensive tests of the matrix effect[2] are required during method development. Ligand-binding assays (immunoassays) are still widely used for quantification of biologics. Innovations in MS instrumentation with much higher mass accuracy have already been applied to smaller MW biologics but still remain unavailable for routine quantification of large proteins (>20kDa) in biomatrices.

Immunoassays require the use of a specific antigen or antibody to capture and/or detect the analyte of interest. Essential reagents such as poly- or monoclonal antibodies might be difficult to obtain in early stages of development. Furthermore, assay development often encounters challenges stemming from interfering residuals in the sample matrix. Dynamic range and linearity, limited in comparison to MS methods, are additional issues that often need to be addressed. Immunoassays are also generally less precise than methods such as MS. Heterogeneity of biologics (e.g. mixtures of differently glycosylated species and various degradation products) can raise specificity problems.

In addition to the PK assay (or mass assay), the activity assay (bioassay) is particularly useful for measuring the neutralizing activity of an ADA, although it was originally developed to measure product efficacy (e.g. for product release). Activity assays might be performed *in vitro* (often human-cell-line based techniques) or *in vivo* (animal models). These assays might suffer from lack of specificity owing to the potentially confounding influence of substances that modulate the biological activity of the compound of interest.[3] They are, however, the only way to determine whether a protein is still intact and active, which cannot be measured by a "usual" PK assay.

How to Estimate Safety Risks of Biologics in Nonclinical Development?

The objectives of the nonclinical safety program for biologics are similar to those for small-molecule drugs (SMDs): to recognize potential toxicities (hazard identification and characterization, and risk assessment), to identify appropriate parameters for clinical monitoring (e.g. biomarkers) and to contribute to first-in-human dose (FIH) selection. This also includes assessing the limitations of nonclinical studies in predicting safety issues for the human situation. Nevertheless, the nonclinical program has to be designed for clinical decision-making. The program for biologics, however, is often

笔记

different from SMD programs because of the nature of the therapeutic protein, its species specificity and its immunogenicity.

Safety risks are generally directly related to uncertainty and are reduced through knowledge and best scientific practices. However, because of the heterogeneity of this compound class and the different approaches needed for different types of biologics, our future nonclinical development programs (NDPs) must be considered largely on a case-by-case basis.

Study Design and Types of Nonclinical Safety Studies

Besides the challenges of species selection for the general toxicity testing of biologics (single- and repeated-dose toxicity studies), there might be even more challenges for specialty studies such as reproductive toxicity, carcinogenicity and immunotoxicity.[4] This is because adequate exposure needed for specific treatment regimens can be hindered by the formation of ADAs with drug neutralization or accelerated clearance. Therefore, toxicology programs with multiple-dose administration of biologics often have less long-term treatments than SMDs. However, this does not mean that a biologic can be developed more rapidly and at lower cost in the nonclinical stage. Special study designs, the use of more sophisticated and costly animal models, longer observations periods owing to ADA response and, especially, the manufacturing complexity for proteins often result in slightly longer and more costly programs, as observed with small molecules.

Word Study

1. affinity [əˈfiniti] *n.* 亲和力，密切关系
2. antibody [ˈæntibɔdi] *n.* 抗体
3. antidrug [ˈænti:drʌg] *adj.* 反对服用麻醉品的
4. antigen [ˈæntidʒən] *n.* 抗原
5. antisense [ˈæntisens] *adj.* 反义的
6. biomarker [ˈbaiɔmɑ:kə] *n.* 生物标记
7. biomatrices [baiɔˈmeitrisi:z]   *n.* 生物基质（单数：biomatrix [baiɔˈmeitriks]）
8. coagulation [kəuˈægjuˈleiʃən] *n.* 凝固，凝结，血凝固，凝结物
9. confound [kənˈfaund] *vt.* 混淆，使（思想等）混乱；使惶惑，使糊涂；挫败（敌人），打破（计划等）；把……毁灭掉
10. cross-reactivity [kˈrɔs ri:ækˈtiviti] *n.* 交叉反应性能
11. cytokine [ˌsaitəˈkain] *n.* 细胞因子
12. dose [dəus] *n.* 剂量，服用量；（一）服，（一）剂；*vt.* 给 ... 服药；
13. endogenous [enˈdɔdʒənəs] *adj.* 内生的，内源的，内生性，内源性
14. fusion [ˈfju:ʒn] *n.* 熔化，结合，融合，融合作用，融合物，
15. heterogeneity [ˌhetərədʒiˈni:iti] *n.* 不均一性，多相性，异质性，不纯一性，不均匀性
16. high-performance liquid chromatography[hai pəˈfɔ:məns likwid ˌkrəuməˈtɔgrəfi] *n.* 高效液相色谱法（HPLC）
17. hybrid [ˈhaibrid] *n.* 混血儿，杂种，混合物，混合词；*adj.* 混合的，杂种的，混合语的
18. immunogenicity [imjunəudʒeˈnisiti] *n.* 免疫原性
19. immunotoxicity [imjunəutɔkˈsisiti] *n.* 免疫毒性
20. inherent [inˈhiərənt] *adj.* 固有的，本来的，生来的
21. interleukin [inˈtəˈlukin] *n.* 白细胞介素

22. intracellular [ˌɪntrəˈseljələ] *adj.* 细胞内的，胞内的

23. ligand [ˈlɪgənd] *n.* 配体，配位子，配位体，配基

24. logistical [lɔˈdʒɪstɪkəl] *adj.* 后勤的

25. mass spectrometry [ˌmæs spekˈtrɔmitri] *n.* 质谱法（MS）

26. mediated [ˈmiːdieitid] *adj.* 介导的

27. molecule [ˈmɔːlikjuːl] *n.* 分子；微点，微小颗粒

28. monoclonal antibody [ˌmɔnəuˈkləunəl ˈæntibɔdi] *n.* 单克隆抗体

29. multiple-dose [ˈmʌltipl dəus] *adj.* 多剂量的，多次给药的

30. neutralization [ˌnjuːtrəlaiˈzeiʃ ən] *n.* 中和（作用），平衡，抵消，使失效

31. neutralize [ˈnuːtrəlaiz] *vt.* 中和，使……中和，使……无效，使……中立

32. nucleic [ˈnjuːkliik] *adj.* 核的

33. oligodeoxynucleotide [ɔligəudiːɔksi nˈjuːkliːəutaid] *n.* 寡聚脱氧核苷酸

34. pegylated [ˈpiːdʒileitid] *adj.* 聚乙二醇化

35. pharmaceutical [ˌfɑːməˈsjuːtikəl] *n.* 药物制剂

36. pharmacokinetics [ˌfɑːməkəukaiˈnetiks] *n.* 药物（代谢）动力学

37. physicochemical property [fizikəuˈkemikəl ˈprɔpəti] *n.* 理化性质

38. predictivity [pridikˈtiviti] *n.* 预测能力，预期性

39. prerequisite [ˌpriːˈrekwəzit] *n.* 先决条件，必要条件，前提；*adj.* 必须预先具备的，先决条件的

40. recombinant [riːˈkɔmbənənt] *n.* 重组体，重组细胞，重组器官

41. residual [riˈzidʒuəl] *n.* 残留，残质，后遗症

42. sponsor [ˈspɑːnsə] *n.* 保证人，发起人，赞助者，教父；*v.* 发起，赞助

43. therapeutic [ˌθerəˈpjuːtik] *adj.* 治疗的，治疗学的

44. toxicology [ˌtɔksiˈkɔlədʒi] *n.* 毒理学，毒物学

Notes

1. immunogenicity 意思是免疫原性，指能够刺激机体形成特异抗体或致敏淋巴细胞的能力。

2. matrix effect 意思是"基质效应"。化学分析中，基质指的是样品中被分析物以外的组分。基质常常对分析物的分析过程有显著的干扰，并影响分析结果的准确性。例如，溶液的离子强度会对分析物活度系数有影响，这些影响和干扰被称为基质效应。

3. These assays might suffer from lack of specificity owing to the potentially confounding influence of substances that modulate the biological activity of the compound of interest. 译为：由于存在目标化合物生物活性的调节物质的潜在混杂性影响，这些检测方法可能受到缺乏特异性的困扰。

4. Besides the challenges of species selection for the general toxicity testing of biologics (single- and repeated-dose toxicity studies), there might be even more challenges for specialty studies such as reproductive toxicity, carcinogenicity and immunotoxicity. 译为：除了存在生物制品一般毒性检测的物种选择的挑战外（单剂量和多剂量毒性试验），还存在诸如生殖毒性、致癌性和免疫毒性等特殊研究的更多挑战。

Exercises

1. Decide whether each of the following statements is true (T) or false (F) according to the passage.

(1) As in the case for small molecules, some toxicological studies have to be performed before first

笔记

use in humans.

(2) Small molecules generally do not necessarily need a PK assay for quantification of the unchanged compound and its (major) metabolite(s).

(3) Sample-clean procedures routinely used for small molecules cannot usually be used for biologics.

(4) Essential reagents such as poly- or monoclonal antibodies might not be difficult to obtain in the early stages of development.

(5) The activity assay is particularly useful for measuring the neutralizing activity of an ADA, although it was originally developed to measure product efficacy.

(6) Tissue cross-reactivity (TCR) studies in a panel of human tissues determining the level of cross-recognition are necessary for targeted biologics such as mAbs.

2.   Questions for oral discussion.

(1) What do you know about biopharmaceuticals? Try to talk about the focus of their current research.

(2) What is the prospect of mAbs products according to this text?

(3) What types of assay are often used in nonclinical development of biologics?

(4) Please discuss the differences between small-molecule drugs and biologics.

3.   Choose the best answer to each of the following questions.

(1) _____ is often referred to all therapeutic, prophylactic, and *in vivo* diagnostic agents produced using live organisms or their functional components.

    A. Biopharmaceutics   B. Biopharmaceutical

    C. Pharmaceutical   D. Pharmaceutics

(2) Chemically, biologics are mainly represented by _____ comprising L-amino acids and various sugar molecules.

    A. glycoproteins   B. monoclonal antibodies

    C. cytokines   D. nucleic acid molecules

(3) As is the case for small molecules, some _____ studies do not necessarily have to be performed before first use in humans but can be performed at later stages.

    A. drug safety   B. pharmacokinetics

    C. clinical sample analysis   D. toxicology

(4) Small molecules generally need a PK assay for _____ of the unchanged compound and its (major) metabolite(s).

    A. quantification   B. qualitation

    C. evaluation   D. characterization

(5) Looking beyond assay technologies, sample-clean procedures routinely used for _____ (e.g. solvent extraction and affinity chromatography) usually cannot be used for biologics.

    A. biologics   B. proteins

    C. small molecules   D. large molecules

(6) The widely used assay for quantification of biologics is _____.

    A. immunoassay   B. crude protein precipitation

    C. PK assay   D. HPLC

(7) _____ is generally directly related to uncertainty and is reduced through knowledge and best scientific practices.

    A. Efficacy   B. Safety

    C. Immunogenicity   D. Specificity

笔记

(8) Because of the _____ of the compound class, our future nonclinical development programs must be considered largely on a case-by-case basis.

A. specificity   B. heterogeneity

C. toxicity   D. safety

(9) Adequate exposure needed for specific treatment regimens can be hindered by the formation of _____ with drug neutralization or accelerated clearance.

A. antibodies   B. antigens

C. antidrug antibodies   D. cytokines

(10) Toxicology programs with _____ administration of biologics often have less long-term treatments than SMDs.

A. single-dose   B. large-dose

C. proper   D. multiple-dose

4. Please give the English equivalents to each of the following.

(1) 毒理学（   ）

(2) 药理学（   ）

(3) 核酸（   ）

(4) 免疫原性（   ）

(5) 基质效应（   ）

(6) 色谱（   ）

(7) 单剂量（   ）

(8) 致癌性（   ）

(9) 清除（   ）

(10) 给药途径（   ）

5. Translate the following sentences and paragraphs into Chinese.

(1) The development of a new therapeutic agent involves a multidisciplinary group in many years of work，and with the development of genetic engineering and the production of monoclonal antibodies it is likely that even more agents will be produced.

(2) Their activity depends on their complicated shape based on secondary, tertiary and quaternary structures. These structures cannot be fully defined with our present set of analytical techniques and approaches for potency testing.

(3) Apart from the intravenous route of drug administration, where a drug is introduced directly into the blood circulation, all other routes of administering systemically acting drugs involve the absorption of drug from the place of administration into the blood.

(4) Biopharmaceuticals are pharmaceutical products consisting of (glyco)proteins, and they have a number of characteristics that set them aside from low molecular weight drugs.

(5) In safety testing and clinical test programs of biopharmaceuticals questions have to be addressed regarding species specific responses, selection of dosing schedules and route of administration, and the possible occurrence of immunogenicity.

(6) Biologics are mostly analyzed without extraction or only with a crude protein precipitation step. Therefore, extensive tests of the matrix effect are required during method development. Ligand-binding assays (immunoassays) are still widely used for quantification of biologics. Innovations in MS instrumentation with much higher mass accuracy have already been applied to smaller MW biologics but still remain unavailable for routine quantification of large proteins (>20kDa) in

笔记

biomatrices.

(7) The objectives of the nonclinical safety program for biologics are similar to those for small-molecule drugs (SMDs): to recognize potential toxicities (hazard identification and characterization, and risk assessment), to identify appropriate parameters for clinical monitoring (e.g.biomarkers) and to contribute to first-in-human dose (FIH) selection. This also includes assessing the limitations of nonclinical studies in predicting safety issues for the human situation. Nevertheless, the nonclinical program has to be designed for clinical decision-making. The program for biologics, however, is often different from SMD programs because of the nature of the therapeutic protein, its species specificity and its immunogenicity.

Text B
Quality Control and Assurance from the Development to the Production of Biopharmaceuticals

Consumer and patient safety have become the prerequisites for (bio)pharmaceutical product development, production and marketing. The ability to provide an effective, pure, safe product is the primary factor determining the product's success. However, with an ever-increasing number of national and international regulations, "quality assurance" has acquired a threatening ring for many project managers. Many think that ensuring and improving quality is expensive, but regulations aid public acceptance. Good manufacturing practice can be developed into a business asset and need not be seen as merely a regulatory hurdle.

Frequently Cited Concerns

Adulteration

The adulteration of drugs can occur for several reasons. Of special interest in this context are all issues connected to good manufacturing practices (GMPs) as defined by, for example, the US Food and Drug Administration (FDA). To ensure that a drug meets the requirements of safety, identity and strength, and meets the quality and purity characteristics that it purports or is represented to possess, the methods used in, or the facilities or controls used for, its manufacture, processing, packing or holding have to conform to or be operated or administered in conformity with current GMP regulations.[1] If these criteria cannot be fulfilled, the drug is deemed to be adulterated.

Changes (variations)

Endangering consumers' (patients') health by changing the product's quality, whether deliberately or otherwise, is a major concern of all regulating authorities. Therefore, any change to the process has to be proved to yield a comparable product. If the product's characteristics have been modified, the resulting product would be considered to be a new product and has to be reevaluated fully.

Wide distribution

As products are increasingly manufactured at specialized production sites, in some cases providing supplies to large areas of the world, a great number of individuals could potentially be affected if the products were defective.

Complex production technology

The metabolic pathways of organisms used in the production of biopharmaceuticals are complex and their responses to changes in the environment are often unpredictable. This means that the

笔记

process parameters must be carefully adjusted and controlled to ensure batch-to-batch reproducibility. The biocompatible chemicals and moderate temperatures and pressures used for production enhance process safety for the operator and the environment but can promote the growth of contaminating microorganisms. Complex downstream-processing steps are normally needed to remove (hazardous) impurities without damaging the product.

Potency

The past few years have seen the advent of a number of biopharmaceuticals (e.g. immune-system modulators, substances with hormone-like action, neuroactive substances) that rival or even surpass traditional chemistry-derived drugs in their potency.

Stability

Chemically derived products tend to be more stable than biopharmaceuticals consisting of proteins or polypeptides, such as cytokines, erythropoietins, plasminogen activators, blood-plasma factors, growth hormones, insulin, monoclonal antibodies and certain types of vaccine. The storage test conditions, study durations, frequency of testing and release, and expiration specifications must therefore all be evaluated carefully. The methods used for purity and molecular characterization must be validated to prove that they can accurately detect changes during storage, including subtle changes that reflect the degradation and loss of biological activity (potency) of the product.

Environmental impact

Most biological agents used in industrial biotechnology have a long history of safe use. In some special cases, such as the production of vaccines with live pathogens, the production organism itself can pose a hazard. There is public concern regarding biological agents with unknown pathogenic or other detrimental traits being unwittingly created by genetic technology and released into the environment; this has resulted in the implementation of various regulations [e.g. by the US National Institute of Health (NIH), the Organization for Economic Cooperation and Development (OECD) and the European Commission (EC)] concerning the application, containment and deliberate release of genetically modified organisms.

Quality management concepts and good manufacturing practice

Much confusion has been created by the varying definitions of five basic terms that are often used in quality management:

- GMP
- Quality control (QC)
- Quality assurance (QA)
- Quality management
- Quality system

GMP is aimed at assuring the quality of the product by assuring the quality of the process. GMP should also: be part of process development (e.g. development reports and approval requirements); proceed through validation, manufacturing, controls and end-product testing; and reach into the distribution network of the product. Process development is often seen as being incompatible with GMP compliance, as development requires flexibility. However, if examined more closely, compliance will always involve process improvement, as GMP regulations actually require procedures and processes to be "state-of-the-art" designs.[2] GMP also applies to research, if activities are aimed at developing recombinant production strains, and to development, if this is aimed at

笔 记

preparing clinical material [3]; it should cover issues such as the testing and systematic documentation of the strains, genes or processes that are used.

GMP compliance for the production of pharmaceuticals, cosmetics and foods is a legal requirement in most national regulatory systems and is enforced through inspections by government investigators. Although there are differences, the content of the various national guidelines is, in fact, very similar and comprises the following elements, representing the major structural categories that make up current GMPs.

- Organization and personnel
- Quality assurance and quality control
- Facilities and equipment
- Production and process controls
- Packaging and labeling
- Storage and distribution
- Complaints and recalls
- Laboratory testing
- Standard operating procedures (SOPs)
- Documentation and document control
- Inspections
- Validation

The standard operating procedure

All procedures that have an impact on product quality need to be identified. A formal written system of documents, including SOPs, must be established. The procedures should describe in detail all the tasks that are to be performed to ensure a certain goal, such as performing analytical tests and organizational matters. SOPs should contain specifications (as needed) and must define the circumstances under which the procedure is deemed to be successful. This is only one element in an array of necessary procedures, such as master production procedures, batch production records and analytical procedures.

Documentation and document control

One of the fundamentals of all quality-assurance concepts is the need for meticulous records of all activities. Activities that have not been recorded are worthless in respect to regulatory compliance as inspecting authorities consider them "not performed" unless they have been recorded. Organizing the documentation structure and maintaining is therefore one of the most important tasks in setting up a QA system, and is the basis of any validation. Documentation has to be adequate to ensure the traceability of the production history of every batch, including all associated issues such as raw materials, cleaning procedures, packaging, labeling and distribution.

Validation

Validation is the action of proving that any material, process, procedure, activity, equipment or mechanism that is used can and does achieve the desired and intended results. Consequently, sufficient scientifically and technically sound data must be provided in writing to show that specifications are met and that the intended results are achieved in a reproducible fashion.

Validating Biopharmaceutical Production

Complete validation of a process can extend from planning and designing an equipment item to

笔记

its routine inspection within production, with the whole cycle incorporating several elements.

- Design qualification (DQ), including user-requirement specifications and detailed functional specifications for engineering design and procurement.

- Installation qualification (IQ), verifying that all key aspects of hardware installation adhere to appropriate codes and approved design intentions.

- Operational qualification (OQ), verifying that subsystems perform as intended with model process materials (e.g. water).

- Performance qualification (PQ) of equipment.

- Process-change control, to ensure that product quality is maintained or optimized after changes have been made to the process.

Facilities

A number of regulatory requirements for biotechnological plants have been developed, including, for example, the requirements for containment measures and equipment systems [e.g. the heating, ventilation and air-conditioning systems (HVAC), water, steam and sterilization systems, material, equipment, product and waste flow, personnel flow, and personnel control]. Requirements are rarely laid down in actual engineering terms but are based on knowledge of the current policies and expectations of the individual regulatory authorities. As technology is constantly in a state of improvement, the guidelines themselves and their interpretation are subject to state-of-the-art technology. Major equipment and facilities are changed or built infrequently, and so individual companies, large or small, rarely have the resources to develop and maintain the necessary in-house knowledge of current engineering compliance.

Equipment

Most biotechnological operations are run under aseptic conditions (i.e. free from viable organisms other than the production organism). The art of aseptic design has developed rapidly, but the need for hygienic design (i.e. the ability of equipment to be cleaned from undesired matter, such as product residues) is often underestimated. The potential carry-over into subsequent products is a major concern, particularly in multipurpose plants. Validation has to ensure that the cleaning procedures are adapted to the equipment and the type of contamination. The hygienic design of fermentation equipment is crucial for cleaning procedures to be successful. Surface finish, "dead legs", alignment of piping and many other criteria affect clean ability and the build-up of contaminating materials. The reproducibility of cleaning procedures can be optimized by designing equipment with automatic cleaning-in-place (CIP) systems, removing the need to dismantle it.

The design of hygienic equipment is based on some very simple criteria. Process validation and GMP production can be achieved by checking for these criteria at a very early stage of the project. All surfaces must be resistant to the product and to cleaning at the full range of operating pressures and temperatures. The surfaces should also be free from crevices, their surface roughness should be 0.5μm or less and they should either be easily accessible for manual cleaning and visual inspection or be validated for CIP. The equipment must be self-draining and dead legs must be avoided or positioned correctly to ensure that CIP procedures reach all surfaces. Hygienic design also extends to the external parts of the equipment, including issues such as adequate insulation to avoid condensation on external surfaces of the equipment, with the insulation sealed with stainless-steel cladding, preferably fully welded, and the equipment and supports either sealed to the building with no gaps or pockets, or with adequate clearance to allow for inspection and cleaning.[4]

Downstream

Purification processes must be validated to prove that they are capable of removing impurities to an acceptable level. In the production of biopharmaceuticals, special emphasis is put on components originating from the host cell (e.g. protein and DNA), media components or substances used during downstream processing (e.g. nutrients, buffer components, stabilizers and chromatography media) and potential external contamination by adventitious agents (e.g. bacteria, viruses and mycoplasmas, as well as scrapie-like agents in cell cultures), which should not be present throughout the process but could accidentally contaminate the culture.

Analytical procedures

Analytical procedures must have their statistical accuracy, precision, sensitivity, robustness (the capacity of a method to remain unaffected by small, deliberate variations in method parameters) and ruggedness (intermediate precision and reproducibility) tested. Validation has to include the evaluation of matrix effects, such as influence of sample pH or protein content. Analytical procedures used to evaluate the quality of the final product have the highest priority for full and comprehensive validation.

Laboratory operations can be streamlined by following a stringent control program. If, for example, analytical equipment is properly selected, set-up and operated using the classical qualification stages (DQ, IQ, OQ and PQ), expensive calibration runs can be reduced. By setting method-specific system-suitability criteria as part of performance qualification, the performance of the equipment's critical components can be monitored. This enables the early detection of trends towards unacceptable performance, helping to reduce equipment downtime. The development of rapid procedures for in-process control can help to identify variations during processing.

Automated systems

As with all other systems used for the production of pharmaceuticals, automated equipment has to be fully documented and validated; both hardware and software must be tested. As is the case for other system components, the installation, operational and performance qualifications have to be performed and test data have to be documented and evaluated. Systems must perform within specified limits (performance test) and cope with certain events, such as erroneous operator inputs and sensor failures, amongst others.

Word Study

1. adulteration [ə,dʌltə'reiʃən] *n.* 掺杂，伪造，劣货，掺假的东西，冒充货
2. adventitious [,ædven'tiʃəs] *adj.* 偶然的，外来的
3. alignment [ə'lainmənt] *n.* 调准，校直，排列，对准
4. blood-plasma factors 血浆蛋白及凝血因子
5. calibration [,kæli'breiʃən] *n.* 校准
6. carry-over ['kæri'əuvə] *n.* 带入
7. clad [klæd] *v.* 包被，覆盖
8. condensation [,kɔnden'seiʃən] *n.* 浓集，压缩，凝缩，缩合，液化
9. containment [kən'teinmənt] *n.* 抑制，遏制，牵制
10. contamination [kən,tæmə'neiʃən] *n.* 污染

笔记

11. crevice ['krevis] *n.* 缝，缝隙，裂缝

12. dead legs *n.* 死角

13. deliberate [di'libərət] *adj.* 审慎的，深思熟虑的，故意的，从容的

14. dismantle [dis'mæntl] *v.* 拆除……的设备，分解，废除，去掉……的覆盖物

15. erythropoietins [əriθrə'pɔiitinz] *n.* 促红细胞生成素

16. expiration [,ekspə'reiʃən] *n.* 断气，死亡，呼气，呼出，期满

17. Food and Drug Administration 美国食品与药品管理局（FDA）

18. good manufacturing practices 药品生产质量管理规范（GMP）

19. holding ['həuldiŋ] *n.* 贮藏，保存

20. hygienic [hai'dʒi:nik] *adj.* 卫生学的，卫生的

21. identity [ai'dentəti] *n.* 同一性，鉴定，鉴别

22. implementation [,implimen'teiʃən] *n.* 完成，器具，实现，履行，执行

23. in-house ['in 'haus] *adj.* 内部的

24. insulation [,insə'leiʃən] *n.* 绝缘，绝缘体，隔离，孤立

25. meticulous [mə'tikjələs] *adj.* 精确的，仔细的

26. modulator ['mɔdʒə,leitə] *n.* 调整基因，调节器

27. mycoplasma [,maikəu'plɑ:zmə] *n.* 支原体

28. packing ['pækiŋ] *n.* 包装

29. plasminogen activator [plæz'minədʒin 'æktiveitə] *n.* 纤溶酶原激活因子

30. polypeptide [,pɔli'pep,taid] *n.* 多肽

31. procurement [prə'kjuəmənt] *n.* 获得，取得

32. purport [pər'pɔ:rt] *n.* 说明，目的，意义，意图

33. reproducibility [riprədju:sə'biliti] *n.* 重现性，再现性

34. robustness [rəu'bʌstnəs] *n.* 稳健性

35. ruggedness ['rʌgidnəs] *n.* 耐用性

36. scrapie ['skreipi] *n.* 绵羊瘙痒病

37. seal [si:l] *n.* 印章，封条，海豹；*v.* 封闭，盖印，猎海豹

38. specifications [spesifi'keiʃnz] *n.* 规格，详述，技术要求，技术条件，详细说明书

39. state-of-the-art 最新水平，技术发展水平，（科技、机电等）最先进的水平

40. sterilization [,sterəlai'zeiʃn] *n.* 灭菌，消毒，绝育

41. strain [strein] *n.* 菌株

42. streamlined ['stri:m,laind] *adj.* ①流线型的；②革新的，现代化的；③合理化的；有效率的；

43. traceability [,treisə'biliti] *n.* 可追溯，可描绘，可描写

44. trait [treit] *n.* 形状，特征，特性

45. unwittingly [ʌn'witiŋli] *adv.* 不知情地，无意地

46. vaccine [væk'si:n] *n.* 疫苗

47. validate ['vælideit] *v.* 使有效，确认，证实

48. ventilation [,venti'leiʃən] *n.* 通风，换气

Notes

1. To ensure that a drug meets the requirements of safety, identity and strength, and meets the quality and purity characteristics that it purports or is represented to possess, the methods used in, or the facilities or controls used for, its manufacture, processing, packing or holding have to conform

笔记

to or be operated or administered in conformity with current GMP regulations. 译为：为了确保一种药物达到安全性、同一性和浓度的要求，并且达到它所说明的或被描述应具备的质量和纯度特性，使用的方法或设施，或者采用的控制方法、生产、加工、包装或贮藏必须符合现行的 GMP 规范，或者在现行的 GMP 规范下进行经营和管理。句中"that it purports or is represented to possess…"意思是"它所说明的或被描述应具备的……"

2. However, if examined more closely, compliance will always involve process improvement, as GMP regulations actually require procedures and processes to be "state-of-the-art" designs. 译为：然而，如果检查的更加严密，顺应性总是会影响到工艺过程的改良，因为 GMP 规程实际上要求操作和过程与工艺水平设计完全相符。句中"state-of-the-art"意思是"工艺水平、工艺状态"。

3. GMP also applies to research, if activities are aimed at developing recombinant production strains, and to development, if this is aimed at preparing clinical material. 译为：如果是针对开发重组生产菌株，GMP 同样也适用于科学研究，如果是针对于制备临床用原料，GMP 也同样适用于研发。

4. Hygienic design also extends to the external parts of the equipment, including issues such as adequate insulation to avoid condensation on external surfaces of the equipment, with the insulation sealed with stainless-steel cladding, preferably fully welded, and the equipment and supports either sealed to the building with no gaps or pockets, or with adequate clearance to allow for inspection and cleaning. 译为：清洁设计也包括设备的外部，诸如以适当的绝缘性避免仪器外表面凝结，采用不锈钢包层绝缘密封，最好是满焊，并且设备和支柱要么无间隙地密封于建筑内，要么保留能够容许检验和清洁的适当间隙。

Supplementary Parts

1. Medical and Pharmaceutical Terms Made Easier (9): Common Suffixes in Medical English Terms

Suffixes	Meaning	Example
-ac	……的	cardiac 心脏的
-al	……的	bronchial 支气管的
-algia	痛	arthralgia 关节痛
-ar	……的	tonsillar 扁桃体的
-arctia	狭窄	bronchiarctia 支气管狭窄
-ary	……的	ciliary 睫状的
-blast	未分化的原始胚细胞	hemocytoblast 成血细胞，原血细胞
-cele	突出、疝气	thyrocele 甲状腺肿
-centesis	外科穿刺吸液	amniocentesis 羊膜穿刺术
-cide	杀，割	germicide 杀菌剂
-clysis	洗	bronchoclysis 支气管灌洗
-cyte	细胞	leukocyte 白血细胞
-eal	……的	esophageal 食管的
-ectasia,-ectasis	扩张，膨胀	nephrectasia 肾扩张
-ectomy	切除	appendectomy 阑尾切除术
-emia	血的情况	leukemia 白血病
-form,-oid	形，样	filiform 线形的
-gram	记录，图	radiogram 放射照片

续表

Suffixes	Meaning	Example
-graphy,-graph	记录	electrocardiography 心电描记术
-ia	条件,情况	anemia 贫血
-iatry,-iatrics	常用于医学分支	podiatry 足医术
-ic	……的	hepatic 肝的
-ist	专家,学者	dermatologist 皮肤病专家
-itis	炎症	hepatitis 肝炎
-ium	部分与整体关系, 与……有关;部位	pericardium 心包
-lith	结石	cholelith 胆结石
-logist	学者和治疗者	urologist 泌尿专家
-logy	学科	pharmacology 药理学
-lysis	溶解	hemolysis 溶血
-malacia	软化	osteomalacia 骨软化
-meter	测量用器具	thermometer 温度计
-metry	测量	pelvimetry 骨盆测量法
-myces	霉菌	streptomyces 链霉菌属
-odynia	痛	cardiodynia 心痛
-oid	类似,像	cystoid 囊样的
-oma	肿胀,肿瘤	sarcoma 肉瘤
-opsy	观	autopsy 尸检
-or(er)	工作者(指人或工具,物)	incisor 切牙,门齿
-osis	异常或病理情况	sclerosis 硬化症
-ous	……的	mucous 黏液的
-pathy	病,病理情况	ophthalmopathy 眼病
-penia	不足,缺少	leukocytopenia 白细胞减少
-pexy	固定,缝于……处	hepatopexy 肝固定手术
-phil	嗜	eosinophil 嗜酸性粒细胞
-phob	惧怕	hydrophobia 恐水症
-plasty	外科整形或修补	osteoplasty 骨成形术
-plegia	麻痹,瘫痪	thermoplegia 热射病,中暑
-ptosis	落下	nephroptosis 肾下垂
-rrhagia	大量流出,出血	gastrorrhagia 胃出血
-rrhaphy	缝合术	herniorrhaphy 疝缝补手术
-rrhea	流出,分泌	diarrhea 腹泻
-rrhexis	破裂	hepatorrhexis 肝破裂
-sclerosis	硬化	arteriosclerosis 动脉硬化
-scope	检查用器具	ophthalmoscope 检眼镜
-scopy	检查,视诊	cystoscopy 膀胱镜检查
-some	体	chromosome 染色体
-stasis	停止,制止	bacteriostasis 制菌作用
-stenosis	变窄,狭窄	arteriostenosis 动脉狭窄
-stomy	开口或吻合	gastrostomy 胃造口术
-tome	切割用器具	arthrotome 关节刀
-tomy	切,切开	craniotomy 颅骨切开术
-uria	尿的情况	hematuria 血尿
-y	情况,动作,过程	splenomegaly 脾大

笔记

(1)   Fill in the blanks with the missing word root, prefix or suffix.

1) _____articular 非关节的，关节外的

2) _____renal 肾上腺的

3) _____ceps 二头肌

4) broncho_____ 支气管灌洗

5) leuk_____ 白血病

6) _____paralysis 偏瘫

7) _____glycemia 高血糖

8) chole_____ 胆结石

9) cardi_____ 心痛

10) hepato_____ 肝固定手术

11) osteo_____ 骨成形术

12) _____synthetic 半合成的

13) arthr_____ 关节痛

14) bronchi_____ 支气管狭窄

15) _____cardia 心动过缓

16) append_____ 阑尾切除术

17) hepat_____ 肝炎

18) _____glossia 巨舌

19) strepto_____ 链霉菌属

20) leukocyto_____ 白细胞减少

21) _____uria 多尿症

22) hepato_____ 肝破裂

23) cysto_____ 膀胱镜检查

24) arterio_____ 动脉狭窄

(2)   Word-matching 1.

1) anabolism	A. 热射病
2) hypoglycemia	B. 心动过速
3) encephalic	C. 肾旁的
4) incoagulability	D. 合成代谢
5) tachycardia	E. 脑的
6) paranephric	F. 修复学
7) chromosome	G. 甲状腺肿
8) thermoplegia	H. 羊膜穿刺术
9) prosthetics	I. 低血糖
10) bacteriostasis	J. 制菌作用
11) thyrocele	K. 染色体
12) amniocentesis	L. 不凝性

(3)   Word-matching 2.

1) antidote	A. 支气管的
2) deoxidation	B. 肉瘤
3) tonsillar	C. 解毒剂

续表

4) endocrine	D. 外胚层
5) ophthalmopathy	E. 关节刀
6) sarcoma	F. 脾大
7) bronchial	G. 动脉硬化
8) ectoderm	H. 内分泌
9) infracostal	I. 肋下的
10) splenomegaly	J. 眼病
11) arthrotome	K. 扁桃体的
12) arteriosclerosis	L. 脱氧

2.　English-Chinese Translation Skills: 药学英语翻译技巧 (5): 长句、复杂句翻译法

英语语言强调形合（hypotactic），结构严密，句子成分逻辑关系强，长句、复杂句较多；汉语语言强调意合（paratactic），结构松散，句子成分的逻辑关系蕴含在词语当中，句式相对简单。药学英语中句式较长、逻辑关系复杂、附加成分多的长句较为常见，其中往往大量使用连词、介词、非谓语动词等。除此之外，药学英语复杂句子也可能由多个抽象名词、多个动词短语表现多层意义，或者为了结构平衡，还出现倒装句子结构。但是无论句子多么长、句式多么复杂，翻译时要抓住主谓（宾）这个核心，理清各成分之间逻辑关系，就可以化繁为简，一目了然。

药学英语长句、复杂句翻译可以采用切分法。所谓切分法，就是翻译时根据句子成分逻辑关系，将长句、复杂句切分成几个意义相对独立的小句。切分长句、复杂句是一种常用的翻译方法，可以使原文错综复杂的逻辑关系用简单的小句表述出来。

例 1: Controlled drug delivery improves bioavailability by preventing premature degradation and enhancing uptake, maintains drug concentration within the therapeutic window by controlling the drug release rate, and reduces side effects by targeting to disease site and target cells.

参考译文：控制药物传递，可以防止药物过早降解和加强药物摄取从而提高生物利用度，可以控制药物释放速率而使药物浓度维持在治疗窗范围内，可以靶向疾病位点和目标细胞从而减少不良反应。

说明：从句子结构看，上面例句不算很复杂，其主要结构是：Controlled drug delivery improves…, maintains…, and reduces…. 每个谓语动词后面又都接了一个 by + v-ing 短语。翻译这样句子，可以直接使用切分法，还要注意每个切分后小句表达前后连贯。参考译文在拆分后的小句前增加了"可以"，使原文中的三个动词短语连成一体。

例 2: To ensure that a drug meets the requirements of safety, identity and strength, and meets the quality and purity characteristics that it purports or is represented to possess, the methods used in, or the facilities or controls used for, its manufacture, processing, packing or holding have to conform to or be operated or administered in conformity with current GMP regulations.

参考译文：为了确保一种药物达到安全性、同一性和浓度的要求，并且达到它所说明的或被描述应具备的质量和纯度特性，使用的方法或设施，或者采用的控制方法、生产、加工、包装或贮藏必须符合现行的 GMP 规范，或者在现行的 GMP 规范下进行经营和管理。

说明：上面例句结构相对比较复杂。翻译时，首先要分析清楚句子主要成分以及各成分之间逻辑关系，然后再将复杂句子结构拆分，用简洁语言表达出来。原英文句子主要结构是：主语是 the methods, or the facilities or controls, its manufacture, processing, packing or holding，谓语是 have to conform to or be operated or administered。在名词 the methods 后有一个动词过去分词 used in 作定语，在名词 the facilities or controls 后面有一个动词过去分词 used for 作定语，在谓语结构后面有一个介词短语。主语之前的动词不定式 To ensure that a drug meets the requirements

笔记

of safety, identity and strength, and meets the quality and purity characteristics that it purports or is represented to possess 作状语，这个状语又有三层结构，首先动词 ensure 后接以 that 引导的宾语从句，这是第一层结构；在 that 引导的从句中，主语是 a drug，后接两个"meets + 名词"并列谓语，这是第二层；在第二个谓语 meets 后面的宾语 the quality and purity characteristics 后面又有一个定语从句 that it purports or is represented to possess，这是第三层结构。

参考译文保持了原文基本结构：状语 + 主句。状语部分的翻译没有拆分，定语从句 that it purports or is represented to possess 正常调整到名词 the quality and purity characteristics 前面；在翻译谓语部分时，采用了拆分法，将连动谓语 conform to or be operated or administered 拆分为两个小句，并且根据表达需要重复了 current GMP regulations。

用切分法翻译药学英语长句、复杂句，不是随意对原句子进行拆分，不能改变原文中句子成分逻辑关系，而且切分后汉语表达要顺畅自然。

Unit Ten　Clinical Pharmacy

Clinical pharmacy is a health science discipline in which pharmacists provide patient care that optimizes medication therapy and promotes health, wellness, and disease prevention. The practice of clinical pharmacy embraces the philosophy of pharmaceutical care; it blends a caring orientation with specialized therapeutic knowledge, experience, and judgment for the purpose of ensuring optimal patient outcomes. As a discipline, clinical pharmacy also has an obligation to contribute to the generation of new knowledge that advances health and quality of life.

Within the system of health care, clinical pharmacists are experts in the therapeutic use of medications. They routinely provide medication therapy evaluations and recommendations to patients and health care professionals. Clinical pharmacists are a primary source of scientifically valid information and advice regarding the safe, appropriate, and cost-effective use of medications.

临床药学是一门有关健康科学的学科,该学科主要内容是药师为患者提供药学服务,包括优化药物治疗、促进健康、保健及预防疾病。临床药学的实践涵盖药学服务的理念;它将服务定位与专业治疗知识、经验、判断相结合,旨在确保患者最佳的治疗效果。作为一门学科,临床药学还有责任促进产生新的医疗知识,以提高健康水平和生活质量。

在医疗保健系统内,临床药师是药物的治疗性使用领域的专家。他们定期向患者和医护人员提供药物治疗的评价和建议。在安全、适当、经济用药这一过程中,临床药师是获取科学有效信息和建议的主要来源。

笔记

Text A
The Practice of Community Pharmacy

(Adapted from *Remington: the Science and Practice of Pharmacy*,
22nd Edition, Chapter 76, 2109-2110)

Distribution and Control of Medication

The pharmacist's role in assuring the safe distribution of medications continues as a major area of responsibility in the community setting, as elsewhere. Pharmacists, as the most readily available healthcare provider, are maintaining this role while becoming more involved clinically. The retail setting was the place of employment for 65% of the nation's 270 000 pharmacists working in 2008. The need for pharmacists in this setting remains high because the percentage of Americans taking prescription medications has increased over the last decade, along with the percentage taking multiple prescription medications. Over $234 billion, or approximately 10% of overall national health expenditures, was spent on retail outlet sales of prescription drugs[1] in 2008, nearly twice the amount spent in the year 2000. In 2010 the number of prescriptions totaled over 3.6 billion, of which approximately 48% were filled in traditional chain pharmacies, 20% in independent pharmacies, 25% in supermarket and mass merchandiser pharmacies combined, and 7% via mail order pharmacy. The same year, generic prescriptions accounted for 71.2% of prescriptions, with 28.8% being brand name drugs[2]. The average price of a prescription had risen to nearly $80 in 2010, up from approximately $64 in 2005, $46 in 2000, and $30 in 1995. The increased use of prescription drugs and associated increase in cost come at a time of a number of changes in the marketplace for outpatient prescription medications. Patients are paying a smaller percentage of prescription drug spending. While out-of-pocket consumer spending for prescription drugs was 56% in 1990, it decreased to 26% by 2001, and declined further to 21% by 2008. At the same time, private health insurance covered 26%, 50%, and 42% of prescription drug costs in 1990, 2001, and 2008, respectively. A steady increase in coverage has occurred in publicly funded programs such as Medicaid, Medicare, and other government programs. In 1990 these programs accounted for 18% of expenditures, rising to 24% in 2001, 28% in 2005, and 37% in 2008. The accelerated rise after 2005 is reflective of the Medicare Part D benefit going into effect and its new function as the primary coverage for beneficiaries having both Medicaid and Medicare[3] drug benefits. With this rise in third party reimbursement for prescription drugs has come with continued pressure from insurance plans and their Pharmacy Benefit Managers (PBMs) to contain medication expense. Strategies such as increasing beneficiary co-payments and establishing co-pay tiers to limit use of non-preferred or expensive drugs, use of formularies to direct therapies to preferred or contracted drug entities and to exclude others, limiting the quantity to be dispensed, and requiring pre-approval of medication selection and reimbursement prior to dispensing have all impacted the community pharmacist in practice.[7] Beyond increasing the complexity of the pricing systems that must be maintained for the many different plans accepted by a community pharmacy, these schemes are also confusing for the beneficiary, and considerable time is spent by pharmacists assisting the patient in both understanding their benefit and working with their providers and the PBM to get the patient the needed medication. Cost

笔记

reduction strategies for the reimbursement of pharmacists for the distribution of the prescription by insurance companies provides another challenge because decreased professional fees must often be accepted by a pharmacist to avoid the loss of patients eligible to receive services from their practice.

These pressures greatly affect the profitability of community pharmacy. Information from the 2010 NCPA (National Community Pharmacists Association) Digest[4] suggests that 21% of independent community pharmacies are operating at a loss, with another 23.4% having just a 0-2% net profit.

In order to most efficiently process prescription orders and attempt to maintain a high level of quality at the lowest cost, community pharmacies are increasingly utilizing technology. The processing of electronic prescriptions and automated refill requests are now becoming part of the daily routine in pharmacies. Utilization of computer systems to facilitate prescription processing is nearly universal because processing of insurance with real time adjudication of claims is the standard of practice. These same systems also assist the pharmacist in screening for drug-disease and drug-drug interactions and therapeutic duplication. They also help with monitoring of adherence to therapy. Importantly, the utility of these database solutions is limited in cases in which fragmentation of care prevents complication of a complete and accurate record of a person's medication history, including nonprescription medications and complementary and alternative medications. The future availability of accessible personal health records should allow for improved functionality in this regard. This is especially true as patients utilize a variety of medication sources to minimize out-of-pocket expenses.

In addition to computer systems to process prescription orders, pharmacists are increasingly making use of other technologies to increase efficiency. Many pharmacies use interactive voice response (IVR) systems to allow patients to request refills on medications using their telephones. This functionality is also available using the internet and with applications on smart phones. A variety of mechanical devices have taken the place of the counting tray in regard to getting the correct number of capsules or tablets into a container for the patient. Stand-alone counting machines have evolved into dedicated counting devices for individual medications. Dispensing system interfaces with banks of these devices was an important step toward the development of robotics, which are practical for the community pharmacy. Many community pharmacies now have one of the several available automated counting or robotic dispensing devices that count the solid dosage forms and place the counted medication into a labeled container. These devices can decrease prescription filling time; however, this improvement doesn't necessarily gain efficiency or assure increased care will be provided. Knowledge on how to best meld technology with human activities in these new environments is still developing. Other technology, such as bar code scanning, allows the pharmacist to better insure accuracy in dispensing by checking ordered medication against product selected, assuring the correct medication is added to counting devices and robots, and performing final verification on filled prescriptions. Software solutions with these systems assist in work flow management, quality assurance, inventory management, and automated ordering. Technology innovation has resulted in many changes in how the basic dispensing functions are completed in a community pharmacy, and, consequently, have produced new management challenges in the day to day practice of pharmacy.

Additional challenges to the practice of community pharmacy grow from other strategies to

笔记

control costs associated with prescription medication. Alternative distribution strategies such as centralized filling of prescription orders with delivery to distribution site pharmacies can change the relationship between the pharmacist and patient. These systems also require a different approach to pharmacy management to assure efficiency. Mail order delivery of prescription services has been a challenge to community pharmacy as established pharmacist-patient relationships are broken, and access to the provision of services for involved patients is limited when plan sponsors and PBMs promote this system as a way to reduce prescription costs. While generally assumed to be a most cost-effective way of delivering prescription drugs, the design of mail order plans and incentives used to promote its use can increase the cost to the plan sponsor. These systems-oriented changes in practice can further fragment the medication-related care a patient receives, and make the provision of pharmacist-provided care, which takes into consideration all of the patients medications, more difficult.

Patients can also complicate the ability of a single pharmacy to have a complete record of their medications. This can occur when patients shop for the lowest prices for their medications. This could occur at other local pharmacies or over the internet. Increasing the risks to the patient from this latter activity go beyond provider knowledge of medications taken by the patient. Studies completed by the FDA and NABP[6] find that many of the prescriptions filled from internet pharmacies are adulterated and do not contain the labeled ingredients. Patients also obtain prescription medications from neighboring countries. In some of these cases, quality also becomes an issue. A relatively recent development to reduce prescription cost to the patient is the offering of $4.00 generic medications by a number of retailers. These patient-initiated methods need to be considered by the pharmacist as they are working with each individual. Other issues, such as the high rate of both initial and ongoing non-adherence with prescribed medication, also reduce the pharmacist's ability to know what a patient is really taking without a detailed medication history.

Areas of Specialty Practice

The Practice of Community Pharmacy has expanded from the conventional role of prescription dispensing to include many other health related services, such as compounding medications, integrating complementary and alternative medications, supplying durable medical equipment, and administering immunizations.

Although compounding medication is not new to the practice of pharmacy, it has gained popularity for the ability to individualize patient medications and produce pharmaceuticals that are not commercially available. Hospice medications, bio-identical hormones, pediatric preparations, veterinary medications, and gluten-free, preservative-free, or dye-free preparations are just a few of the examples of commonly compounded pharmaceuticals. Thousands of community pharmacies offer compounded medications; however, the volume of compounded prescriptions varies from practice to practice. Some pharmacies may base their primary business on compounded medications alone. Pharmacies that specialize in compounding may choose to become certified by the Pharmacy Compounding Accreditation Board[5].

Complementary and alternative medication (CAM), which also has roots in early pharmacy practice, is becoming more widely used in the United States as an option to prevent and treat health conditions. According to the 2007 National Health Interview Survey, 38.3% of Americans used some form of CAM. This category of treatment encompasses a wide range of therapies, including herbals

笔记

and other natural products, acupuncture, meditation, chiropractic care, or massage. Many herbals and natural products have become a mainstay in the community pharmacy and these pharmacists are positioned to help patients safely integrate CAM therapy with traditional medications to assist in patient self-care efforts.

Another expanded community pharmacy service beyond the prescription counter is durable medical equipment (DME). The Medicare Modernization Act of 2003, which established Durable Medical Equipment, Prosthetics, Orthotics, and Supplied (DME-POS) Quality Standards, requires suppliers of these products to become accredited in order to bill Medicare. Some pharmacies may be exempt from this accreditation, such as those with DME sales billed to Medicare of less than 5% of the total pharmacy sales. Accreditation must be from a CMS (Centers for Medicare & Medicaid Services)-approved, independent national Accreditation Organization, and accreditation can cost more than $3000 for a three-year period.

As of 2010 all states allow pharmacists to immunize; however, each state differs in their laws and regulations for pharmacist immunization administration. Many local, state, and national programs are available to pharmacists to obtain training on vaccine administration. Accessibility to the community pharmacy allows pharmacist-administered immunizations to make a positive impact on public health and improved vaccination rates.

Word Study

1. accessibility [əkˌsesəˈbiləti] *n.* 可获得性，可及性
2. accredited [əˈkreditid] *adj.* 认可的
3. adjudication [əˌdʒuːdiˈkeiʃn] *n.* 裁定
4. adulterate [əˈdʌltəreit] *v.* 掺假
5. beneficiary [ˌbeniˈfiʃəri] *n.* 受益人
6. capsule [ˈkæpsjuːl] *n.* 胶囊
7. complexity [kəmˈpleksəti] *n.* 复杂性
8. complicate [ˈkɔmplikeit] *v.* 使复杂化
9. compounding [ˈkɔmpaundiŋ] *adj.* 组合的，混合的
10. co-payment [ˈkəupˈeimənt] *n.* 共同支付
11. duplication [ˌdjuːpliˈkeiʃn] *n.* 复制
12. exempt [igˈzempt] *adj.* 被免除的
13. expenditure [ikˈspenditʃə] *n.* 支出，开支
14. hospice [ˈhɔspis] *n.* 临终关怀，善终
15. incentive [inˈsentiv] *n.* 激励
16. inventory [ˈinvəntri] *n.* 存货，库存
17. meld [meld] *v.* 融合，合并
18. orthotics [ɔːˈθɔtiks] *n.* 矫正学，矫正体
19. out-of-pocket [aut əv ˈpɔkit] *adj.* 现款支付的，自费的
20. profitability [ˌprɔfitəˈbiləti] *n.* 赢利，收益
21. prosthetics [prɔsˈθetiks] *n.* 修复学，假体
22. reimbursement [ˌriːimˈbəːsmənt] *n.* 退还，报销
23. robotics [rəuˈbɔtiks] *n.* 机器人技术
24. tablet [ˈtæblət] *n.* 药片，片剂

笔记

Notes

1. "retail outlet sales of prescription drugs"的意思是处方药在零售店的销售。
2. "generic drug"和"brand name drug"的意思分别是非专利药（仿制药）和专利药（原厂药）。
3. "medicaid and medicare"是美国政府出台的两个为特殊人群设立的医疗保险补助项目。Medicaid 针对的是低收入及残疾人群，而 medicare 针对的是老年人群。
4. "NCPA Digest"是美国社区药师协会文摘，NCPA-National Community Pharmacists Association）。
5. "Pharmacy Compounding Accreditation Board"的意思是药房配药认证委员会。
6. "NABP"是国家药房委员会协会，National Association of Boards of Pharmacy。
7. Strategies such as increasing beneficiary co-payments and establishing co-pay tiers to limit use of non-preferred or expensive drugs, use of formularies to direct therapies to preferred or contracted drug entities and to exclude others, limiting the quantity to be dispensed, and requiring pre-approval of medication selection and reimbursement prior to dispensing have all impacted the community pharmacist in practice. 译为：很多策略都对社区药师的实践有影响，例如：增加受益人共同支付和建立共同支付层级，以限制使用非优选或昂贵的药物；使用处方集引导治疗，以选用最佳或合约规定的药物，并停用其他药物；限制分配数量；以及在分配之前要求对药物选择和报销进行预先审批。

Exercises

1. Decide whether each of the following statements is true (T) or false (F) according to the passage.

(1) The average price of a prescription has fallen over the last twenty years.

(2) Computer system is utilized to facilitate prescription processing, which has become nearly universal.

(3) Studies have shown that many of the prescriptions filled from Internet pharmacies are adulterated, and do not contain the labeled ingredients.

(4) Compounding pharmacy is not new to the practice of pharmacy, but it has never been popular over the years.

(5) Community pharmacy is reluctant to encompass complementary and alternative medication due to the declined use of these products.

(6) Community pharmacists are not authorized to perform immunization.

2. Questions for oral discussion.

(1) Why does the need for community pharmacist remain high?

(2) Please discuss various ways that could potentially impact the community pharmacist in practice.

(3) Why is community pharmacy motivated to utilize technology?

(4) Besides prescription dispensing, the practice of community pharmacy has now been successfully expanded into many other health-related services. Please name a few areas of specialty practice.

3. Choose the best answer to each of the following questions.

(1) What is the main responsibility of a pharmacist in the community settings?

A. safe distribution of medication

B. ability to develop a business-practice plan

C. perform periodic needs assessments

笔记

D. advocacy for healthcare policies

(2) Community pharmacists are facing the following challenges, except _____.

    A. complexity of the pricing system associated with different insurance plans

    B. more time spent assisting patients in understanding their benefit

    C. decreased professional fees accepted by pharmacists

    D. remote locations

(3) Which of the following statements best describes the profitability of community pharmacy?

    A. All the community pharmacies operate at a gain.

    B. All the community pharmacies are operated at a loss.

    C. About 20% of all the community pharmacies operate at a loss.

    D. About 50% of all the community pharmacies operate at a gain.

(4) Utilization of computer system to facilitate prescription processing becomes _____.

    A. impossible

    B. universal

    C. possible in some states

    D. possible in the near future

(5) In the US, requesting refills of prescription has been made through a variety of different ways, except _____.

    A. interactive voice response (IVR)　　　B. telephones

    C. the Internet　　　D. WeChat

(6) Studies conducted by the FDA and NABP find that many of the prescriptions filled from Internet pharmacies are _____.

    A. in good quality　　　B. not packaged well

    C. adulterated　　　D. from either Canada or India

(7) Compounded medications gain their popularity due to _____.

    A. their ability to individualize patient medications

    B. their much lowered price

    C. their greater extend of advertising power

    D. all of the above

(8) Which of the following products is considered as a complementary and alternative medication (CAM)?

    A. herbals and other natural products　　　B. medication products

    C. chiropractic care products　　　D. all of the above

(9) What is the significance of including complementary and alternative medication (CAM) in pharmacy practice?

    A. It is used as a supplement.

    B. It targets a special population with low income.

    C. It is to prevent and treat health conditions.

    D.It is used mainly as placebos.

(10) As of 2010, all states in the US allow pharmacists to immunize, which has made a positive impact on public health and _____.

    A. boosted public satisfaction

    B. improved vaccination rates

笔记

C. cut down cost

D. increased profit

4. Match the words with the Chinese versions.

1) affordable	A. 学术的
2) pertinent	B. 倡导
3) sustained	C. 接种疫苗
4) pharmacotherapy	D. 相关的，中肯的
5) practitioner	E. 令人费解的
6) humanistic	F. 药物疗法
7) advocacy	G. 从业者
8) vaccination	H. 人道主义的
9) academic	I. 持久的
10) perplexing	J. 负担得起的

5. Translate the following sentences and paragraphs into Chinese.

(1) Community pharmacy continues to evolve in its ability to provide medication-related patient care services.

(2) The image of what was once considered community pharmacy practice has been blurred both by the multiple types of practice and by the speed of change now occurring.

(3) The use of technicians in community pharmacy has increased considerably as pharmacists try to maximize efficiency in prescription processing while maintaining high quality standards.

(4) The pharmacy is staffed with English speaking licensed pharmacists capable of solving medication and health care related issues for expatriates.

(5) We feature a variety of professional services such as prescription filling, health and drug information, medication review and referral.

(6) The practice of pharmacy has changed significantly in response to organizational standards, patient safety, growth of technology and informatics, and increasingly complex medication regimens. The American College of Clinical Pharmacy defines clinical pharmacists as "someone who takes care of patients in any setting" and clinical pharmacy as "that area of pharmacy concerned with the science and practice of rational medication use." As such, all pharmacists are involved in clinical pharmacy services.

(7) The practice of health-system pharmacy has changed dramatically over the past 20 years. Years ago, the practice centered on preparation, compounding, and distribution of medications. Slowly, the practice of "clinical pharmacy" emerged in the 1980s. The term "clinical services" refers to the practice of providing medications to patients in the most safe, effective, and rational manner possible, while individualizing care to the recipient.

Text B
Standards of Practice for Clinical
Pharmacists: The Time Has Come

[Abridged from the original paper by American College of Clinical

Pharmacy. Pharmacotherapy, 2014, 34(8):794-797]

This document sets forth American College of Clinical Pharmacy's[1] expectations for clinical pharmacists within the United States and countries around the world where clinical

笔记

pharmacy is emerging. It is also intended to serve as a reference for those designing and assessing clinical pharmacy education and training programs. In addition to articulating the clinical pharmacist's process of care and documentation, the eight standards below address the clinical pharmacist's involvement in collaborative, team-based practice and privileging; professional development and maintenance of competence; professionalism and ethics; research and scholarship; and other professional responsibilities. The standards define for the public, health professionals, and policy-makers what they can and should expect of clinical pharmacists.

1. Qualifications

Clinical pharmacists are practitioners who provide comprehensive medication management and related care for patients in all health care settings. They are licensed pharmacists with specialized advanced education and training who possess the clinical competencies necessary to practice in team-based, direct patient care environments. Accredited residency training or equivalent post-licensure experience is required for entry into direct patient care practice. Board certification is also required once the clinical pharmacist meets the eligibility criteria specified by the Board of Pharmacy Specialties (BPS).

2. Process of Care

Clinical pharmacists work in collaboration with other providers to deliver comprehensive medication management that optimizes patient outcomes. Care is coordinated among providers and across systems of care as patients transition in and out of various settings.

The clinical pharmacist's process of care comprises the following components.

A. Assessment of the patient

The clinical pharmacist assesses medication related needs by:

● Reviewing the medical record using a problem-oriented framework (e.g., interpreting and analyzing subjective and objective information) to determine the clinical status of the patient;

● Meeting with the patient/caregivers to obtain and document a complete medication history to identify all of the patient's current medications (including regimens and administration routes), medication-taking behaviors, adherence, allergies, and attitudes and experiences with medication therapy;

● Obtaining, organizing, and interpreting patient data;

● Prioritizing patient problems and medication-related needs.

B. Evaluation of medication therapy

The clinical pharmacist identifies strategies to optimize medication therapy by:

● Assessing, with other members of the health care team, the appropriateness of current medications on the basis of health conditions, indication, and the therapeutic goals of each medication;

● Evaluating the effectiveness, safety, and affordability of each medication;

● Assessing medication-taking behaviors and adherence to each medication;

● Identifying medication-related problems and evaluating collaboratively with other members of the health care team the need for intervention.

C. Development and implementation of a plan of care

The clinical pharmacist develops and implements, collaboratively with the patient and his/her health care providers, a plan for optimizing medication therapy by:

笔记

- Reviewing the patient's active medical problem list to inform and guide the development of an individualized assessment and plan for optimizing medication therapy;
- Formulating a comprehensive medication management assessment and plan in collaboration with the health care team and implementing this plan to achieve patient-specific outcomes;
- Educating the patient/caregivers (both verbally and in writing) to ensure understanding of the care plan, to optimize adherence, and to improve therapeutic outcomes;
- Establishing patient-specific measurable parameters and time frames for monitoring and follow-up in collaboration with other members of the health care team.

D. Follow-up evaluation and medication monitoring

The clinical pharmacist performs follow-up evaluations in collaboration with other members of the health care team to continually assess patient outcomes by:

- Coordinating with other providers to ensure that patient follow-up and future encounters are aligned with the patient's medical and medication-related needs;
- Revisiting the medical record to obtain updates on the clinical status of the patient and then meeting with the patient/caregivers to obtain an updated medication history to identify, assess, and document any new medication-related needs or problems;
- Conducting ongoing assessments and refining the plan of care to optimize medication therapy and ensure that individual goals are achieved;
- Monitoring, modifying, documenting, and managing the plan of care in collaboration with the patient/caregivers and his/her other health care providers.

3. Documentation

Clinical pharmacists document directly in the patient's medical record the medication-related assessment and plan of care to optimize patient outcomes. This documentation should be compliant with the accepted standards for documentation (and billing, where applicable) within the health system, health care facility, outpatient practice, or pharmacy in which one works. Where applicable, accepted standards must be considered as they relate to the use of electronic health records (EHRs), health information technology and exchange systems, and e-prescribing.

The following components of the encounter are essential to include in the documentation, which may be communicated in the form of a traditional SOAP (subjective data, objective data, assessment, plan)[2] note or other framework consistent with the standards of documentation within the practice setting.

A. Medication history

- A brief summary of the patient's past medication use and related health problems as an introduction to the documentation that will follow;
- A list of all current medications that includes information regarding actual use, adherence, and attitudes toward therapy;
- A list of medication-related allergies and any adverse drug events that may affect prescribing and monitoring or preclude the future use of a medication.

B. Active problem list with assessment of each problem

- A list of current health conditions and supporting data for the status of each condition, emphasizing associated medications and medication-related problems that may have an impact on desired goals;
- A list of any additional medication-related problems or other medical issues that may be

unrelated to current health conditions.

  C. Plan of care to optimize medication therapy and improve patient outcomes

  ● The specific medication therapy plan that has been or will be implemented collaboratively by the health care team, including drug, dose, route, frequency, and relevant monitoring parameters;

  ● The collaborative plan for follow-up evaluation and monitoring as well as future visits.

4. Collaborative, Team-Based Practice and Privileging

  Clinical pharmacists work with other health professionals as members of the health care team to provide high-quality, coordinated, patient-centered care. They establish written collaborative drug therapy management (CDTM)[3] agreements with individual physicians, medical groups, or health systems and/or hold formally granted clinical privileges from the medical staff or credentialing system of the organization in which they practice. These privileging processes, together with the applicable state pharmacy practice act, confer certain authorities, responsibilities, and accountabilities to the clinical pharmacist as a member of the health care team and contribute to the enhanced efficiency and effectiveness of team-based care.

5. Professional Development and Maintenance of Competence

  Clinical pharmacists maintain competence in clinical problem-solving, judgment, and decision-making; communication and education; medical information evaluation and management; management of patient populations; and a broad range of therapeutic knowledge domains. Clinical pharmacists maintain competency through:

  A. Certification and maintenance of certification in the appropriate specialty relevant to their practice, including those specialties recognized by the Board of Pharmacy Specialties (BPS)[4] or other nationally recognized multiprofessional certifications;

  B. Consistent participation in continuing professional development (CPD)[5] activities that enhance direct patient care practice abilities;

  C. Maintenance of active licensure, including required continuing pharmacy education activities, through the appropriate state board(s) of pharmacy.

  Clinical pharmacists also pursue professional and career development by participating in formal and informal activities that enhance research and scholarship, teaching, leadership, and/or management.

6. Professionalism and Ethics

  Clinical pharmacists have a covenantal, "fiducial" relationship with their patients. This relationship relies on the trust placed in the clinical pharmacist by the patient and the commitment of the clinical pharmacist to act in the best interest of individual patients and patient populations, within the context of legal and ethical parameters. Clinical pharmacists exhibit the traits of professionalism: responsibility, commitment to excellence, respect for others, honesty and integrity, and care and compassion. They subscribe to the pharmacy profession's code of ethics and adhere to all pharmacist-related legal and ethical standards.

7. Research and Scholarship

  Clinical pharmacists support and participate in research and scholarship to advance human health and health care by developing research questions; conducting or participating in clinical, translational, and health services research; contributing to the evolving literature in evidence-based pharmacotherapy; and/or disseminating and applying research findings that influence the quality of

笔记

patient care.

8. Other Responsibilities

Clinical pharmacists serve as direct patient care providers, but they may also serve as educators, researchers, clinical preceptors/mentors, administrators, managers, policy developers, and consultants. As the clinical pharmacy discipline grows, it must continue to familiarize more patients, families, caregivers, other health professionals, payers/insurers, health care administrators, students, and trainees with the full range of clinical pharmacists' responsibilities.

Word Study

1. address [əˈdres] *v.* 说明，讲述
2. code of ethics [kəud əv ˈeθiks] *n.* 道德规范
3. collaborative [kəˈlæbərətiv] *adj.* 合作的
4. commitment [kəˈmitmənt] *n.* 承诺，保证
5. competence [ˈkɔmpitəns] *n.* 能力，胜任
6. covenantal [ˌkʌvəˈnæntəl] *adj.* 盟约的
7. disseminate [diˈsemineit] *v.* 散布，传播
8. eligibility [ˌelidʒəˈbiliti] *n.* 合格
9. encounter [inˈkauntə] *n.* 接触，见面
10. fiducial [fiˈdjuːʃəl] *adj.* 信托的
11. implement [ˈimplimənt] *v.* 实施
12. preceptor [priˈseptə] *n.* 指导教师
13. prioritize [praiˈɔrətaiz] *v.* 优先考虑
14. privilege [ˈprivəlidʒ] *n.* 特权
15. professionalism [prəˈfeʃənəlizəm] *n.* 职业精神
16. residency [ˈrezidənsi] *n.* 实习培训

Notes

1. "ACCP"的全称是"**American College of Clinical Pharmacy**"（美国临床药学会）。这是一个以职业发展和相关临床药学科学研究并重的学会，官方网站为 http://www.accp.com。目前在全美有 19 个不同的分会，为临床药师的教育培训、资源共享以及新理念的推广提供平台。

2. "SOAP"由"**S**ubjective data, **O**bjective data, **A**ssessment, **P**lan"的首字母组成。这是临床药师进行临床药历书写过程中的四个核心要素，包括有关患者的主观信息、客观信息、病情评价和治疗计划。

3. "CDTM"的全称是"**C**ollaborative **D**rug **T**herapy **M**anagement"（以合作共享为基础建立的药物治疗管理方案）。在这一新理念倡导下，临床药师成为治疗团队中的一部分，以自身的优势，与临床医生及不同临床部门共同合作，提供更高质量的以患者为中心的医疗服务。

4. "BPS"的全称"**B**oard of **P**harmacy **S**pecialties"（药学专业委员会）。自 70 年代以来，在美国临床药师相继出现了专业的细化，例如核药学、营养药学、药物治疗学、肿瘤药学等不同的分支，这些分支都是由不同方向的药学专业委员会来管理的。

5. "**C**ontinuing **P**rofessional **D**evelopment (CPD)"的意思是继续职业教育，是针对临床药师在临床实践工作中专业知识的更新完善，可通过不定期的授课、讲座、培训等形式多样的方式进行。

笔记

Supplementary Parts

1. Medical and Pharmaceutical Terms Made Easier (10): Common Morphemes of Numbers in Medical & Pharmaceutical English Terms

Number	Greek & Latin Morphemes	Number	Greek & Latin Morphemes
1/2	hemi-, semi-	27	heptacosa
1	mono-, haplo-, uni-	28	octacosa
2	di-, bi-, duo-, bis-	29	nonacosa
3	tri-, triplo-, ter-	30	triaconta
4	quarto-, tetra-, quadri-	31	hentriaconta
5	pento-, quinque-	40	tetraconta
6	hexa-, sex(i)-	50	pentaconta
7	hepta-, septi-	60	hexaconta
8	octa-	70	heptaconta
9	nona-, novem-	80	octaconta
10	deca-, decem-	90	enneaconta
11	undeca, hendeca	10^{18}	exa- (E)
12	dodeca	10^{15}	peta- (P)
13	trideca	10^{12}	tera- (T)
14	tetradeca	10^{9}	giga- (G)
15	pentadeca	10^{6}	mega- (M)
16	hexadeca	10^{3}	kilo- (k)
17	heptadeca	10^{2}	hecto- (h)
18	octadeca	10^{1}	deca- (da)
19	nonadeca	10^{-1}	deci- (d)
20	eicosa	10^{-2}	centi- (c)
21	heneicosa	10^{-3}	milli- (m)
22	docosa	10^{-6}	micro- (μ)
23	tricosa	10^{-9}	nano- (n)
24	tetracosa	10^{-12}	pico- (p)
25	pentacosa	10^{-15}	femto- (f)
26	hexacosa	10^{-18}	atto- (a)

2. English-Chinese Translation Skills: 药学英语翻译技巧 (6)：被动句翻译

药学英语中大量使用被动结构，以动作对象作为主语，将动作发出者隐退，强调过程和结果。翻译被动句时，可根据句子整体结构、使用语境以及汉语表达习惯，采用恰当的方法。一般说来，药学英语被动句翻译可以有以下三种方法：①将被动句译成汉语的主动句；②将被动句译成汉语的无主句；③将被动句译成汉语的被动句。

1.　将被动句译成汉语的主动句　英语中被动结构常常用 in、by 等介词将动作发出者表示出来，将英文句子被动结构翻译成汉语主动结构，是一种常见的翻译策略。如：

例 1：A good number of the products found in a grocery or drug store are regulated by the FDA.

参考译文：许多在食品店和药店中可以找到的产品都由 FDA 管理。

有时候英语原句中动作发出者没有出现，将被动句翻译成主动句时，可以根据具体情况加上一个主语。如：

例 2：Significant efforts through genomic approaches have been dedicated towards the identification of novel protein interactions as promising therapeutic targets for indications such as Alzheimer's disease, Parkinson's disease and neuropsychiatric disorders.

参考译文：科学家针对识别新型蛋白质相互作用的基因组学方法做出了大量研究工作，这些新型蛋白质相互作用可为如阿尔兹海默病、帕金森病、神经精神紊乱等疾病提供较有希望的治疗方法。

说明：上面例句是一个简单句，主句是被动结构，主语是 significant efforts through genomic approaches，译文根据上下文增加了主语"科学家"，将原被动句改成了主动句，并且利用重复 novel protein interactions，将原句拆分成两个小句，表达顺畅自然。

2. 将被动句译成汉语的无主句

例3：A drug such as neomycin will not be absorbed when given orally and will appear in the feces unchanged.

参考译文：像新霉素这类药物口服不吸收，原形在粪便中排出。

说明：此例句中有两个被动结构，分别出现在谓语部分和时间状语从句中，译文很好地理解原句成分的结构关系，将被动结构用主动式表述出来。

例4：Many fundamental biological processes, such as regulation of blood pressure, learning and memory, defence against microorganisms and tumors are now known to be dependent upon the formation of metal nitrosyl complexes.

参考译文：现在已经知道，诸如血压的调节、学习和记忆、微生物及肿瘤的预防等许多基本生物过程都依赖于金属亚硝基络合物的形成。

说明：根据英语和汉语语言表达习惯，例句中原文被动结构在翻译成汉语时变成了主动结构，在原被动结构无法准确确定动作发出者的情况下，可以用无主句陈述。

英语中有一种结构，比如 It has been established that… 在翻译成汉语时往往都译成无主句。

例5：It has been pretty well established that the increase in strains of bacteria resistant to an antibiotic correlates directly with the duration and extent of use of that antibiotic in a given location.

参考译文：现在已经确定在一些地区抗生素广泛和长期的使用与细菌耐药性增加有直接的相互关系。

类似这样的英语结构还有：it is reported…It has been accepted that…It is estimated that… 等等，有时候这样的结构还可以加个主语，译成"人们……"。

3. 将被动句译成汉语的被动句   有时候，出于表达效果需要，英语中被动句也被译成汉语被动句。如：

例6：Medications for food producing animals, often mixed with feeds, are closely monitored because remaining drug residues in the animal tissue are ultimately consumed at dinner tables.

参考译文：食用动物使用的药物经常和饲料混合在一起，也是受到严密监督的，因为在动物组织中的药物残留物最终会在餐桌上被吃掉。

说明：原文中有两个被动结构 are closely monitored 和 are consumed 出现在主句和从句中，译文用"受到……""被……"等保留了它们的被动结构，分别译成"受到严密监督""被吃掉"，突显了被动动作，更好地表述了原文的意思。

笔记

Unit Eleven Drug Safety and Efficacy

The concepts of efficacy and safety have not been suddenly discovered or created. They have always existed in medical thought. In an intuitive sense, an efficacious and safe medical technology is one that "works" and causes no undue harm. That statement may sound naive to individuals working in the field of health today. However, for a major portion of the history of medicine, efficacy and safety were measured by that intuitive standard. Furthermore, that intuitive standard still lies at the heart of medical practice, but the meaning and measurement of those concepts have evolved with increased sophistication of scientific methods in medicine.

Measurement of efficacy and safety is in essence an examination of interventions in the processes by which various phenomena affect health and disease. Neither these phenomena (whether they be biological, psychological, or social) nor the interventions (often, technologies) need be thought of as having a fully predictable mechanistic effect. A probabilistic view of effects—that is, when an event occurs, there is a range of possibilities that other events will occur—is more useful. The concept of probability is used to summarize the effects of causal variables which are unknown or not taken into account. Thus, we can speak of estimating or evaluating efficacy and safety, but not exactly determining them. Specific technologies have certain probabilities of effects; therefore, efficacy and safety information is normally expressed in terms of probabilities.

效能与安全的概念并非突然发现或创造的，它们一直存在于医学思维中。凭直观感觉而言，一种有效并安全的医疗技术是指它"奏效了"且造成的伤害不大。这种表述如今在健康领域工作的人看来显得粗浅幼稚。然而，在相当长的医学历史中，效能与安全性均凭直观标准判断，而且这种直观标准依然存在于医疗实践中。不过那些概念的含义和测定随着医学科学方法的日益精密复杂而不断演化。

效能与安全性的测定本质上是对治疗干预的检验，在这一过程中各种因素都会影响健康和疾病。这些因素（无论是生理、心理或社会的）和治疗干预（通常是技术）均不需要被认为具有完全可预测的机械效应。采用发生概率来考察效应更为有效，亦即当一个事件发生时，有一定的可能性其他事件将会发生。概率的概念用来总结未知的或未纳入考虑的因果变量的效应。因此，我们可以说估计或评估效能和安全性，但无法精确地测定它们。特定技术有产生一定作用的概率，因此，效能和安全性信息通常是用发生概率来表示。

笔记

Text A
Drug Safety and Efficacy

Obviously, a drug (or any medical treatment) should be used only when it will benefit a patient. Benefit takes into account both the drug's ability to produce the desired result (efficacy) and the type and likelihood of adverse effects (safety). Cost is commonly also balanced with benefit.

Efficacy and Effectiveness

Efficacy is the capacity to produce an effect (e.g., lower BP). Efficacy can be assessed accurately only in ideal conditions (ie, when patients are selected by proper criteria and strictly adhere to the dosing schedule). Thus, efficacy is measured under expert supervision in a group of patients most likely to have a response to a drug, such as in a controlled clinical trial.

Effectiveness differs from efficacy in that it takes into account how well a drug works in real-world use; often, a drug that is efficacious in clinical trials is not very effective in actual use. For example, a drug may have high efficacy in lowering BP but may have low effectiveness because it causes so many adverse effects that patients stop taking it. Effectiveness also may be lower than efficacy if clinicians inadvertently prescribe the drug inappropriately (e.g., giving a fibrinolytic drug to a patient thought to have an ischemic stroke, but who had an unrecognized cerebral hemorrhage on CT scan). Thus, effectiveness tends to be lower than efficacy.

Patient-oriented outcomes, rather than surrogate or intermediate outcomes, should be used to judge efficacy and effectiveness.

Patient-oriented outcomes

Patient-oriented outcomes are those that affect patients' well being. They involve the following:
- Prolongation of life
- Improved function (e.g., prevention of disability)
- Relief of symptoms

Surrogate outcomes

Surrogate or intermediate outcomes involve things that do not directly involve patients' well being. They are often such things as physiologic parameters (e.g., BP) or test results (e.g., concentrations of glucose or cholesterol, tumor size on CT scan) that are thought to predict actual patient-oriented outcomes. For example, clinicians typically presume that lowering BP will prevent the patient-oriented outcome of uncontrolled hypertension[1] (e.g., death resulting from MI or stroke). However, it is conceivable that a drug could lower BP but not decrease mortality, perhaps because it has fatal adverse effects. Also, if the surrogate is merely a marker of disease (e.g., HbA_{1c}) rather than a cause of disease (e.g., elevated BP), an intervention might lower the marker by means that do not affect the underlying disorder. Thus, surrogate outcomes are less desirable measures of efficacy than patient-oriented outcomes.

On the other hand, surrogate outcomes can be much more feasible to use, for example, when patient-oriented outcomes take a long time to appear (e.g., kidney failure resulting from uncontrolled hypertension) or are rare. In such cases, clinical trials would need to be very large and run for a long

笔记

time unless a surrogate outcome (e.g., lowered BP) is used. In addition, the main patient-oriented outcomes, death and disability, are dichotomous (i.e., yes/no); whereas surrogate outcomes are often continuous, numerical variables (e.g., BP, blood glucose). Numerical variables, unlike dichotomous outcomes, may indicate the magnitude of an effect. Thus, use of surrogate outcomes can often provide much more data for analysis than can patient-oriented outcomes, allowing clinical trials to be done using many fewer patients.

However, surrogate outcomes should ideally be proved to correlate with patient-oriented outcomes. There are many studies in which such correlation appeared reasonable but was not actually present. For example, treatment of certain postmenopausal women with estrogen and progesterone resulted in a more favorable lipid profile but failed to achieve the hypothesized corresponding reduction in MI or cardiac death. Similarly, lowering blood glucose to near-normal concentrations in patients with diabetes in the ICU resulted in higher mortality and morbidity (possibly by triggering episodes of hypoglycemia) than did lowering blood glucose to a slightly higher level. Some oral antihyperglycemic drugs lower blood glucose, including HbA_{1c}^{2} concentrations, but do not decrease risk of cardiac events. Some antihypertensive drugs decrease BP but do not decrease risk of stroke.

Adverse Effects

Similarly, clinically relevant adverse effects are patient-oriented outcomes; examples include the following:

- Death
- Disability
- Discomfort

Surrogate adverse effects (e.g., alteration of concentrations of serum markers) are often used but, as with surrogate efficacy outcomes, should ideally correlate with patient-oriented adverse effects. Clinical trials that are carefully designed to prove efficacy can still have difficulty identifying adverse effects if the time needed to develop an adverse effect is longer than the time needed for benefit to occur or if the adverse effect is rare. For example, cyclooxygenase-2 (COX-2) inhibitors[3] relieve pain quickly, and thus their efficacy can be shown in a comparatively brief study. However, the increased incidence of MI caused by some COX-2 inhibitors occurred over a longer period of time and was not apparent in shorter, smaller trials. For this reason, and because clinical trials may exclude certain subgroups and high-risk patients, adverse effects may not be fully known until a drug has been in widespread clinical use for years.

Many drug adverse effects are dose-related.

Balancing Benefits and Adverse Effects

Whether a drug is indicated depends on the balance of its benefits and harms. In making such judgements，clinicians often consider factors that are somewhat subjective, such as personal experience, anecdotes, peer practices, and expert opinions.

The **number needed to treat (NNT)** is a less subjective accounting of the likely benefits of a drug (or any other intervention). NNT is the number of patients who need to be treated for one patient to benefit. For example, consider a drug that decreases mortality of a certain disease from 10% to 5%, an absolute risk reduction of 5% (1 in 20). That means that of 100

笔记

patients, 90 would live even without treatment, and thus would not benefit from the drug. Also, 5 of the 100 patients will die even though they take the drug and thus also do not benefit. Only 5 of the 100 patients (1 in 20) benefit from taking the drug; thus, 20 need to be treated for 1 to benefit, and the NNT is 20. NNT can be simply calculated as the inverse of the absolute risk reduction; if the absolute risk reduction is 5% (0.05), the NNT = 1/0.05 = 20. NNT can be calculated for adverse effects also, in which case it is sometimes called the number needed to harm (NNH)[4].

Importantly, NNT is based on changes in *absolute* risk; it cannot be calculated from changes in *relative* risk. Relative risk is the proportional difference between two risk levels. For example, a drug that decreases mortality from 10% to 5% decreases absolute mortality by 5% but decreases relative mortality by 50% (i.e., a 5% death rate indicates 50% fewer deaths than a 10% death rate). Most often, benefits are reported in the literature as relative risk reductions because these make a drug look more effective than the absolute risk reductions (in the previous example, a 50% reduction in mortality sounds much better than a 5% reduction). In contrast, adverse effects are usually reported as absolute risk increases because they make a drug appear safer. For example, if a drug increases the incidence of bleeding from 0.1% to 1%, the increase is more likely to be reported as 0.9% than 1000%.

When balancing NNT against NNH, it is important to weigh the magnitude of specific benefits and harms. For example, a drug that causes many more harms than benefits may be worth prescribing if those harms are minor (e.g., reversible, mild) and the benefits are major (e.g., preventing mortality or morbidity). In all cases, patient-oriented outcomes are best used.

Genetic profiling[5] is increasingly being used to identify subgroups of patients that are more susceptible to the benefits and adverse effects of some drugs. For example, breast cancers can be analyzed for the HER2[6] genetic marker that predicts response to particular chemotherapy drugs. Patients with HIV/AIDS can be tested for the allele HLA-B*57:01, which predicts hypersensitivity to abacavir, reducing the incidence of hypersensitivity reactions and thus increasing NNH. Genetic variations in various drug-metabolizing enzymes help predict how patients respond to drugs and also often affect the probability of benefit, harm, or both.

Therapeutic index

One goal in drug development is to have a large difference between the dose that is efficacious and the dose that causes adverse effects. A large difference is called a wide therapeutic index, therapeutic ratio, or therapeutic window. If the therapeutic index is narrow (e.g., < 2), factors that are usually clinically inconsequential (e.g., food-drug interactions, drug-drug interactions, small errors in dosing) can have harmful clinical effects. For example, warfarin has a narrow therapeutic index and interacts with many drugs and foods. Insufficient anticoagulation increases the risk of complications resulting from the disorder being treated by anticoagulation (e.g., increased risk of stroke in atrial fibrillation), whereas excessive anticoagulation increases risk of bleeding.

Word Study

1.　abacavir [æbækæ'viə] *n.* 阿巴卡韦（抗病毒药）
2.　allele [ə'li:l] *n.* 等位基因
3.　anecdote ['ænikdəut] *n.* 轶事，奇闻

笔记

4. antihypertensive [ˈænti:haipəˈtensiv] *adj.* 抗高血压的，降压的

5. causal   [ˈkɔːzl] *adj.* 原因的，关于因果的

6. conceivable [kənˈsiːvəbl] *adj.* 想得到的，可想像的，可能的

7. dichotomous [daiˈkɔtəməs] *adj.* 分成两个的，叉状分枝的

8. estrogen [ˈestrədʒən] *n.* 雌激素

9. evolve [iˈvɔlv] *v.* （使）逐步形成，（使）逐步演变，进化

10. fibrinolytic [faibrinəuˈlitik] *adj.* 纤维蛋白溶解的

11. hemorrhage [ˈheməridʒ] *n.* 出血，溢血，失控的行为

12. hypoglycemia [ˌhaipəuglaiˈsiːmiə] *n.* [医] 血糖过低，低血糖症

13. inadvertently [inədˈvəːrtəntli] adv. 不注意地，疏忽地，非故意地

14. intuitive [inˈtuːitiv] *adj.* 直觉的

15. progesterone [prəˈdʒestərəun] *n.* 孕酮，黄体酮

16. surrogate [ˈsəːrəgət] *n.* 代理人，代用品，代孕者；*adj.* 替代的

17. undue [ˌʌnˈduː] *adj.* 过分的，不适当的

Notes

1. uncontrolled hypertension: 顽固性高血压

2. HbA$_{1c}$: hemoglobin A$_{1c}$，糖化血红蛋白 A$_{1c}$

3. cyclooxygenase-2 (COX-2) inhibitors: 环氧化酶 -2 抑制剂

4. the number needed to harm (NNH) : 出现伤害事件时所需的受治人数，NNH 愈大，则药物愈安全。

5. Genetic profiling: 遗传识别，基因图谱，即基于鉴定身份的目的对人体组织或体液样品进行 DNA 分析的过程。

6. HER2 : human epidermal growth factor receptor 2，人表皮生长因子受体 2

Exercises

1. Decide whether each of the following statements is true (T) or false (F) according to the passage.

(1) The intuitive standard used for the measurement of efficacy and safety in medical history are no longer used today.

(2) Unlike effectiveness, efficacy cannot be evaluated accurately even in an ideal environment.

(3) Surrogate outcomes are preferred measures of efficacy than patient-oriented outcomes, because they can be much more feasible to use.

(4) Adverse effects may only be fully known after a drug has been in widespread clinical use for a long time.

(5) Even a drug that causes many more harms than benefits, it may still be worth prescribing to patients.

(6) A drug with wide therapeutic window is often safer than those with narrow ones.

2. Questions for oral discussion.

(1) Are efficacy and effectiveness the same thing?

(2) What do surrogate or intermediate outcomes involve?

(3) Tell us something about the advantage of surrogate outcomes.

(4) What kind of risk do you know is used when reporting adverse effects? And why?

笔记

3. Choose the best answer to each of the following questions.

(1) _____should be used to judge efficacy and effectiveness.

A. Surrogate and intermediate outcomes　　B. Surrogate outcomes

C. Patient-oriented outcomes　　D. Intermediate outcomes

(2) Surrogate or intermediate outcomes involve things that do not directly involve patients'

_____.

A. life　　B. function

C. symptom　　D. well being

(3) Lowering blood glucose to a _____ higher level in patients with diabetes resulted in lower mortality and morbidity than did lowering blood glucose to near-normal concentrations.

A. much　　B. slightly

C. very　　D. rather

(4) If the adverse effect is_____, a clinical trial that is designed to prove efficacy may have difficulty identifying adverse effects.

A. common　　B. moderate

C. severe　　D. rare

(5) Which of the following statements is TRUE?

A. Patients with HIV/AIDS can be tested for the allele HLA-B*57:01, which predicts hypersensitivity to abacavir, reducing the incidence of hypersensitivity reactions and thus decreasing NNH.

B. Some patients may be hypersensitive to abacavir.

C. Abacavir might reduce the incidence of hypersensitivity reactions.

D. Patients with HIV/AIDS are not suggested to take abacavir if they are not hypersensitive to it.

(6) The increased incidence of MI occurred over a longer period of time and was not noticed in shorter, smaller trials of _____.

A. drugs　　B. progesterone

C. COX-2 inhibitors　　D. chemotherapy drugs

(7) _____ increases risk of bleeding.

A. Insufficient warfarin

B. Insufficient anticoagulation

C. Excessive warfarin

D. Excessive coagulation

(8) Which of the following statements is TRUE?

A. Drugs that are efficacious in clinical trials may not be very effective in clinical uses.

B. A drug that is proved effective in a clinical trial will have similar effectiveness in actual use.

C. A drug that is efficacious in clinical trials will always be not very effective in actual use.

D. A drug will certainly be efficacious in actual use if it was already proved in clinical trials.

(9) Which of following elements is not involved in Patient-oriented outcomes?

A. prolongation of life

B. prevention of disability

C. concentrations of cholesterol

D. relief of symptoms

(10) Clinicians often consider factors that are somewhat_____, such as personal experience,

笔记

anecdotes, peer practices, and expert opinions.

A. objective

B. subjectively

C. subjective

D. objectively

4. **Fill in each of the following blanks with an appropriate word or expression according to the meaning of the sentence(s).**

> subjective; adverse; absolute; relative; insufficient; dichotomous; wide; inadvertently; benefit; naive

(1) The statement that an efficacious medical technology is one that "works" and causes no undue harm may sound _____ to health workers today.

(2) The number of patients who need to be treated for one patient to_____ is defined as NNT.

(3) Effectiveness may be lower than efficacy if clinicians_____ prescribe the drug inappropriately.

(4) The main patient-oriented outcomes, such as death and disability, are_____.

(5) The number needed to treat is a less _____ accounting of the likely benefits of a drug.

(6) A lot of drug _____effects are dose-related.

(7) It is important that NNT cannot be calculated from changes in _____ risk.

(8) Adverse effects of drugs are often reported as _____ risk increases because they make a drug appear safer.

(9) Usually, a large difference is called a _____therapeutic index or therapeutic window.

(10) _____anticoagulation increases the risk of complications resulting from the disorder being treated by anticoagulation

5. **Translate the following sentences and paragraphs into Chinese.**

(1) A drug may have high efficacy in lowering lipid level but may have low effectiveness because it causes fatal adverse effects that stop patients from taking it.

(2) Because numerical variables may indicate the magnitude of an effect, use of surrogate outcomes can often provide more data than patient-oriented outcomes, allowing clinical trials to be done using fewer patients.

(3) Efficacy may be assessed accurately when patients are selected by proper criteria and strictly adhere to the dosing schedule.

(4) Obviously, kidney failure resulting from uncontrolled hypertension is not a surrogate outcome.

(5) Many studies in which the correlation that surrogate outcomes correlated with patient-oriented outcomes appeared rather reasonable but was not actually present.

(6) Most often, benefits are reported in the literature as relative risk reductions because these make a drug look more effective than the absolute risk reductions. In contrast, adverse effects are usually reported as absolute risk increases because they make a drug appear safer. For example, if a drug increases the incidence of bleeding from 0.1% to 1%, the increase is more likely to be reported as 0.9% than 1000%.

(7) The main patient-oriented outcomes, death and disability, are dichotomous (i.e., yes/no), whereas surrogate outcomes are often continuous, numerical variables. Numerical variables, unlike dichotomous outcomes, may indicate the magnitude of an effect. Thus, use of surrogate outcomes can often provide more data for analysis than patient-oriented outcomes, allowing clinical trials to be done using fewer patients.

笔记

Text B
Drug Safety and Efficacy: Two Sides of the Same Coin

This year, the 110th Congress of the United States will consider a drug safety legislation that could have a direct effect on the entire biomedical community. The legislation could affect the ease with which drugs can be developed, proven safe and effective, and reach the public in a timely manner[1]. The Food and Drug Administration (FDA) plays a pivotal role in analyzing the benefits and risks of new therapies and also must ensure continued monitoring of products once they reach the market. Without an optimally functioning FDA, new therapies discovered by some of the world's most talented researchers and developed by our pharmaceutical industry will have little chance to reach patients in a timely manner. A new legislation must be carefully considered to prevent negative unintentional consequences. Instead, the legislation must effectively improve drug safety, ensure access to new drugs, and foster the development of innovative new treatments. Efforts to increase the effectiveness and efficiency of FDA are important and well justified. The agency is currently facing the challenge of strengthening the review of product safety at both pre-approval and post-marketing stages. Several months ago, a committee of academic scientists and clinicians, research advocates, and representatives of the patient community was convened to recommend ways in which policy makers in the Congress and FDA could further strengthen product evaluation. The resulting report, Drug Safety and Drug Efficacy: Two Sides of the Same Coin, released on March 9th, is a proposal for improving drug safety, ensuring new drug access and strengthening the FDA. In the view of this committee, drug efficacy and safety should continue to be evaluated simultaneously by the existing FDA division that is most familiar with the product under review, rather than by a separate center or agency. Furthermore, an expanded and systematic approach to safety surveillance should be implemented. Post-marketing surveillance should utilize a variety of sources to routinely identify and obtain accurate data, have the computational and statistical ability to analyze large-scale information sets, and incorporate emerging scientific tools to improve the methods of distinguishing and describing safety and efficacy signals. FDA currently lacks the resources and personnel to fully integrate the science and technology necessary to develop a systematic approach to safety surveillance. To ensure that FDA has adequate resources, there must be an appropriate commitment of public funds by congress and not exclusively through increases in funds required from the pharmaceutical industry. In addition to resources, FDA will require employee training programs and a commitment to the advancement of science through the Critical Path Initiative[2] to strengthen safety monitoring. Although the current passive surveillance method does provide useful information, it is not as efficient as it could be in detecting emerging safety and efficacy data; it should be strengthened. In addition, an automated post-marketing system of drug monitoring should be created using existing public and private databases. Such a system will improve the agency's ability to identify risks of new marketed products in a timelier manner and to evaluate risks along with the health benefits provided by the product. A benefit-risk approach across a product life cycle is the cornerstone of drug development and should be the foundation of drug regulation as

笔记

well. This is particularly true with regard to drugs for serious and life-threatening diseases like cancer, refractory cardiovascular disease, and neurodegenerative diseases. To focus solely on drug safety without consideration of drug benefit, the severity of the underlying disease, the effectiveness of the product, and the availability of alternative therapies, risks creating a chilling effect on the development of new treatments for patients most in need of innovation.[3] As Congress considers drug safety legislation, it is an opportunity to strengthen and increase the capabilities and efficiency of FDA in all phases of its work. Simply stated, Congress must invest more in the FDA if it expects it to properly carry out its mandate. Whereas recent policy recommendations contain elements that would provide assistance to an over-burdened[4] agency, proposals focused on increasing FDA authority and regulatory oversight do not fully address ways to insure innovation and improvements in overall public health. The goal of the report commissioned by the committee is to provide lawmakers with a balanced perspective from a broad group of physician investigators and advocates who have extensive experience in the field of drug development for patients with serious diseases. The new legislation must achieve the goals of enhancing the drug approval and monitoring process and optimizing the productivity of FDA. Unintentional consequences, such as restricting or slowing patient access to life-saving treatments, or discouraging innovative product development, would be detrimental for the American public. Over-regulation and subsequent slowing of the drug approval process increases the cost of medical care, thereby decreasing access to medications because of their expense. To best position FDA for continued success, the committee encourages members of Congress and FDA officials to implement policies to address the following recommendations:[5]

1. Continually and simultaneously evaluate safety and efficacy when determining public access to and marketing of new products

1.1. Ensure that the regulatory process reflect the essential balance of benefit and risk that is fundamental to all medical decision making;

1.2. Discourage new policies that duplicate existing mechanisms or unnecessarily slow FDA evaluations of new agents;

1.3. Ensure that up-to-date information is accessible to patients and healthcare providers at the time a prescription is written.

2. Improve information technology and increase training to strengthen the effectiveness of the FDA

2.1. Improve informatics systems within FDA;

2.2. Increase training of FDA personnel to enhance agency effectiveness and standards;

2.3. Capitalize on the unique expertise at FDA;

2.4. Minimize future leadership gaps at FDA.

3. Enhance existing infrastructure for adverse event reporting and analysis to improve post-market safety monitoring

3.1. Improve the existing tools for adverse event reporting to enable systematic post-market surveillance;

3.2. Engage public-private partnerships to aid in safety monitoring and data management;

3.3. Examine electronic medical records as a potential data source to enhance widespread systematic tracking for the Adverse Event Reporting System;

笔记

3.4 Equitably share funding for programs to ensure the safety and efficacy of new products between public and private sources.

4.   Advance current scientific opportunities to create a stronger, safer, and science-based FDA

4.1. Increase support for the Critical Path Initiative to modernize FDA;

4.2. Prioritize discovery, evaluation, validation, and clinical application of new biomarkers to improve drug evaluation and refine drug prescribing.

It is the view of the report's authoring committee that with proper advancement, support, and leadership, FDA can move into the 21st century and firmly remain the gold standard of science-based drug review and safety monitoring.[6]

Word Study

1.   advocate ['ædvəkeit] *n.* 提倡者；律师；辩护者

2.   convene [kən'viːn] *vi.* 集合 *vt.* 集合；召集；召唤

3.   cornerstone ['kɔːnəstəun] *n.* 隅石；奠基石

4.   foster [fɔstə] *vt.* 促进；鼓励

5.   legislation [ˌledʒis'leiʃn] *n.* 法律；法规；立法

6.   neurodegenerative [ˌnjuːrəudi'dʒenərətiv] *adj.* 神经变性的

7.   pivotal ['pivətl] *adj.* 重要的；关键的；轴的

8.   refractory [ri'fræktəri] *adj.* 执拗的；难治疗的

Notes

1.   in a timely manner：及时

2.   The Critical Path Initiative (CPI)：关键路径计划，是美国 FDA 在 21 世纪初建立的一个战略项目，旨在推动医药产品在开发、评价、生产等过程中的科学创新。

3.   To focus solely on drug safety without consideration of drug benefit, the severity of the underlying disease, the effectiveness of the product, and the availability of alternative therapies, risks creating a chilling effect on the development of new treatments for patients most in need of innovation. 译为：仅着眼于药品安全性而忽略药品带来的益处、基础疾病的严重性、产品的有效性、替代疗法的实用性以及为患者开发新的治疗手段时产生寒蝉效应的风险，这种做法最迫切需要改革。其中 chilling effect 为美国英语，意为"寒蝉效应"（阻碍言论自由的行为或局面）；"令人寒心、失望的效应"。此句强调不能片面关注安全性。

4.   over-burdened：超负荷，负担过重

5.   To best position FDA for continued success, the committee encourages members of Congress and FDA officials to implement policies to address the following recommendations. 译为：为使 FDA 获得最佳定位取得持续成功，该委员会在劝说审定政策的国会议员和 FDA 官员时提出了如下建议。句中 position 为动词，意为"把……放在适当位置"；implement 意为"使……生效""使实行起来"。

6.   It is the view of the report's authoring committee that with proper advancement, support, and leadership, FDA can move into the 21st century and firmly remain the gold standard of science-based drug review and safety monitoring. 译为：报告起草委员会认为，通过适当的促进、支持和领导，FDA 能在迈进 21 世纪时依然坚定地保持基于科学的药品审查和安全监测的黄金标准。

笔记

Supplementary Parts

1. Medical and Pharmaceutical Terms Made Easier (11): Irregular Singular and Plural Forms of Greek & Latin Endings in Nouns

Singular	Plural	Example (Singular)	Example (Plural)	Meaning
-a	-ae	antenna	antennae	触角，天线
		aqua	aquae	水（剂）
		conjunctiva	conjunctivae	结膜
		cornea	corneae	角膜
		mucosa	mucosae	黏膜
		formula	formulae	公式
-is	-es	analysis	analyses	分析
		dermatosis	dermatoses	皮肤病
		diagnosis	diagnoses	诊断
		hydrolysis	hydrolyses	水解
		paralysis	paralyses	麻痹
-ix	-ices	appendix	appendices	阑尾，附录
		cervix	cervices	颈
-ex,	-ices	cortex	cortices	皮质
-ax	-aces	thorax	thoraces	胸
-ma	-mata	carcinoma	carcinomata	癌
		fibroma	fibromata	纤维瘤
-um	-a	bacterium	bacteria	细菌
		cerebrum	cerebra	大脑
		myocardium	myocardia	心肌
		spectrum	spectra	光谱
-us	-i	fungus	fungi	真菌
		bacillus	bacilli	杆菌
		focus	foci	病灶
-on	-a	phenomenon	phenomena	现象
		protozoon	protozoa	原虫

Write down the plural forms of the following words.

1) formula   _____

2) analysis   _____

3) appendix   _____

4) thorax   _____

5) fibroma   _____

6) cerebrum   _____

7) bacillus   _____

8) phenomenon   _____

2. English-Chinese Translation Skills: 药学英语翻译技巧 (7)：定语从句翻译

定语从句在句子结构中属于次要成分，但在语言表达功能上却占有重要地位。药学英语中大量使用定语从句，有长有短，结构有繁有简，对先行词的限制有强有弱，起着补充说明作用。汉语中定语成分，包括定语从句都是在所修饰名词之前，少有结构复杂、描述性强的定语从句用在名词前面。因此翻译英语定语从句时，不能一律把它们译成前置定语。药学英语英译汉

笔记

中，定语从句有时候不一定译成定语，根据实际情况还可以译成表示目的、让步、条件状语等。从技巧上看，翻译定语从句可以采用拆分法、转译法等。

例 1：This review summarizes these studies with an emphasis on major natural antioxidants found in three categories of plant-based foods (fruits, vegetables and legume) and mechanisms that these antioxidants may use in promoting cardio-health.

参考译文：本文对这些实验进行了综述性总结，并着重强调了植物性食物即水果、蔬菜、豆类中发现的三种主要天然抗氧剂，以及这些抗氧剂促进心血管健康的作用机制。

说明：例句中 mechanisms 后面有一个定语从句，译文直接根据汉语表达习惯将定语从句前置，这种处理法是英汉语翻译中常见的方法，符合英汉两种语言特点。但是在药学英语翻译中大多数定语从句翻译则要视具体情况而定。

例 2：Green tea is a widely consumed beverage that has attracted more attention in the recent years due to its health benefits like antioxidant, antimicrobial, anticarcinogenic and anti-inflammatory properties.

参考译文：绿茶饮料由于具有抗氧化、抗菌、抗癌和抗炎等特性，近年来消费量极大，受到人们越来越多的关注。

说明：例句原文主句是 Green tea is a widely consumed beverage. 在 beverage 后面有一个 that 引导的定语从句。译文根据实际情况，没有将定语从句提前到名词之前做前置定语，而是将定语从句拆分开来，单独成句，与主句并列，从整体看，并没有改变原句意思，符合汉语表达习惯。

一般来讲，翻译非限定性定语从句时要用拆分法，但要注意被拆分小句与原来主句之间顺序，而且往往要重复被修饰的名词。如：

例 3：Inhaled insulin, which could replace shots for millions of people with diabetes, won approval Friday from the Food and Drug Administration, making it the first new form of insulin since the hormone was discovered nearly 90 years ago.

参考译文：吸入胰岛素可以代替成百万糖尿病患者所采用的注射方式，它在星期五获得了(美国)食品与药品管理局的许可，这使它成为发现该激素近 90 年以来第一种新形式的胰岛素。

说明：例句原文中，which 引导的非限定性定语从句修饰前面 inhaled insulin。译文采用了拆分法将定语从句和主句分译成两个小句，根据原文的意思，将定语从句小句放在前面，并将原主句的主语用"它"表示，译文顺畅自然，符合汉语言表达习惯。但有时候非限定性定语从句采用拆分法翻译时，表达效果不是很好，这个时候可以将非限定性定语从句糅合到主句当中，增加主句信息容量，如：

例 4：Pharmacognosy is a study of drugs that originate in the plant and animal kingdoms.

参考译文：生药学研究动植物界中的药物。

在有些情况下，英语中定语从句可以翻译成汉语中状语从句，但转译从句功能前提是不能改变原句意义，并且要符合汉语言表达习惯。如：

例 5：When some of the structures and functions of the body deviate from the norm to the point where the ability to maintain homeostasis is destroyed or threatened or where the individual can no longer meet environmental challenges, disease is said to exist.

参考译文：当机体的某些结构和功能偏离正常值，维护内环境的能力受到破坏或受到威胁时，或者是个体再也不能面对环境的挑战时，就可以说患病了。

说明：例句中 to the point 后面有两个 where 引导的定语从句，表示程度，但细致分析原文结构和意思，这里的定语从句具有表示时间的意思，因此译文将两个 where 引导的定语从句处理成时间状语从句，跟前面 when 引导的时间状语从句并列，没有改变原文意思，也使译文自然流畅。

Unit Twelve Drug Regulation

Drug laws and regulations aims to regulate all activities pertaining to drug R&D, manufacture, distribution, use and surveillance. They function to ensure drug quality, safeguard the safety and efficacy of medications and crack down the manufacture and sale of adulterants and counterfeits. Different categories of laws and regulations are required upon manufacturers, distributors, non-clinical safety evaluation research institutions and clinical trials institutions. The main categories can be summarized as: laws and regulations for drug R&D, such as GLP and GCP; laws and regulations for drug manufacture, such as GMP; laws and regulations for drug distributions, such as GSP; laws and regulations for medication use and pharmaceutical administration, such as Controlled Substances Act.

药事法规是规范药品研发、生产、经营、使用和监督管理的法规,对于保证药品的质量,保障人民用药安全、有效,打击制售假药、劣药发挥着重要作用。需对药品生产企业、经营企业、药品非临床安全性评价研究机构和临床试验机构分别实行不同的法律法规。药品管理法律法规主要可归纳为以下几个方面:药品研发领域法律法规,例如《药物非临床研究质量管理规范》(GLP)与《药物临床试验质量管理规范》(GCP);药品生产领域法律法规,例如《药品生产质量管理规范》(GMP);药品流通领域法律法规,如《药品经营质量管理规范》(GSP);药品使用领域法律法规及药品监督领域法律法规,例如《特殊管制药物法案》。

笔记

Text A
Good Manufacturing Practices (GMP)

GMP is probably the most widespread quality system followed across the pharmaceutical industry as a whole. GMP compliance is a requirement within the R&D environment for the manufacture and testing of clinical trial materials (both drug product and API[1]) and for commercial manufacture and testing of these materials for human and animal consumption. R&D facilities performing these operations may be subject to audit for compliance to GMP; commercial facilities will be audited by the appropriate regulatory authority, possibly without prior warning.

1. USA/ GMP Regulations

The USA Food, Drugs and Cosmetics Act (FD&C Act)[2] states that "All drugs shall be manufactured, processed and packaged in accordance with current good manufacturing practice". No distinction is drawn between the manufacture of drug products (secondary manufacture) and the manufacture of APIs (primary manufacture). It is also noted in the preamble to the FD&C Act that the act applies to all drugs for human use, and this therefore includes the requirement for both APIs and drug products manufactured for clinical trials, to be manufactured according to Current Good Manufacturing Practice (cGMP).

The requirements for compliance to cGMP are laid down in the following Code of Federal Regulations (21CFR)[3]:

Part 210 Current Good Manufacturing Practice in manufacturing, processing, packing or holding of drugs;

Part 211 Current Good Manufacturing Practice for finished pharmaceuticals.

It must be noted that the US regulations refer to current GMP. The regulations as detailed in 21CFR parts 210 and 211, give the pharmaceutical manufacturer plenty of scope to interpret the requirements appropriately for his specific facility and process, but in doing this, the regulations require the manufacturer to adopt best current practice. The onus is placed upon the manufacturer to keep current with what the industry is doing (best practice), with what the current interpretations of the regulations are, and what the US FDA's expectations are.

Although the FD&C Act requires all drugs (products and APIs) to be manufactured to cGMP, the regulations 21CFR parts 210 and 211 are only mandatory for the manufacture of drug products and not APIs. In the past, the onus has been on the pharmaceutical industry to interpret these requirements with respect to the manufacture of APIs. FDA has published guidelines in the form of guides for FDA investigators, to assist industry to meet compliance to cGMP and to place their interpretation on cGMP requirements for APIs and a number of other key areas such as impurities in new drugs, allowable solvent residues and stability testing. Guides issued by International Conference on Harmonization of Technical Requirements for Registration of Pharmaceuticals for Human Use (ICH) have now supplemented most of these guidelines and these, along with other FDA guidelines, will be discussed in more detail later.

These regulations and guidelines may not always be appropriate for the manufacture of clinical trial materials. Although most of the regulations are reasonably applicable in an R&D drug product environment, they may become inappropriate where attempts are made to apply them to

笔记

the early manufacture of clinical APIs within an R&D environment. It is only with the issue of the International Conference on Harmonization (ICH), Harmonized Tripartite Guideline ICH Q7 A—Good Manufacturing Practice Guide for *Active Pharmaceutical Ingredients* in November 2000, that the worldwide pharmaceutical industry finally received detailed guidance for manufacture of APIs for both commercial and R&D purposes.

If one looks at the major headings of 21CFR part 211, the similarity with other quality systems becomes apparent. The following areas of these regulations that will be most important for a pharmaceutical analyst will be:

Organization and personnel—this includes the requirement to have a Quality Control (QC) unit having responsibility and authority to approve and reject all starting materials, drug product containers, closures, in-process materials, packaging materials, labeling and drug products and the authority to review production records to assure that no errors have occurred or, if errors have occurred, that they have been fully investigated. Further requirements cover laboratory facilities and the responsibility of the quality unit for approving or rejecting all materials, specifications and procedures.[4] The responsibilities of the quality unit must be described in written procedures.

Laboratory controls—this part covers mainly calibration of equipment, testing and release procedures, stability testing, reserve samples, laboratory animals and penicillin contamination.

Records and reports—this part describes the key records that require to be retained. These include starting materials and container/closure records, labeling records, production records, production record review, laboratory records, distribution records and complaint files.

These requirements can be further compared with the ICH guidelines for API manufacture later when discussing worldwide harmonization.

In conclusion, the USA cGMP regulations apply to interstate commerce within the USA and to any facility worldwide, that exports pharmaceutical materials (drug products, APIs, or components of these products) to the USA or, wishes to perform clinical trials in the USA. These facilities are open to inspection for cGMP compliance by US FDA inspectors and for those facilities found to be in non-compliance with these requirements the material will be deemed adulterated with respect to identity, strength, quality, and purity. Products from these facilities will be refused entry for sell or use within the USA. Data from these facilities may not be accepted in support of regulatory filings.

2. EU/UK GMP Requirements

Two European directives lay down the principles and guidelines for GMP in the EU, one for medicinal products for human use and the other for veterinary products. These directives have been incorporated in the national law of member states. The European Commission has issued nine volumes of *the rules governing medicinal products in the EU*. The latest edition was issued in 1998. Volume four covers GMP for medicinal products for human and veterinary use. These are now used as a basis for inspection by the various national regulatory authorities [e.g. Medicines and Healthcare Products Regulatory Agency (MHRA) in the UK].

If one looks at the requirement of the EU GMP rule, the similarity with 21 CFR part 211 is clear, as is the consistency with other quality systems.

3. USA/EU GMP Differences

Historically, there have been distinct and fundamental differences between USA regulation and

笔记

EU/UK requirements for GMP. As discussed previously, the US required all drugs to be made to GMP requirements and performed inspections throughout the world in support of these requirements. In the UK, only drug products and biological manufacturers (not APIs, except some specified antibiotics) were inspected by the regulatory authority for compliance to GMP. Other EU countries, such as France and Italy, did require audits of API manufacturers, but the requirements and standards varied widely throughout the EU.

Although drug product manufacturers have always been audited by the UK authorities, the UK GMP guideline (The Orange Guide) was not mandatory and did not have the force of law. The original European Directive defined a medicinal product as "Any substance or combination of substances presented for treating or preventing disease in human beings or animals." This applied to finished pharmaceutical dosage forms (drug products) only.

There are fundamental differences between a drug product and API that makes the application of many GMP drug product requirements difficult or inappropriate. An API is normally prepared by chemical processes that involve purification at each stage of manufacture, and early raw materials and processing stages may not have much influence over the quality of the final API. Impurities that are present in the final API will not be removed and will still be present in the manufactured drug product. Similarly, if the morphic form of the API is changed through unassessed changes in the API manufacture, this could have a considerable effect on the bioavailability of the drug product. To use the API based on end-product testing, as previously discussed, is not in keeping with the principles of Quality Assurance (QA).

Historically, in the UK and Europe, there has been no legal requirement to manufacture drug products or APIs to GMP for use in clinical trials (investigational medicinal products, IMPs[5]). This has always been a requirement under the USA FD&C Act.

The situation in the EU with respect to APIs and IMPs is now changing with the requirement for consistent standards throughout the EU and the wish to harmonize inspection standards and other regulatory requirements with other countries. The lack of GMP controls for APIs and IMPs has been seen as a major barrier to harmonization with the USA. Harmonization with the US through a Mutual Recognition Agreement (MRA) is seen as a big saving of inspection resources to both the EU and the USA, through mutual acceptance of facility inspection reports.

Word Study

1. closure [ˈkləuʒə] *n.* 密封件
2. morphic [ˈmɔːfik] *adj.* 形态(上)的
3. onus [ˈəunəs] *n.* 义务,职责,责任
4. preamble [priˈæmbl] *n.* 前文,序文,前言
5. residue [ˈrezidu:] *n.* 残渣,残留
6. strength [streŋθ] *n.* 效力,浓度

Notes

1. API: active pharmaceutical ingredient 活性药物成分,即法规中通常所说的原料药。
2. Food, Drugs and Cosmetics Act (FD&C Act): 美国联邦食品、药品、化妆品法案。A set of laws passed by Congress in 1938 giving authority to the U.S. Food and Drug Administration (FDA) to oversee the safety of food, drugs, and cosmetics.

笔记

3. Code of Federal Regulations (21CFR):　联邦法规。The codification of the general and permanent rules published in the Federal Register by the executive departments and agencies of the Federal Government; 50 titles totally and the 21st title pertaining to food and drug.

4. Further requirements cover laboratory facilities and the responsibility of the quality unit for approving or rejecting all materials, specifications and procedures. 译为：更进一步的要求包括实验室设施，以及质量部门批准或拒收所有物料、质量标准和规程的职责。

5. investigational medicinal products, IMPs：临床研究用药物，注意 "investigational" 一词的使用。

Exercises

1. Decide whether each of the following statements is true (T) or false (F) according to the passage.

(1) GMP compliance is a requirement only for the manufacture of drug products.

(2) According to FD&C Act, only drug products shall be manufactured in accordance with cGMP.

(3) ICH Q7 A is a worldwide guidance for the manufacture of drug products for both commercial and R&D purposes.

(4) Same as that in the USA, all drug products are inspected by the regulatory authority for compliance to GMP in the UK.

(5) Impurities in the final API will be removed because it will influence the quality of drug products.

(6) Each stage of API production will influence the quality of final API.

2. Questions for oral discussion.

(1) Please state briefly the scope that GMP is applied to.

(2) Please discuss the development of regulations and guide in the USA for the manufacturing of APIs.

(3) Please describe the differences between the US regulations and EU requirements for GMP.

(4) What are the characteristics of APIs?

3. Choose the best answer to each of the following questions.

(1) GMP are regulating activities in the _____ of drugs.

　　A. manufacturing　　　　　　　　B. distribution

　　C. clinical trials　　　　　　　　D. non-clinical trials

(2) GMP compliance is a requirement for the manufacture of _____

　　A. APIs　　　　　　　　　　　　B. investigational medicinal products

　　C. drug products　　　　　　　　D. all of the above

(3) GMP compliance requirement is stated in _____.

　　A. FD&C Act　　　　　　　　　　B. CFR

　　C. ICH　　　　　　　　　　　　　D. MRA

(4) Which of the following is not appropriate for the interpretation of the word "current"?

　　A. keeping current with the best practice of pharmaceutical industry

　　B. keeping current with the interpretations of the regulations

　　C. keeping current with FDA's expectations

　　D. keeping current with the requirements of patients.

(5) ICH Q7 A is a guideline for the manufacture of _____.

　　A. drug products　　　　　　　　B. APIs

　　C. raw materials　　　　　　　　D. biologics

笔记

(6) The cGMP of the US applies to the following except _____.

　　A. interstate commerce within the USA

　　B. any facility worldwide which exports pharmaceutical material to the USA

　　C. any facility wishes to import pharmaceutical material from the USA

　　D. any facility wishes to perform clinical trials in the USA

(7) _____ is the drug regulatory agency in the UK.

　　A. FDA　　　　　　　　　　　　　B. MHRA

　　C. EMA　　　　　　　　　　　　　D. CFDA

(8) Which of the following statements about the US and the UK requirements on GMP is NOT true?

　　A. The US required all drugs should be manufactured according to GMP requirements.

　　B. The UK only inspected drug products and biological manufacturers.

　　C. The UK GMP was mandatory.

　　D. The US GMP has the force of law.

(9) Which of the following statements on the manufacture of API is NOT true?

　　A. An API is normally prepared by chemical processes.

　　B. Impurities present in final API will be removed.

　　C. The manufacturing processes involve purification at each stage.

　　D. The impurities in API will not influence the quality of drug product.

(10) "Starting material" includes _____

　　A. raw material　　　　　　　　　　B. excipients

　　C. both A and B　　　　　　　　　　D. packaging material

4. Please choose appropriate word from a list of word bank to complete the following sentences

> compliance; FD&C Act; ICH Q7A; non-clinical; impurities; bioavailability;
> mandatory; current; investigational; APIs

(1) That all drugs shall be manufactured in accordance with cGMP is specified in _____.

(2) It is only with the issue of _____ that the pharmaceutical industry finally received the guidance for the manufacture of APIs.

(3) _____ GMP is the practice adopted by pharmaceutical industry in the US.

(4) GLP is a practice regulating activities in _____ process.

(5) _____ present in final API will not be removed.

(6) In the UK, GMP guideline was not _____ and only drug products manufacturers, not _____, were inspected to comply with GMP.

(7) If there is a change in the morphic form of API, a considerable effect on _____ will be the result.

(8) GMP _____ is also required within the R&D environment for the manufacture and testing of _____ medicinal products.

5. Translate the following sentences and paragraphs into Chinese.

(1) GMP compliance is a requirement within the R&D environment for the manufacture and testing of clinical trial materials (both drug product and API) and for commercial manufacture and testing of these materials.

(2) It is only with the issue of ICH Q7 A that the worldwide pharmaceutical industry finally received detailed guidance for manufacture of APIs for both commercial and R&D purposes.

(3) Any facility wishes to perform clinical trials in the US should be inspected for GMP compliance.

笔记

(4) QC unit has responsibility and authority to approve and reject all starting materials, drug product containers, closures, in-process materials, packaging materials, labeling and drug products.

(5) Harmonization with the US through a Mutual Recognition Agreement (MRA) is seen as a big saving of inspection resources to both the EU and the USA, through mutual acceptance of API facility inspection reports.

(6) There have been distinct and fundamental differences between USA regulation and EU/UK requirements for GMP. The US required all drugs to be made to GMP requirements and performed inspections throughout the world in support of these requirements. In the UK, only drug products and biological manufacturers (not APIs. except some specified antibiotics) were inspected by the regulatory authority for compliance to GMP.

(7) An API is normally prepared by chemical processes and even if purification is involved at each stage of manufacture, impurities in APIs cannot be removed thoroughly. Therefore, trace impurities are allowed to be present in drug product to a limited extent. If the morphic form of the API is changed through unassessed changes in the API manufacture, this could have a considerable effect on the bioavailability of the drug product.

Text B
Opioid Risk Management in the US

(Adapted from *Foundations of Opioid Risk Management*)

Affecting at least 75 million Americans each year, acute and chronic pain remain inadequately treated, despite the availability of effective treatment options for many sufferers. Opioids play a central and incontrovertible role in the management of acute pain and pain secondary to cancer. Indeed, accumulated evidence indicates that opioid analgesics yield well-tolerated and adequate pain relief in 70% to 90% of patients with cancer pain. Government agencies involved in healthcare policy, such as the US Department of Health and Human Services (HHS)[1] and the Agency for Healthcare Research and Quality, and professional organizations, such as the American Pain Society and American Academy of Pain Medicine, recognize the benefits of adequate pain management and the pivotal palliative role for opioids in the treatment of chronic cancer pain and moderate to-severe acute pain.

A 1986 case series study revealed that long-term opioid therapy, in some cases lasting more than 7 years, can be a safe and effective treatment option in selected patients with noncancer pain. Other, more recent studies, have confirmed these findings in chronic noncancer pain populations, including subpopulations with neuropathic pain. In carefully selected patients, opioid therapy can provide at least partial analgesia without intolerable side effects or the development of aberrant drug-related behaviors. Yet, many primary care physicians and specialists remain uncomfortable prescribing opioid analgesics, a potential barrier to the effective treatment of chronic pain.

Physician lack of comfort may be related to insufficient understanding about the abuse potential and side effects of the agents, insufficient methods for detection of possible diversion and abuse by patients, or concern with the criminal justice aspects of interdiction with abuse and diversion. Additional factors may include limited data on the long-term safety and efficacy of opioid analgesics, including the risk of addiction, creating legitimate uncertainties about the risk-benefit ratio[2] of long-term opioid therapy.

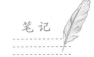 笔记

In recent years, the expanded use of opioid analgesics for the treatment of chronic noncancer pain and the introduction of high-dose, extended-release[3] opioid formulations with high oral bioavailability have, while improving access to analgesia for many patients, magnified opportunities for diversion and abuse. As the legitimate and clinically prudent use of prescription opioid analgesics has grown, 2-fold for fentanyl and 4-fold for oxycodone, prescription opioid abuse as a percentage of all drug abuse cases has also increased. Prescription opioid abuse has become an increasingly significant public health issue, with an abuse incidence now surpassing that for most conventional street drugs, including heroin. The total financial costs associated with prescription opioid abuse, including healthcare costs and lost productivity, has been estimated at approximately $10 billion annually.

Efforts to address prescription opioid abuse may have the undesirable consequence of diminishing legitimate access to opioids; conversely, actions to improve access to opioids for legitimate pain may fuel the prescription opioid abuse problem. The risks for opioid diversion and abuse must be addressed in an effective and medically prudent manner, coordinated among the various stakeholders, without hindering the legitimate use of opioid analgesics for patients in whom this modality has demonstrated benefits—the so-called "balanced" approach. The same considerations apply to efforts to promote greater access to analgesics for the treatment of pain.

No single governmental or private entity has responsibility for overseeing opioid risk reduction programs. Instead, this responsibility is spread among disparate groups. Chief among them are federal and state agencies, as well as the pharmaceutical industry and healthcare payers, and, finally, clinicians and patients themselves. Each of these stakeholders has different goals and responsibilities with regard to opioid risk management. These goals and responsibilities are often split between those oriented toward optimizing pain relief and those oriented toward minimizing opioid abuse and diversion.

For more than 90 years, the federal government has exerted an important influence on opioid analgesic use. The US Food and Drug Administration (FDA) and the US Drug Enforcement Administration (DEA) share the primary federal regulatory authority and responsibility for opioid risk management. The US Substance Abuse and Mental Health Services Administration (SAMHSA), which includes the Center for Substance Abuse Treatment, plays a key role in surveillance of drug abuse and supports delivery of addiction treatment services, and the US National Institute on Drug Abuse (NIDA) supports drug abuse research.

FDA

FDA's essential mandate is to protect public health, which includes regulating the marketing of prescription drugs. The statutory foundation for FDA's responsibilities related to drug safety in this area springs from the Federal Food, Drug, and Cosmetics (FD&C) Act, especially as amended in 1962[4]. The FD&C Act does not provide authority for FDA to regulate the practice of medicine, which is a responsibility of the states. Based on the FD&C Act of 1962, FDA exercises critical oversight over prescription drugs by regulating approval for marketing based on efficacy and safety data—including their potential for abuse—submitted by the drug's sponsor, usually the manufacturer. In the development of a new drug, FDA evaluates a drug's potential for abuse based on a composite profile of the drug's chemistry, pharmacology, clinical actions, and similarity to other drugs in its class. If evidence of abuse potential emerges, FDA requires the sponsor to provide all data relevant to abuse at the time of New Drug Application submission. If the benefits of a new drug are deemed to outweigh the risks, and if the labeling instructions permit the safe use of the product in the indicated treatment population, FDA typically considers the drug safe for marketing.

DEA

The Controlled Substances Act (CSA)[5] of 1970 charges the DEA with regulating the production and distribution of controlled substances to control their nonmedical use. Under the provisions of the CSA, the DEA schedules controlled substances; sets production quotas; regulates prescribers, dispensing pharmacies, manufacturers, distributors, importers, researchers, etc.; and plays a role in law enforcement activities to stem drug abuse and diversion. The CSA is not intended to supersede the FD&C Act. The CSA provides for a closed system of distribution, encompassing manufacturers, distributors, pharmacies, and physicians, by which the distribution of prescription drugs with the potential for abuse can be controlled.

All drugs with a potential for abuse, termed controlled substances, are placed into one of 5 schedules (schedules I to V) based on their medical usefulness and potential for abuse. Schedule I drugs (eg, heroin, LSD[6]) manifest a high potential for abuse and no medically recognized therapeutic value in the US. Prescription drugs with a potential for abuse, that is, controlled substances with approved medical uses, are placed into schedules II to V, based on their abuse potential. Schedule II includes those pharmaceuticals with the highest potential for abuse. The placement of a drug into a particular schedule is not irrevocable; controlled drugs can move from one schedule to another, based on new information related to abuse. The DEA, HHS, or private petitioners, including the drug's manufacturer, can each initiate proceedings to add, delete, or change the schedule of a specific drug. By statute, FDA and DEA consider many factors when determining whether a drug will be scheduled or removed from scheduling. HHS has the power to veto scheduling of a drug.

State Regulation

Neither FDA nor the DEA has statutory authority to regulate medical practice. This responsibility lies with the individual states under the sections of state constitutions intended to protect public health and safety. States can require that a drug prescription be filled within a specified amount of time after it is written, and they can classify drugs at a higher level of abuse risk than the CSA schedule or place the drug on a state controlled substance list if not on the CSA list. Similar to federal law, state-controlled substance laws prohibit nonmedical use of controlled substances; yet, unlike federal laws, many state regulations have not recognized the clinical benefits of controlled substances, including opioid analgesics, or the need to ensure their availability for medical purposes.

Excessive state regulation and monitoring has the potential to hinder the appropriate management of pain by raising the specter of regulatory scrutiny and discipline for "inappropriate" prescribing, a recognized barrier to treatment. Indeed, 40% of physician members of the American Pain Society have indicated that regulatory, not medical, concerns have dissuaded them from prescribing opioids for chronic noncancer pain.

Optimal pain treatment necessarily involves the appropriate use of opioid analgesics and the prevention and management of opioid abuse and diversion. In recent years, considerable progress has been made toward achieving a balance between the benefits and risks of opioid analgesic therapy; yet, much remains to be done. As the appropriate use of opioid therapy has laudably increased, the parallel increased risk for opioid abuse and diversion has been an unwelcome companion that

笔记

raises regulatory scrutiny and physician and patient fears. Although certain beneficial trends have emerged in recent years, they represent a growing recognition of the therapeutic importance of opioid analgesia in selected patients and critical steps toward a balanced approach to the effective management of chronic pain that should continue into the future.

Word Study

1. aberrant [æ'berənt] *adj.* 脱离正道的
2. analgesia [ˌænəl'dʒiːʒə] *n.* 止痛，痛觉缺失
3. disparate ['dispərət] *adj.* 不同的
4. fentanyl ['fentənil] *n.* 芬太尼（止痛药）
5. interdiction [ˌintə'dikʃn] *n.* 封锁，禁止
6. irrevocable [i'revəkəbl] *adj.* 不可挽回的，不能变更的
7. mandate ['mændeit] *n.* 命令
8. modality [məu'dæləti] *n.* 模式
9. neuropathic [ˌnjurə'pæθik] *adj.* 神经病的
10. opioid [əu'piːəuid] *n.* 阿片类
11. oxycodone [ˌɔksi'kəudəun] *n.* 羟考酮
12. palliative ['pæliətiv] *adj.* 缓和的
13. petitioner [pə'tiʃənə] *n.* 请愿人
14. veto ['viːtəu] *v.* 否决

Notes

1. the US Department of Health and Human Services (HHS)：美国卫生和公众服务部。The Department of Health and Human Services is the United States government's principal agency for protecting the health of all Americans and providing basic human services.
2. risk-benefit ratio：利弊比，利弊关系。It's the key principle for FDA's new drug approval. Only when benefits outweigh the risks can FDA consider the drug is safe enough to be marketed.
3. extended-release：缓释的。
4. …especially as amended in 1962. It refers to amendment to FD&C Act in 1962, in which pharmaceutical manufacturer firstly was required to show a drug's effectiveness before marketing.
5. The Controlled Substances Act (CSA)：管制药品法案。It is the statute prescribing federal U.S. drug policy under which the manufacture, importation, possession, use and distribution of certain substances is regulated.
6. LSD: Lysergic acid diethylamide, D- 麦角酸二乙胺。It is a powerful semi-synthetic hallucinogen.

Supplementary Parts

1. Medical and Pharmaceutical Terms Made Easier (12): Morphemes from Latin and Greek in Medical and Pharmaceutical English Terms

在医药英语术语中，我们经常可以发现表达某一个含义的词素不止一个。这往往是由于它们分别来自希腊语、拉丁语等不同语言。一般来说，来自希腊语的词素往往出现在更为专业的术语中，来自拉丁语的词素往往出现在相对基础的专业术语中。在此，我们通过下表中列举的部分词根来加以提醒：

Latin	Greek	English Meaning	Chinese Meaning	Examples
ventro-	coelio-, laparo-	belly (abdomen)	腹	ventrodorsad 向腹背 coeliotomy 腹部切开术 laparoscope 腹腔镜
bili-	chole-	bile	胆	bilirubin 胆红素 cholecyst 胆囊
vesico-	cysto-	bladder	膀胱	vesicotomy 膀胱切开术 cystolith 膀胱结石
sangui-	em- hemo- hemato-	blood	血	sanguinopoietic 造血的 anemia 贫血 hemoperitoneum 腹腔积血 hematemesis 吐血；咯血
os(se)o-	osteo-	bone	骨	osseous 骨的，骨质的 osteomyelitis 骨髓炎
mammo-	masto-	breast	乳	mammography 乳房 X 线照相术 mastoid 乳头状的
auri-	oto-	ear	耳	auricular 耳状的 otitis 耳炎
oculo-	ophthalmo-	eye	眼	binocular 用两眼的 ophthalmology 眼科学
palpebro-	blepharo-	eyelid	睑	palpebral conjunctiva 睑结膜 blepharitis 睑炎
lip-	steato-	fat	脂肪	lipemia 脂血 steatorrhea 脂肪泻
gingivo-	ulo-	gum	龈	gingivitis 牙龈炎 ulorrhagia 牙龈出血
cord-	cardi-	heart	心	cordiform 心形的 cardiology 心（脏）病学
reno-	nephro-	kidney	肾	renal 肾的 nephrectomy 肾切除术
labio	cheilo-	lip	唇	labionasal 唇鼻音，唇鼻音的 cheiloschisis 唇裂（畸形）
pulmo-	pneumo-	lung, air	肺，气	pulmonary 肺部的 pneumothorax 气胸
oro-	stomato	mouth	口	orolingual 口与舌的 stomatology 口腔病学
ungui-	onychi-	nail	甲	unguis 爪，蹄 onychia 甲床炎
nerv-	neuro-	nerve	神经	nervous 神经的 neuroblast 成神经细胞
naso-	rhino-	nose	鼻	nasopharynx 鼻咽 rhinology 鼻科学
palato-	urano-	palatine	腭	palatitis 腭炎 uranoschisis 腭裂
cutano-	derm(at)o-	skin	皮	cutaneous 皮肤的，影响皮肤的 dermoid 皮样的，皮状的
lieno-	spleno	spleen	脾	lienectomy 脾切除术 splenomegaly 脾肿大

笔记

续表

Latin	Greek	English Meaning	Chinese Meaning	Examples
lacrimo-	dacryo-	tear	泪	lacrimal 泪腺的，泪的 dacryocyst 泪囊
denti-	odonto-	tooth	牙齿	dentistry 牙科 odontodynia 牙痛
omphalo-	umbilico-	umbilicus	脐	omphalitis（幼小动物患的）脐炎 umbilical hernia 脐疝
vagino-	colpo-	vagina	阴道	vaginorrhaphy 阴道缝合术 colposcope 阴道镜
veno-	phlebo-	vein	静脉	venograft 静脉移植 phlebitis 静脉炎
vaso-	angio-	vessel	血管	vasomotor 血管收缩的 angiography 血管造影术，
utero-	hystero- metro-	womb, uterus	子宫	uterine 子宫的 hysteroscope 子宫镜 endometrium 子宫内膜

(1) Fill in the blanks with certain Latin affix, Greek affix or its English meaning according to the given Chinese meaning.

Chinese meaning	Latin affix	Greek affix	English meaning
Sample: 腹	ventro-	coelio-, laparo-	belly (abdomen)
静脉	veno-		vein
神经	nerv-		
心		cardi-	heart
骨			bone
膀胱	vesico-		

(2) Fill in the blanks with the missing word root, prefix or suffix.

1) _____rubin 胆红素
2) _____nopoietic 造血的
3) _____cular 耳状的
4) bin_____ 用两眼的
5) _____emia 脂血
6) _____rrhagia 牙龈出血
7) _____ectomy 肾切除术
8) _____logy 口腔病学
9) _____pharynx 鼻咽
10) _____megaly 脾大
11) _____cyst 泪囊
12) _____graphy 血管造影

2. English-Chinese Translation Skills: 药学英语翻译技巧 (8)：状语从句翻译

药学英语语篇较多使用状语从句，表示时间、原因、条件、让步、目的、结果等意义。状语从句通常可以直接翻译，但需要注意的是在翻译过程中如何正确处理状语从句与主句的位置。由

笔记

于英汉两种语言表达形式不同,翻译状语从句要根据汉语言表达习惯灵活处理。

状语从句翻译也要看句子具体情况而定,并非所有状语从句都要直接翻译出来,有时候状语从句也可以跟主句糅合在一起。比如:

例1:There are two types of diabetes. Type 1 occurs when the body doesn't produce any insulin. People with type 2 diabetes don't produce enough insulin or their cells ignore the insulin.

参考译文:糖尿病分为两型。1型是指人体不制造胰岛素。2型是指人体未制造足够多的胰岛素或是人体细胞不识别胰岛素。

说明:译文很好地将时间状语从句 when the body doesn't produce any insulin 与主句 Type 1 occurs 糅合在一起,没有改变原句意思,汉语表述简洁流畅。

翻译状语从句时,要正确划分主句和从句,理清楚主句与从句之间的逻辑关系。例如在翻译原因状语从句时,要根据句子内容出发确定好哪个是"因",哪个是"果",比如:

例2:Isolation of natural products differs from that of the more commonly occurring biological macromolecules because natural products are smaller and chemically more diverse than the relatively consistent proteins, nucleic acids and carbohydrates, and isolation methods must take this into account.

参考译文:天然产物的分离不同于通常出现的生物大分子,因为天然产物与常见的组成成分蛋白质、核酸和碳水化合物相比,分子量小且更具化学多样性,所以分离方法也要将这些因素考虑在内。

说明:例句原文由三个小句组成,结构并不复杂,正确理解和翻译的关键是判断 because 引导的原因状语从句到哪里结束,这是翻译药学英语状语从句较为重要的环节。根据原文意思并结合药学基础知识,译文通过增加连词"所以",很好地界定了原文三个小句之间的逻辑关系。

有时候,状语从句与主句之间的逻辑关系并不是十分明显,翻译时可以将主从句关系处理成并列关系。

例3:A few antibiotics have such toxic effects that their usefulness is strictly limited.

参考译文:有些抗生素有毒性作用,其应用受到严格限制。

说明:例句中 such…that… 结构表示"如此……以至于……",是结果状语从句,译文将这种显然的"因果"关系处理成两个并列小句,没有改变原句意思。

有时候不同逻辑关系状语从句也可以因为表达需要而进行转换,前提当然还是不能够改变原句意思。如:

例4:Drugs with such serious potential dangers as these should be used only if life is threatened and nothing else will work.

参考译文:这些有严重危险的药物只有在生命受到威胁或其他药物无效时才使用。

说明:原例句中 only if 引导条件状语从句,译文在没有改变原句意思的情况下将这个从句处理成时间状语从句。再如:

例5:All the possible troubles that can result from antibiotic treatment should not keep anyone from using one of these drugs when it is clearly indicated. Nor should they discourage certain preventive uses of antibiotics which have proved extremely valuable.

参考译文:由于有些抗生素疗效确切,因此使用抗生素所带来的所有可能的麻烦也不能阻止任何人用任何一种抗生素,对于被证明是有效的抗生素,人们不会不鼓励它们的使用。

说明:例句有两个小句。第一句中,主句是 All the possible troubles should not keep anyone from using one of these drugs,从句是 when 引导的时间状语从句。译文没有将 when 引导的从句翻译成时间状语从句,而是译成原因状语从句:"由于有些抗生素疗效确切",并没有改变原句意思。第二句中没有状语从句,只有 which 引导的定语从句修饰 antibiotics,但是译文将这个定语从句处理成了状语:"对于被证明是有效的抗生素"。从整个句子来看,参考译文虽有将从句功能进行转译,但没有改变原文意思,而且符合汉语言表达习惯。

笔记

Unit Thirteen Pharmacopoeia

Pharmacopoeia is an official compendium containing drug standard and specifications in a country. Pharmacopoeia is usually compiled and implemented under the supervision of the health administration department of the country and the international pharmacopoeia is compiled under the negotiation of the publicly recognized organizations and countries. Setting drug standards plays a crucial role in regulating the drug quality, ensuring the quality and safety of medication and guaranteeing the people's health. Drug standard is the most important component in drug modern production and the quality regulation, and is also the statutory basis jointly followed by the departments of drug production, drug supply and drug use and the supervision and management departments. Drug standard usually includes official name, description, identification, purity test, content (potency or activity) assay, dosage, strength, storage and preparation etc. Some important pharmacopoeias include United States Pharmacopoeia/National Formulary, British Pharmacopoeia, European Pharmacopoeia, and Japanese Pharmacopoeia.

药典是一个国家记载药品标准、检测项目的法典，一般由国家卫生行政部门主持编纂、颁布、实施，国际性药典则由公认的国际组织及有关国家协商编订。制定药品标准对加强药品质量的监督管理、保证质量、保障用药安全、有效维护人民健康起着十分重要的作用。药品标准是药品现代化生产和质量管理最重要的组成部分，是药品生产、供应、使用和监督管理部门共同遵循的法定依据。药品标准一般包括以下内容：法定名称、性状、鉴别、纯度检查、含量（效价或活性）测定、剂量、规格、贮藏、制备等。现在世界上主要药典有：《美国药典/国家处方集》《英国药典》《欧洲药典》以及《日本药局方》。

笔记

Text A
The United States Pharmacopoeia

The United States Pharmacopoeia (USP)—the National Formulary (NF) is published in continuing pursuit of the mission of United States Pharmacopoeia Convention (USPC): To improve the health of people around the world through public standards and related programs that help ensure the quality and safety of medicines and foods.

This text from USP-NF provides background information on the United States Pharmacopoeia Convention (USPC), as well as general information about the 38th revision of the United States Pharmacopeia (USP 38) and the 33rd edition of the National Formulary (NF 33).

1. History of USP—NF

On January 1st, 1820, 11 physicians met in the Senate Chamber of the U.S. Capitol building to establish a pharmacopoeia for the United States. These practitioners sought to create a compendium of the best therapeutic products, gave them useful names, and provided recipes for their preparation. Nearly a year later, on December 15th, 1820, the first edition of The Pharmacopoeia of the United States was published. Over time, the nature of the United States Pharmacopeia (USP) changed from being a compendium of recipes to a compendium of documentary standards that increasingly are allied with reference materials, which together establish the identity of an article through tests for strength, quality, and purity. The publishing schedule of the USP also changed over time. From 1820 to 1942, the USP was published at 10-year intervals; from 1942 to 2000, at 5-year intervals; and beginning in 2002, annually.

In 1888, the American Pharmaceutical Association published the first national formulary under the title *The National Formulary (NF) of Unofficial Preparations*. Both the USP and the NF were recognized in the Federal Food and Drugs Act of 1906 and again in the Federal Food, Drug, and Cosmetic Act of 1938. In 1975, USP acquired the National Formulary (NF), which now contains excipient standards with references to allied reference materials. Today, USP continues to develop USP and NF through the work of the Council of Experts into compendia that provide standards for articles based on advances in analytical and metrological science. As these and allied sciences evolve, so do USP and NF.[1]

USP's governing, standards-setting, and advisory bodies include the USP Convention, the Board of Trustees, the Council of Experts and its Expert Committees, Advisory Panels, and staff. Additional volunteer bodies include Stakeholder Forums, Project Teams, and Advisory Groups, which act in an advisory capacity to provide input to USP's governing, standards-setting, and management bodies.[2]

2. Legal Recognition

Recognition of USP-NF—USP-NF is recognized by law and custom in many countries throughout the world. In the United States, the Federal Food, Drug, and Cosmetic Act (FD&C Act) defines the term "official compendium" as the official USP, the official NF, the official Homeopathic Pharmacopeia of the United States, or any supplement to them. The Food and Drug Administration (FDA) may enforce compliance with official standards in USP-NF under the adulteration and misbranding provisions of the FD&C Act. These provisions extend broad authority to the FDA to prevent entry or to remove designated products from the United States market on the basis of

笔记

standards in the USP-NF.

The identity of an official article, as expressed by its name, is established if it conforms in all respects to the requirements of its monograph and other relevant portions of the compendia. The FD&C Act stipulates that an article may differ in strength, quality, or purity and still have the same name if the difference is stated on the article's label. The FDA requires that names for articles that are not official must be clearly distinguishing and differentiating from any name recognized in an official compendium. Official preparations (a drug product, a dietary supplement including nutritional supplements, or a finished device) may contain additional suitable ingredients.

Drugs   USP's goal is to have substance and preparation (product) monographs in USP-NF for all FDA-approved drugs, including biologics, and their ingredients. USP also develops monographs for therapeutic products not approved by the FDA, e.g., pre-1938 drugs, dietary supplements, and compounded preparations. Although submission of information needed to develop a monograph by the Council of Experts is voluntary, compliance with a USP-NF monograph, if available, is mandatory.

Biologics   In the United States, although some biologics are regulated under the provisions of the Public Health Service Act (PHSA), provisions of the FD&C Act also apply to these products. For this reason, products approved under the PHSA should comply with the adulteration and misbranding provisions of the FD&C Act at Section 501(b) and 502(g) and, thus, should conform to applicable official monographs in USP-NF.

Medical Devices   Section 201(h) of the FD&C Act defines a device as an instrument, apparatus, similar article, or component thereof recognized in USP-NF. There is no comparable recognition of USP's standards-setting authority and ability to define a medical device as exists for other FDA-regulated therapeutic products.

Dietary Supplements   The Dietary Supplement Health and Education Act of 1994 *amendments* to the FD&C Act name USP-NF as the official compendia for dietary supplements. The dietary supplement must be represented as conforming to a USP-NF dietary supplement monograph.

Compounded Preparations   Preparation monographs provide information or standards applicable in compounding. Standards in USP-NF for compounded preparations may be enforced at both the state and federal levels, e.g., if a practitioner writes a prescription for a compounded preparation that is named in a USP-NF monograph, the preparation, when tested, must conform to the stipulations of the monograph so named.

3. Pharmacopoeial Discussion Group's (PDG) Harmonious Activities

A pharmacopoeial monograph for an active ingredient or excipient, preparation, or other substance used in the manufacture or compounding of a medicinal product generally provides a name, definition, description, and sometimes packaging, labeling, and storage statements. Thereafter, the monograph provides tests, procedures, and acceptance criteria that constitute the specification. For frequently cited procedures, a monograph may refer to a general chapter for editorial convenience. The PDG works to harmonize excipient monographs and general chapters. This will reduce manufacturers' burden of performing analytical procedures in different ways, using different acceptance criteria. The PDG, which includes representatives from the European, Japanese, and United States pharmacopoeias, and WHO (as an observer), harmonizes pharmacopoeial excipient monographs and General Chapters. At all times, the PDG works to maintain an optimal level of science consistent with protection of the public health.[3]

4. Revision of USP–NF

USP-NF is continuously revised. Revisions are presented annually, in twice-yearly Supplements, in Interim Revision Announcements (IRAs), and in Revision Bulletins on the USP website.

USP-NF Revision Processes Include:

Public Participation　Although USP's Council of Experts is the ultimate decision-making body for USP-NF standards, these standards are developed by an exceptional process of public involvement and substantial interaction between USP and its stakeholders, both domestically and internationally. Participation in the revision process results from the support of many individuals and groups and also from scientific, technical, and trade organizations.

Requests for revision of monographs, either new monographs or those needing updating, contain information submitted voluntarily by manufacturers and other interested parties. At times USP staff may develop information to support a monograph Request for Revision. USP has prepared a document titled Guideline for Submitting Requests for Revision to USP-NF available USP official website. Via Pharmacopoeial Forum (PF), USP solicits and encourages public comment on these monographs, General Chapters, and other draft documents. USP scientific liaisons to Expert Committees review these responses and create draft proposals that are provided to the Council of Experts. These drafts become official when Expert Committees ballot to make them official in USP-NF. Thus, the USP standards-setting process gives those who manufacture, regulate, and use therapeutic products the opportunity to comment on the development and revision of USP-NF standards.

Working with the FDA　As specified in U.S. law, USP works with the Secretary of the Department of Health and Human Services in many ways.[4] Principal agencies in the Department for this work are the Food and Drug Administration and the Centers for Medicare and Medicaid Services. The FDA Liaison Program allows FDA representatives to participate in Expert Committee meetings, enabling continuing interactions between the FDA scientific staff and Expert Committee activities. Staff in the FDA Centers who are responsible for review of compendial activities provide specific links and opportunities for exchange of comments.

5. USP–NF Publications

Print and Electronic Presentations　All USP-NF publications are available in print form. In addition, USP-NF and its two annual Supplements are available in compact disc (CD) and online versions. The CD version makes USP-NF accessible to users on their computer hard drives. The online format allows individual registered users to access the online format through the Internet.[5] Both electronic formats provide access to official USP-NF content, along with extensive search options. The electronic formats are cumulatively updated to integrate the content of Supplements. Searchable electronic versions of PF and of the USP Dictionary also are available.

6. General Introduction of USP 38–NF 33

USP 38-NF 33 refers to the 38th revision of the United States Pharmacopeia (USP 38) and the 33rd edition of the National Formulary (NF 33). USP 38-NF 33 text is official on May 1, 2015, unless otherwise noted. USP-NF contains official substance and preparation (product) monographs. The terms official substance and official preparation are defined in the General Notices of this Pharmacopeia. With few exceptions, all articles for which monographs are

笔记

provided in USP 38-NF 33 are legally marketed in the United States or are contained in legally marketed articles.

A USP-NF monograph for an official substance or preparation includes the article's definition; packaging, storage, and other requirements; and a specification. The specification consists of a series of universal (description, identification, impurities and assay) and specific tests, one or more analytical procedures for each test, and acceptance criteria. Ingredients are defined as either drug substances or excipients. An excipient is any component, other than the active substance(s), intentionally added to the formulation of a dosage form. Excipients are not necessarily inserted. Drug substances and excipients may be synthetic, semisynthetic, drawn from nature (natural source), or manufactured using recombinant technology. Larger molecules and mixtures requiring a potency test are usually referred to as biologicals or biotechnological articles.

USP 38-NF 33 contains approximately 4900 monographs and more than 220 General Tests and Assays (General Chapters numbered 1,000 and below) and USP General Information Chapters (numbered above 1,000). General Chapters provide frequently cited procedures, sometimes with acceptance criteria, in order to compile into one location repetitive information that appears in many monographs.

Word Study

1. ally ['ælai] *n.* 与……联合，与……结盟
2. amendment [ə'mendmənt] *n.* （对法律或协议的）修订，修正
3. applicable [ə'plikəbl] *adj.* 合适的，可用的
4. ballot ['bælət] *v.* 投票，抽签
5. biologicals [baiə'lɔdʒikl] *n.* 生物制品，生物制剂
6. biotechnological [ˌbaiəuˌteknə'lɔdʒikəl] *adj.* 生物技术的，生物工艺的
7. by-law *n.* 细则，附则，（机构的）内部章程．
8. capitol ['kæpitl] *n.* the Capitol（美国）国会大厦
9. chamber ['tʃeimbə] *n.* 大厅，（尤指）会议厅
10. citation [sai'teiʃn] *n.* 引证，引用
11. compendial [kəm'pendiəl] *adj.* 与药典相关的
12. compendium [kəm'pendiəm] *n.* 概略，概要，汇编（复数 compendia）
13. convention [kən'venʃn] *n.* 惯例，习俗；（国际）公约；大会，会议
14. cumulative ['kjuːmjələtiv] *adj.* 累积的，渐增的
15. designated ['dezigneitid] *adj.* 指定的，标出的
16. documentary [ˌdɔkju'mentri] *adj.* 文献的，书面的
17. eligible ['elidʒəbl] *adj.* 符合条件的，合格的
18. entrust [in'trʌst] *v.* 委托，交托
19. exceptional [ik'sepʃənl] *adj.* 超常的，独特的
20. excipient [ik'sipiənt] *n.* [药学] 赋形剂，辅料 [同 vehicle= 载体]
21. guideline ['gaidlain] *n.* 指导方针，准则，指标
22. homeopathic [həumjə'pæθik] *adj.* 顺势疗法的
23. incorporate [in'kɔːpəreit] *v.* 纳入，合并
24. interim ['intərim] *adj.* （只用在名字前面）临时的，过渡性的
25. liaison [li'eizn] *n.* 通讯，联络

26. Medicare ['medikeə(r)] n. [美国] 国家老年医疗服务制度, 医疗保障方案

27. meterological [,mi:tiərə'lɔdʒikl] adj. 计量的

28. misbrand ['mis'brænd] v. 标示不符, 贴错标签

29. monograph ['mɔnəɡrɑ:f] n. (药典中的) 各论, 专著

30. pharmacist ['fɑ:məsist] n. 药师

31. pharmacopoeia [,fɑ:məkə'pi:ə] n. (同 pharmacopeia) 药典

32. pharmacopoeial [,fɑ:məkə'pi:əl] adj. (同 pharmacopeial) 药典的

33. recipe ['resəpi] n. 处方, 食谱, 烹调法

34. semisynthetic ['semisin'θetik] adj. 半合成的

35. senate ['senət] n. the Senate (美国) 参议院

36. solicit [sə'lisit] v. 恳求, 征求

37. stakeholder [s'teikhəuldə] n. 股东, 利益相关者

38. stipulate ['stipjə,leit] v. 约定, 规定

39. substantial [səb'stænʃəl] adj. 大量的, 多的; 真实的, 实际的

40. thereof [,ðeər'ɔv] adv. 其, 在其中, 关于那

41. trustee [trʌ'sti:] n. 受托人, 托管小组成员

Notes

1. As these and allied sciences evolve, so do USP and NF. 意思是"有了这些工作和科学的进展, USP 和 NF 也得到发展。"这个句子是一个固定结构: As + 主语 + 动词, so + 倒装结构, 意思是"有了……, 就有……"。如: As you sow, so will you reap. 种瓜得瓜, 种豆得豆。

2. Additional volunteer bodies include Stakeholder Forums, Project Teams, and Advisory Groups, which act in an advisory capacity to provide input to USP's governing, standards-setting, and management bodies. 意思是"其他志愿机构包括: 股东论坛、项目团队和顾问小组, 他们以顾问身份给《美国药典》的管理、标准制定和经营机构提供信息。"in an advisory capacity: 以顾问身份。相比较 as an advisor (作为一个顾问), 这是一个比较正式的说法, 又如: in professional/personal/advisory capacity (正式): 以专家 / 个人 / 顾问身份)。

3. 在理解"At all times, the PDG works to maintain an optimal level of science consistent with protection of the public health. "这个句子的时候, 要注意它的结构, "consistent with protection of the public health"是个形容词短语, 做定语修饰前面的"an optimal level of science"。这个句子的意思是: "药典讨论小组的工作始终就是维持最理想的科学水平, 以及保护公共健康"。"at all times"的意思是"总是, 一直"; "be consistent with"的意思是"始终如一的, 与……一致的"。

4. As specified in U.S. law, USP works with the Secretary of the Department of Health and Human Services in many ways. 译为: 根据美国法律规定, 美国药典委员会在许多方面与卫生及公共服务部秘书处有工作关系。注意"As specified in U.S. law"这个结构, 在"as"后面省略了"is/was"; 在意思理解上, as 就代表后面的句子。又如: As stated in the package insert: 正如药品说明书所说。

5. The CD version makes USP-NF accessible to users on their computer hard drives. The online format allows individual registered users to access the online format through the Internet. 译为: CD 版可让用户在电脑硬盘上使用 USP-NF; 个人注册用户可以通过网络使用网络版。"make…accessible to sb."意思是"使某人能够使用 / 得到……"; "allow sb access" 意思是"允许……使用 / 进入"; "registered users": "注册用户"。

笔记

Exercises

1. Decide whether each of the following statements is true (T) or false (F) according to the passage.

(1) In the United States, the Federal Food, Drug, and Cosmetic Act (FD&C Act) defines the term "official compendium" as the official USP, the official NF, the official Homeopathic Pharmacopeia of the United States, but the supplements to them are not included.

(2) The FD&C Act stipulates that the article different in strength, quality, or purity may still have the same name if the difference is stated on the article's label.

(3) If a practitioner writes a prescription for a compounded preparation that is named in a USP-NF monograph, the preparation, when tested, must conform to the stipulations of the monograph so named.

(4) USP-NF is continuously revised. Revisions are presented annually, in twice-yearly Supplements, in IRAs, and in Revision Bulletins on the USP website.

(5) USP-NF and its two annual Supplements are available in print form, and in compact disc (CD) and online versions.

(6) An excipient is any component, including the active substance(s), intentionally added to the formulation of a dosage form, and excipients are the necessarily inert in USP. They may be synthetic, semisynthetic, drawn from nature (natural source), or manufactured using recombinant technology.

2. Questions for oral discussion.

(1) What is the mission of USPC? Can you explain how it pursues it?

(2) What is the legal status of USP in the United States and in the world? Why?

(3) What do you think of USP's revision processes? Which process do you think is the most crucial one?

(4) What is the relationship between USP-NF and Supplements? Are they both official?

3. Choose the best answer to each of the following questions.

(1) The _____ designates the USP–NF as official compendia for drugs marketed in the United State.

A. United States Pharmacopoeia Convention   B. U.S. Federal Food, Drug, and Cosmetics Act

C. Pharmacopoeial Discussion Group   D. Food and Drug Administration

(2) A drug product in the U.S. market must conform to the standards in_____to avoid possible charges of adulteration and misbranding.

A. USP–NF   B. United States Pharmacopoeia

C. National Formulary   D. International Pharmacopoeia

(3) USP–NF is a book of public pharmacopoeial standards for chemical and biological drug substances, dosage forms, and _____.

A. compounded preparations   B. excipients

C. medical devices   D. dietary supplements

(4) _____ and the PDG, harmonizes pharmacopoeial excipient monographs and General Chapters.

A. FDA   B. WHO

C. The Federal Government   D. CFDA

(5) Although _____ is the ultimate decision-making body for USP-NF standards, these standards are developed by an exceptional process of public involvement and substantial interaction between USP and its domestic stakeholders.

笔记

A. Pharmacopoeial Forum   B. Pharmacopoeial Discussion Group

C. USP's Council of Experts   D. United States Pharmacopoeia Convention

(6) Tests and procedures referred to in multiple monographs are described in detail in the USP–NF

_____.

A. general notices   B. general chapters

C. excipient   D. compendial notice

(7) USP-NF contains official substance and preparation (product) monographs and all the texts in

USP38-NF33 are official on _____.

A. May 1, 2012   B. May 1, 2013

C. May 1, 2014   D. May 1, 2015

(8) An_____is any component, other than the active substance(s), intentionally added to the

formulation of a dosage form.

A. excipient   B. placebo

C. addictives   D. ingredient

(9) _____in pharmacopoeia set forth the article's name, definition, specification and other

requirements related to packaging, storage, and labelling.

A. General chapters   B. National Formulary

C. Monographs   D. USP dictionary

(10) The_____is an official compendium containing drug standard and specifications in a country.

A. General chapters   B. National Formulary

C. Monographs   D. Pharmacopoeia

4. **Fill in the blanks in the following sentences with the words given in the box. Change the forms of the words if necessary.**

> molecular weight, official name, trade name, molecular formula, graphic formula, chemical name, brand name, chemical abstract registry number, molecular weight, identification, monograph, test, assay, British Pharmacopoeia, Japanese Pharmacopoeia, United States Pharmacopoeia/National Formulary

(1)

> Aspirin ①
>
> H_3C HO O O ②
>
> $C_9H_8O_4$ ③   180.16 ④
>
> Benzoic acid, 2-(acetyloxy)-Salicylic acid acetate ⑤   [50-78-2] ⑥

① _____   ② _____   ③ _____

④ _____   ⑤ _____   ⑥ _____

(2) To control the quality of drugs, the monograph of a particular drug in Pharmacopoeia must

include _____ item to identify the quality, _____ item to know the purity, and _____ to

determinate the quantity of the drug.

笔记

(3) The _____ and the European Pharmacopoeia are two official compendia within the United Kingdom.

5. Translate the following sentences and paragraphs into Chinese.

(1) The U.S. Pharmacopoeial Convention (USPC) is a scientific nonprofit organization that sets standards for the identity, strength, quality, and purity of medicines, food ingredients, and dietary supplements manufactured, distributed and consumed worldwide.

(2) USP–NF is published in continuing pursuit of the mission of U.S. Pharmacopeial Convention: To improve global health through public standards and related programs that help ensure the quality, safety, and benefit of medicines and foods.

(3) USP–NF is a combination of two compendia, the United States Pharmacopeia (USP) and the National Formulary (NF). Monographs for drug substances, dosage forms, and compounded preparations are featured in the USP. Monographs for dietary supplements and ingredients appear in a separate section of the USP. Excipient monographs are in the NF.

(4) Medicinal ingredients and products will have the stipulated strength, quality, and purity if they conform to the requirements of the monograph and relevant general chapters.

(5) Drug substances and excipients may be synthetic, semi-synthetic, drawn from nature (natural source), or manufactured using recombinant technology. Larger molecules and mixtures requiring a potency test are usually referred to as biologicals or biotechnological articles.

(6) A USP-NF monograph for an official substance or preparation includes the article's definition; packaging, storage, and other requirements; and a specification. The specification consists of a series of universal (description, identification, impurities and assay) and specific tests, one or more analytical procedures for each test, and acceptance criteria.

(7) All USP-NF publications are available in print form. In addition, USP-NF and its two annual Supplements are available in compact disc (CD) and online versions. The CD version makes USP-NF accessible to users on their computer hard drives. The online format allows individual registered users to access the online format through the Internet.

Text B
An Illustrated Guide to USP Standards Using the Acetaminophen Monograph

1. **Acetaminophen**[1]

HO—〈benzene ring〉—N(H)—C(=O)—CH₃

$C_8H_9NO_2$ 151.17

Acetamide, *N*-(4-hydroxyphenyl)-.4'-Hydroxyacetanilide [103-90-2].

2. >>Acetaminophen contains not less than 98.0 percent and not more than 101.0 percent of $C_8H_9NO_2$, calculated on the anhydrous basis.[2]

3. **Packaging and storage**—Preserve in tight, light-resistant containers.

4. **USP Reference standards** <11>—*USP Acetaminophen RS.*

5. **Identification**—[3]

A: *Infrared Absorption* <197K>

B: *Ultraviolet Absorption* <197U>

Solution: 5 μg per ml.

Medium: 0.1N hydrochloric acid in methanol (1 in 100).

C: it responds to *Thin-layer Chromatographic Identification Test* <201>, a test solution in methanol containing about 1 mg per ml and a solvent system consisting of a mixture of methylene chloride and methanol (4:1) being used.

6. **Melting range** <741>: between 168℃ and 172℃.

7. **Water,** *Method I* <921>: not more than 0.5%.

8. **Residue on ignition** <281>: not more than 0.1%.

9. **Chloride** <221>—[4] Shake 1.0 g with 25 ml of water, filter, and add 1 ml of 2 *N* nitric acid and 1 ml of silver nitrate TS: the filtrate shows no more chloride than corresponds to 0.20 ml of 0.020 *N* hydrochloric acid (0.014%).

    Sulfate <221>—Shake 1.0 g with 25 ml of water, filter, add 2 ml of 1 *N* acetic acid, then add 2 ml of barium chloride TS: the mixture shows no more sulfate than corresponds to 0.20 ml of 0.020 *N* sulfuric acid (0.02%).

    Sulfide—Place about 2.5 g in a 50-ml beaker. Add 5 ml of alcohol and 1 ml of 3 *N* Hydrochloric acid. Moisten a piece of lead acetate test paper with water, and fix to the underside of a watch glass. Cover the beaker with the watch glass so that part of the lead acetate paper hangs down near the pouring spout of the beaker. Heat the contents of the beaker on a hot plate just to boiling: no coloration or spotting of the test paper occurs

10. **Heavy metals**[5], *Method II* <231>: 0.001%.

11. **Free *p*-aminophenol**[6]—Transfer 5.0 g to a 100-ml volumetric flask, and dissolve in about 75 ml of a mixture of equal volumes of methanol and water. Add 5.0 ml of alkaline nitroferricyanide solution (prepared by dissolving 1 g of sodium nitroferricyanide and 1 g of anhydrous sodium carbonate in 100 ml of water), dilute with a mixture of equal volumes of methanol and water to volume, mix, and allow to stand for 30 minutes. Concomitantly determine the absorbances of this solution and of a freshly prepared solution of *p*-aminophenol, similarly prepared at a concentration of 2.5 μg per ml, using the same quantities of the same reagents, in 1-cm cells, at the maximum at about 710 nm, with a suitable spectrophotometer, using 5.0 ml of alkaline nitroferricyanide solution diluted with a mixture of equal volumes of methanol and water to 100 ml as the blank: the absorbance of the test solution does not exceed that of the of standard solution, corresponding to not more than 0.005% of p-aminophenol.

    Limit of *p*-chloroacetanilide—Transfer 1.0 g to a glass-stoppered, 15-ml centrifuge tube, add 5.0 ml of ether, shake by mechanical means for 30 minutes, and centrifuge at 1000 rpm for 15 minutes or until a clean separation is obtained. Apply 200 μL of the supernatant, in 40-μL portions, to obtain a single spot not more than 10 mm in diameter to a suitable thin-layer chromatographic plate (see *Chromatography* <621>) coated with a 0.25-mm layer of chromatographic silica gel mixture. Similarly apply 40 μL of a Standard solution in ether containing 10 μg of *p*-chloroacetanilide per ml, and allow the spots to dry. Develop the chromatogram in an unsaturated chamber, with a solvent system consisting of a mixture of solvent hexane and acetone (75:25), until the solvent front has moved three-fourths of the length of the plate. Remove the plate from the developing chamber, mark the solvent front, and allow

笔 记

the solvent to evaporate. Locate the spots in the chromatogram by examination under short-wavelength ultraviolet light: any spot obtained from the solution under test, at an R_f value corresponding to the principal spot from the Standard solution, is not greater in size or intensity than the principal spot obtained form the Standard solution, corresponding to not more than 0.001% of *p*-chloroacetanilide.

12. **Readily carbonizable substances** <271>—Dissolve 0.50 g in 5 ml of sulfuric acid TS: the solution has no more color than *Matching Fluid A*.

13. **Assay**—[7] Dissolve about 120 mg of Acetaminophen, accurately weighed, in 10 ml of methanol in a 500-ml volumetric flask, dilute with water to volume, and mix. Transfer 5.0 ml of this solution to a 100-ml volumetric flask, dilute with water to volume, and mix. Concomitantly determine the absorbances of this solution and of a Standard solution of USP Acetaminophen RS, in the same medium, at a concentration of about 12 μg per ml in 1-cm cells, at the wavelength of maximum absorbance at about 244 nm, with a suitable spectrophotometer, using water as the blank. Calculate the quantity, in mg, of $C_8H_9NO_2$ in the Acetaminophen，taken by the formula: $10C(A_U/A_S)$, in which C is the concentration inμg per ml, of USP Acetaminophen RS in the Standard solution, and A_U and A_S are the absorbances of the solution of Acetaminophen and the Standard solution, respectively.

Word Study

1. acetaminophen [ə,si:tə'minəfen] [药] 对乙酰氨基酚（一种替代阿司匹林的解热镇痛药）
2. absorbance [əb'sɔ:rbəns] *n.* 吸光度
3. infrared absorption [,infrə'red əb'sɔ:rpʃn] *n.* 红外吸收
4. nitroferricyanide [naitrəuferisa'iənaid] *n.* 硝基氰铁酸盐 , 硝基铁氰化物
5. *p*-aminophenol ['pi: 'æminɔfinɔl] *n.* 对氨基苯酚
6. *p*-chloroacetanilide ['pi: klərəusi:'teinilaid] *n.* 对氯苯乙酰胺
7. residue on ignition ['rezidju: ɔn ig'niʃn] *n .* 炽灼残渣
8. sulfate ['sʌl,feit] *n.* 硫酸盐
9. sulfide ['sʌlfaid] *n.* 硫化物
10. ultraviolet [,ʌltrə'vaiələt] *adj.* 紫外线的；*n.* 紫外线

Notes

1. 药典各论中所收载的原料药以法定名称开头,法定名称采用美国采用的名称（USAN）,然后给出药物的描述性信息,包括结构式,化学式,分子量,化学名称和化学文摘（CAS）登记号。

2. 各论中第一项由粗面双 V 形符号引入（>>）,是药物的定义。在定义中,规定药物的含量。它通常根据含量测定项给出药物化学式的百分比,以无水或干燥品来计。合成药物的测定含量通常应不低于 98.0% 且不大于 102.0%。含量限度的数值范围取决于所用测定方法的精密度以及不增加不合理的费用时生产高纯度药物的能力。对一些纯度较低的药物,如来源于天然资源或发酵工艺,以及一些生物制品,它们的含量可以表示为每毫克中所占的毫克数或者以每毫克为单位。

3. 鉴别试验提供了帮助判断药物真伪的一种手段。红外吸收光谱是鉴别药物真伪的最确凿方法。除少数例外,对于某个给定的化合物而言,其官能团的红外吸收带特征往往具有唯一性。如果同时符合红外吸收和紫外吸收两个检查要求"被检测样品的真伪几乎是毋庸置

笔记

疑的"。如果无法获得合适的红外光谱图,薄层色谱鉴别检查也可以是一个不错的替代方法,但必须确保色谱系统能使药物和它密切相关的其他药物成分相分离。

4. 本各论中对氯化物、硫酸盐和硫化物的检查是一类常规检查,各论中对其限量进行了详细说明。

5. 当药物的生产工艺中有可能引入有毒金属时都需要作重金属检查。重金属的限量检查,实际上测定了相对于铅标准溶液的重金属含量。随着现代合成方法的使用以及对酸类物质实施现代化的供应,发达国家对于这项检查的需要有所减少,因此在很多药物各论中,往往会降低重金属存在的允许量。

6. 药物合成或降解过程产生的毒性杂质,具有有害的生物学性质,称为特殊杂质。这些有害杂质必须通过合适的检查方法控制在用药安全的水平。药物生产商必须通知 USP 关于这类杂质的存在,并且需要提供限度检查的方法和论证资料。适宜的限度检查方法可采用色谱法或专属、灵敏的光谱分析法和化学法。

7. 定义项下的含量限度是建立在含量测定项基础之上的,所以含量测定应当力求准确。含量测定项并不需要表明稳定性,但是从各论这一整体来看,应确保能通过色谱或其他专属的方法检测到任一降解产物,并且来限定其含量。理想的组合是色谱试验检查常规杂质外加准确的滴定分析法。只要有可能,HPLC 法应取代抗生素的微生物检查法。然而,对于有多重活性成分构成的抗生素,微生物检查法仍然是一种优选方法,有时可以结合色谱实验来定量单个组分含量。生物制品、蛋白和多肽等药物需要更专业的生物分析法来测定其含量。

Supplementary Parts

1. **Medical and Pharmaceutical Terms Made Easier (13): Common Morphemes in English Terms for Chemistry**

Morpheme	Meaning	Example
chem	化学	biochemistry 生物化学
chrom	铬	chromic 铬的
bar	钡	barium 钡
arg	银	argentaffin 嗜银的
kal	钾	hyperkalemia 高钾血症
natr	钠	hypernatremia 血钠过高
magnes	镁	magnesium 镁
sider	铁	sideropenia 铁(质)缺乏
ferr	铁	ferrated 含铁的
ferro	(二价)铁	ferrous 亚铁的,二价铁的
ferri	(三价)铁	ferric 高铁的,三价铁的
calc	钙	calcium 钙
mercur	汞	mercury 汞,水银
bor	硼	borax 硼砂,硼酸钠
silic	硅	silicon 硅
thi	硫	thiacetazone 氨硫脲
sulf	硫	sulfur 硫
carb	碳	carbon 碳
arsen	砷	arsenic 砷的;含砷的
iod	碘	iodide 碘化物

笔记

续表

Morpheme	Meaning	Example
bromo	溴	bromide 溴化物
hal	卤素	halide 卤化物
fluor	氟	fluorine 氟
hydr	氢	hydrogen 氢
oxy	氧	oxygen 氧
oxid	氧	oxidant 氧化剂
deoxy	脱氧	deoxycytidylic acid 脱氧胞苷酸
desoxy	脱氧	desoxymorphine 脱氧吗啡
chlor	氯	chlorine 氯
nitr	氮，硝基	nitrogen 氮
amin	氨	amine 胺
ammon	氨	ammonia 氨
cyan	氰	cyanide 氰化物
anthrac	炭	anthracosis 炭末沉着病，炭肺
hydr	水	hydragogue 水泻剂
meth	甲基	methane 甲烷，沼气
methyl	甲基	methyl 甲基
ethyl	乙基	ethyl 乙基；乙烷基
acet	乙基	acetaldehyde 乙醛
acyl	酰基	acylase 酰基转移酶
acetyl	乙酰基	acetylcholine 乙酰胆碱
amyl	戊基	amyl 戊基
phen	苯基	phenacetin 乙酰对氨苯乙醚（非那西汀）
phenyl	苯基	phenylalanine 苯丙氨酸
benzyl	苯甲基，苄基	benzyl 苄基，苯甲基
alkyl	烷基	alkylation 烷化
keto	酮基	ketogenesis 酮生成
aceton	丙酮基	acetonuria 丙酮尿
phenol	酚基	phentolamine 酚妥拉明
hydroxy	羟基	hydroxyamphetamine 羟苯丙胺
carboxyl	羧基	carboxylase 羧化酶
prote	蛋白质	protease 蛋白酶
globulin	球蛋白	globulinuria 球蛋白尿
hemoglobin	血红蛋白	hemoglobinopathy 血红蛋白病
fibrin	纤维蛋白	fibrinogen 纤维蛋白原
pept	肽	dipeptide 二肽
zym	酶	zymogen 酶原
glyc	糖	glycogen 糖原
acchar	糖	saccharide 糖类，糖化物
carbohydro	糖	carbohydrate 碳水化合物，糖类
gluc	葡萄糖	glucagon（胰）高血糖素
fruct	果糖	fructosuria 果糖尿
rib	核糖	ribosome 核糖体
amyl	淀粉	amyloid 淀粉样的

续表

Morpheme	Meaning	Example
lip	脂肪	lipid 脂类，油脂
adip	脂肪	adipose 脂肪的
glycer	甘油	glycerin 甘油，丙三醇
salicyl	水杨酸	salicylic acid 水杨酸
phosph	磷酸	phosphagen 磷酸肌酸
chlorhydr	盐酸	chlorhydric acid 盐酸，氢氯酸
hydrochlor	盐酸	hydrochloric acid 盐酸，氢氯酸
glycin	甘氨酸	glycinate 甘氨酸盐
uric	尿酸	uricacidemia 尿酸血症
bas	碱	basophil 嗜碱细胞
alkal	碱	alkali 碱，强碱
ald	醛	aldehyde 醛
formal	甲醛	formalin 甲醛，福尔马林
sorb	山梨醇	sorbitol 山梨醇
sulf	磺胺	sulfonamide 磺胺
cyt	胞苷	cytidine 胞苷
quin	喹啉	quinine 奎宁
quinon	醌	quinone 醌，苯醌
erg	麦角	ergometrine 麦角新碱
pyrazin	吡嗪	pyrazinamide 吡嗪酰胺
pyrazon	唑酮	sulfinpyrazone 磺吡酮
pyrim	嘧啶	pyrimidine 嘧啶
uracil	尿嘧啶	fluorouracil 氟尿嘧啶
uridine	尿苷	floxuridine 氟尿苷
lys	分解	lysin 溶素，溶解素
solv, solut	分解，溶解	solution 解决；溶液；溶解
tox	毒	toxemia 毒血症
coll	胶体	colloid 胶体，胶质
gel	凝胶	gelatin 明胶

(1)   Fill in the blanks with the missing word root, prefix or suffix.

1) hyper_____mia 血钠过高

2) _____ated 含铁的

3) _____ium 钙

4) _____ide 碘化物

5) _____ant 氧化剂

6) _____osis 炭末沉着病

7) _____agogue 水泻剂

8) _____ation 烷化

9) _____genesis 酮生成

10) _____acidemia 尿酸血症

11) _____ophil 嗜碱细胞

12) _____metrine 麦角新碱

笔记

(2)   Word-matching.

1) chromic	A. 嘧啶
2) silicon	B. 奎宁
3) mercury	C. 苄基
4) methyl	D. 蛋白酶
5) pyrimidine	E. 甲醛
6) formalin	F. 铬的
7) quinine	G. 汞，水银
8) magnesium	H. 甲基
9) protease	I. 戊基
10) benzyl	J. 甲烷，沼气
11).methane	K. 镁
12) amyl	L. 硅

2.   English-Chinese Translation Skills: 药学英语翻译技巧 (9)：名词性从句翻译

英语中名词性从句包括主语从句、表语从句、宾语从句、同位语从句等，由于汉语句子结构相对松散，这类名词性从句在汉语中一般没有固定格式。名词性从句大量使用在药学英语语篇中。翻译名词性从句本身没有什么特别之处，最重要的是要考虑这类从句在复合句中的位置。在英译汉过程中，大多数语序可以不变，即可按原文顺序翻译，但有时也需要一些其他处理方法。

例 1：The FD&C Act stipulates that an article may differ in strength, quality, or purity and still have the same name if the difference is stated on the article's label.

参考译文：《食品、药品及化妆品法案》规定品种在规格、质量或者纯度方面可以有不同，而且只要在品种标签上注明可以用同样的名称。

说明：例句中谓语动词 stipulate 后面有一个 that 引导的宾语从句，翻译这类句子时，只需要按照正常顺序表述即可。

例 2：What stated above obviously indicates that Pharmacy Services Quality is in urgent need of improving.

参考译文：上述内容明显地表明了药学监护质量亟待提高。

说明：例句中 what stated above 是一个主语从句，译文没有调整原句子顺序，采用顺译法翻译，很好地表达了英语原句意思，也符合汉语表达习惯。但有时候名词性从句在翻译过程中需要调整顺序。如：

例 3：This is supported by the fact that secondary metabolites are often unique to a particular species or group of organisms and, while many act as antifeedants, sex attractants, or antibiotic agents, many have no apparent biological role. It is likely that all these concepts can play some part in understanding the production of the broad group of compounds that come under the heading of secondary metabolite.

参考译文：事实表明次级代谢产物通常对特殊物种或某些有机体是独一无二的，有一些常用作拒食剂、性引诱剂、抗生素等，还有很多并没有明显的生物作用。这些概念很有可能在理解在次级代谢旺盛期大量各种化合物的产生方面起重要作用。

说明：上面例句有两个名词性从句。一个是在 fact 后面 that 引导的同位语从句，另一个构成英语中的特殊结构：It is likely that + 从句。译文在处理这两个名词性从句时没有简单教条地按照英语结构形式来表达，而是跳出英语原来的结构，将原句意思用流畅得体的汉语结构表述出来。第一句的主要结构是 This is supported by the fact that…，为了意义表达需要译文将主句

笔记

This is supported by the fact 省略，直接将名词性从句独立成句，语言简洁流畅。第二句是英语中特有的句子结构，汉语中没有。译文直接按照汉语表达结构译成："很有可能……"，通顺自然。翻译这类套用英语固定结构的名词性从句时，可以直接使用对应的汉语表达结构，再如：

例 4：It is worth bearing in mind that the relationship between the degrees of purity achieved in a natural product extraction, and the amount of work required to achieve this, is very approximately exponential.

参考译文：值得记住的是天然产物提取过程中要达到的纯度和所需要工作量之间关系接近于指数关系。

说明：例句也是英语中一个句型：It is worth *v*-ing that+ 名词性从句，翻译这样句子可以直接采用汉语表达结构："值得……是……"。同样是类似句型，在翻译过程中有时候需要适当添加一些成分，如：

例 5：It is also probably true to say that this exponential relationship also often holds for the degree of purity achieved versus the yield of natural product.

参考译文：我们或许真的可以说所得到的纯度与天然产物的产量之间也是指数关系。

翻译名词性从句本身没有特别技巧，只要正确理解并表述从句意义即可，但是名词性从句往往都跟英语特定句型连在一起使用，处理好名词性从句与句型之间的位置关系则显得更加重要。

Unit Fourteen Drug Instructions

If you don't feel well, probably you will go to a hospital. When you get the prescription filled in the pharmacy, the pharmacist usually gives you some additional written information, or you may receive a very detailed "package insert" filled with information provided by the drug manufacturer and approved by the U.S. Food and Drug Administration (FDA). Such package inserts are available for all prescription medications approved by the FDA. Similar information is available for nonprescription medicines and for some herbal medicines and dietary supplements as well. The package insert is a good source of information to be used in addition to instructions your doctor or nurse may have given you. It's a good idea to review the package insert for any new medicine and to look at it again if anything about your health changes after taking the medicine. If it raises any questions in your mind, contact your doctor or nurse for an explanation.

The package insert follows a standard format for every medication, and written in technical language. After the brand name, chemical name and molecular formula of the product, the following sections appear: Description，Microbiology and Clinical Pharmacology, Indications and Usage, Contraindications, Warnings, Precautions, Adverse Reactions, Overdosage, Dosage and Administration, Pregnancy and Lactation, Interaction with other Drugs, Pharmacological and Toxicological Properties, Pharmacokinetic Properties, Storage, Package, and Shelf Life etc.

如果你不舒服,你可能就会去医院看病。在药房用处方取药的时候,药师一般也会给你一些书面的用药信息,或者你会拿到一个详细的"药品说明书",上面有药厂提供的经过美国食品药品管理局(FDA)批准的内容。FDA批准的所有处方药都附有药品说明书。非处方药、一些草药和膳食补充剂也有说明书。除了医生或者护士给你的用药指导以外,药品说明书也是一个很好的信息来源。使用任何新药都要看说明书,如果用药后身体发生了变化要及时再看看说明书。如果有什么疑惑,要询问医生或者护士。

药品说明书都遵循一个标准格式,并且用技术语言书写。在介绍商品名、化学名和分子式之后,还包括其他信息,如:性状、微生物学和临床药理学、适应证和用法、禁忌证、警告、注意事项、不良反应、药物过量、用法用量、孕妇及哺乳期妇女用药、药物相互作用、药理毒理、药动学、贮藏、包装和有效期等。

笔记

Text A
The New Drug Package Insert-Implications for Patient Safety

The package insert contains detailed drug information compiled and distributed by the drug manufacturer after the FDA's review and approval. The purpose of the package insert is to provide complete and unbiased prescribing and safety information to health professionals. In 1968, a two line warning placed on the isoproterenol inhaler package is considered as the first patient package insert. Although in 1970 the FDA mandated that a separate patient package insert detailing risk and benefits accompany each package of birth control pills, it was not until 1979 that the FDA promulgated the content and format of physician prescribing information inserts (also known as the package insert).[1] Within the Warnings section of this document, the term "boxed warning" (black box warning) was used for the first time in the FDA labeling requirements. Since then, the volume and detail of the package insert had increased significantly. In the 1980s, the FDA acknowledged that the information included in the package insert had become so lengthy, detailed, and complex that it was difficult for health practitioners to find specific information and to distinguish critical information from less important issues.

To address the problem, the FDA conducted a research to assess how prescription drug labeling was used by health care practitioners, and to determine which labeling information was considered the most important. The studies documented that many practitioners usually find the information they need, but that the process was often time-intensive and clinically inefficient. In addition, the package insert format disproportionately stressed the occurrence of extremely rare clinical events. As a result, the FDA developed a new package insert format that had three major sections: ① "The Highlights of Prescribing Information"; ② "Full Prescribing Information Table of Contents"; and ③ "The Full Prescribing Information" (FPI). This new organization of information improved access to critical information and made the label more user-friendly. The new label format proposal was issued in December 2000 and, after public meetings and comment by practitioners, a final version became official in June 2006. A transition to the new format will not be mandatory for drugs that received the FDA's approval more than 5 years before the final ruling in June 2006. However, pharmaceutical companies may elect to reformat the package insert for these older drugs. Drugs approved within the 5-year window must resubmit the package insert in the revised label format during a 3-7-year phase—in period to comply with the new FDA standards. Here list some sections selected in the new drug package insert.

1. Highlights of Prescribing Information

Most of the information included in the "Highlights of Prescribing Information" section communicates risks or warning information. A succinct summary of critical clinical information is presented in a bulleted format that is cross-referenced to the FPI section for more in depth explanation. The organization of the section reflects the priorities and most common patterns of product insert usage as expressed by practitioners during the FDA reformatting studies.

2. Black Box Warning

The black box warning is set apart as the most prominent information included in a product insert. Any warning elevated to the status of a black box warning must be bolded (only the heading must be in all capitals, not the text of the warning) and "boxed" by a solid black line on all four sides.

笔记

A black box warning is indicated in the following three situations, but may be used in other situations to highlight warning information that is particularly important to the prescriber:

(1) There is an adverse reaction so serious in proportion to the potential benefit from the drug that it is essential that it be considered in assessing the risks and benefits of using the drug.[2] This includes potentially life threatening or permanently disabling adverse reactions.

(2) There is a serious reaction that can be prevented or reduced in frequency or severity by patient selection, careful monitoring, avoiding certain concomitant therapy, addition of another drug or managing patient in a specific manner, or avoiding use in a specific clinical situation.

(3) The FDA has approved the drug with restrictions on use and distribution to assure safe use.

A black box warning has implications for the manufacturer, health care provider, and patients. Manufacturer implications include a restriction on the degree of advertising, a potentially negative impact on sales, a decreased use of the drug, and an increased risk of litigation. From the provider's and patients' perspective, the substitution of a drug without a black box warning may actually entail greater expense and exposure to another set of side effects than the use of the drug with a black box warning. Further, in the absence of patients' awareness of the potential dangers of a drug, when untoward events are precipitated by the drug, there is also an increased risk of litigation.

3. Recent Major Changes, Indications and Usage, Dosage and Administration, Dosage Forms and Strengths

The "Recent Major Changes" section lists only major changes in the boxed warning, indications and usage, dosage and administration, contraindications and warnings, and precautions sections. The three sections following Recent Major Changes are practical information giving indications and usage, dosage and administration, and dosage forms and strengths. These informational sections placed after the most serious warning issues have been identified to facilitate practical use of the label, whose major purpose is to provide dosage information for routine use.

The sections following the routine use information are warning or risk information of high importance. These sections include contraindications, warnings and precautions, adverse reactions, drug interactions, and use in specific populations.

4. Contraindications

A drug is classified as contraindicated in the clinical situation for which the risks outweigh any possible therapeutic benefit of the drug. Only known hazards, and not theoretical possibilities, can be listed. If there are no known contraindications for a drug, "none" must be designated in this section. The order in which the contraindications are presented in the text reflects the relative public health risk. The significance of the contraindications is based on the likelihood of occurrence and the size of the population potentially affected.

5. Warnings and Precautions

When an adverse reaction is considered clinically significant, or when the reaction risk is serious, it will be included in the "Warning and Precautions" section. There must be reasonable evidence of a causal relationship between the drug and the reaction. The order of the list of adverse reactions (ADRs) reflects their relative public health significance. The relative seriousness of the reaction and the ability to prevent or mitigate its occurrence are prioritized in this section. A description of the reaction and outcome, including time to resolution, significant sequelae, estimated risk of ADRs, and discussion of any known risk factors for the reaction, are required. Treatment or management strategies for the ADRs and discussion of any possible steps to reduce the risk, shorten the duration, or minimize the

笔记

severity of a reaction are included in this section.

Observed ADRs and expected ADRs are included in the Warnings and Precautions section. Observed ADRs are those events that have been observed in association with the use of the drug and that are serious or are otherwise clinically significant. "Clinically significant" means that the ADRs may require:

- adjustment of the drug dosage or regimen;
- discontinuation of the drug;
- supplement treatment with an additional drug;
- appropriate patient selection to avoid the ADRs;
- avoidance of concomitant therapy which triggers the ADRs;
- evaluation of the patient for medication compliance;
- use of alternative laboratory tests.

Expected ADRs are events that can be anticipated to occur with a drug, based on observations from other members of the drug class or animal studies. Expected ADRs are appropriate for warnings and precautions if the reaction is clinically serious, indicating that it could have an outcome of death, life-threatening illness, or require hospitalization to treat.

6. Drug Interactions

The "Drug Interactions" section includes concise information about the potential for interaction with other drugs or foods. These include both pharmacokinetic (e.g., food effects, enzyme induction and inhibition) and pharmacodynamic effects (e.g., meperidine with monoamine oxidase inhibitors).

7. Use in Specific Populations

This section on "Use in Specific Populations" lists clinically significant or important differences in patient response or the use of a drug in specific populations of patients.

8. FPI Contents

The purpose of the table of contents is to reference all the sections and subsections included in the FPI, some of which will not be cross-referenced in the Highlights. The Highlights contains cross-references to the FPI, which contains the full explanatory text for the bulleted summaries and is easily accessed by practitioners to encourage its use and discourage use of the Highlights section as the sole source of information. The sections of the FPI coincide with the order of the sections covered in the Highlights section. Also, similar to the Highlights, the most crucial dosing and warning sections are at the beginning of the FPI text. The sections dealing with risk information are grouped together. The informational sections not dealing with risk are grouped collectively. Additional sections in this part of the package insert include drug abuse and dependence, over-dosage, description, clinical pharmacology, non-clinical toxicology, clinical studies, references, how supplied/storage and handling, and patient counseling information.

Hospital-based medication errors and preventable adverse drug reactions occur at a rate of 400,000 per year according to a recent Institute of Medicine (IOM) study. These errors are reported to translate into an annual cost of $3.5 billion in extra hospital expense. The new format changes the landscape of drug information, and the FDA has expressed the hope that these changes would increase effective use of prescription of drugs and decrease medication errors.

Word Study

1. concomitant [kənˈkɔmətənt] *adj.* 相伴的，相随的
2. contraindication [ˌkɔntrəˈindiˌkeiʃən] *n.* [医] 禁忌证，禁忌证候

笔记

3. cross-referenced [ˈkrɔːs ˈrefərənst] *adj.* 互相参照的，交叉引用的

4. designate [ˈdezigneit] *v.* 指定，标明，表示

5. disproportionately [ˌdisprəˈpɔːʃənətli] *adv.* 不成比例地

6. elevate [ˈeliveit] *v.* 提高，提升

7. entail[inˈteil] *v.* 使成为必要，导致

8. enzyme [ˈenzaim] *n.* 酶

9. highlight [ˈhailait] *n.* 最重要的细节或事件；*v.* 强调，使……突出

10. indication [ˌindiˈkeiʃn] *n.* 适应证

11. inhale [inˈheil] *v.* 吸气，吸入

12. inhibition [ˌinhiˈbiʃn] *n.* 抑制，阻止

13. inpatient [ˈinpeiʃnt] *n.* 住院病人（反义词为 outpatient [ˈautpeiʃnt] *n.* 门诊病人）

14. isoproterenol [aisəuprəˈterənɔl] *n.* 异丙肾上腺素

15. litigation [ˌlitiˈgeiʃn] *n.* 诉讼，起诉

16. mandate [ˈmændeit] *v.* 命令，规定，颁布（法律）

17. meperidine [məˈperədin] *n.* 哌替啶，度冷丁

18. mitigate [ˈmitigeit] *v.* 减轻，缓和

19. monoamine [ˌmɔnəuəˈmiːn] *n.* 单胺

20. oxidase [ˈɔksədeis] *n.* 氧化酶

21. pharmacodynamic [fɑːməkəudaiˈnæmik] *adj.* 药效的，药效学的

22. pharmacokinetic [ˌfɑːməkəukiˈnetik] *adj.* 药动的

23. precipitate [priˈsipiteit] *v.* 使（尤指坏事）发生，促成

24. promulgate [ˈprɔːmlgeit] *v.* 发布，颁布，传播（观点等）

25. reformat [ˌriːˈfɔːmæt] *v.* 重新制定格式

26. regimen [ˈredʒimən] *n.* 养身之道，疗程，方案

27. sequelae [siˈkwiːliː] (*pl.*) *n.* 后遗症 (*sig.*) sequela [siˈkwiːlə]

28. severity [siˈverəti]   *n.* 严重，严重性

29. succinct [səkˈsiŋkt] *adj.* 言简意赅的，简明的

30. unbiased [ʌnˈbaiəst] *adj.* 公正的

Notes

1. 在"Although in 1970 the FDA mandated that a separate patient package insert detailing risk and benefits accompany each package of birth control pills, it was not until 1979 that the FDA promulgated the content and format of physician prescribing information inserts (also known as the package insert)."句中，although 引导让步状语从句，动词 accompany 前面省略了 should。

2. 在理解"There is an adverse reaction so serious in proportion to the potential benefit from the drug that it is essential that it be considered in assessing the risks and benefits of using the drug."这个句子的结构时，首先要知道，这个句子的主要结构是：There is an adverse reaction. 后面的"so serious in proportion to the potential benefit from the drug that it is…"都是做定语修饰"an adverse reaction"。另外，在理解这个很长的定语部分时，要注意 3 个问题：①构成"so…that…"结构的是第一个"that"，表示"如此……以至于……"；②这个"that"引导的结果状语从句是一个句型：it is essential that it be considered in assessing the risks and benefits of using the drug，在这个句型中，第一个"it"是形式主语，真正的主语是后面"that it be considered

笔记

in assessing the risks and benefits of using the drug."在这个主语中，"it"代表的是前面的"an adverse reaction"；③在"…that it be considered…"的"be"前面，省略了"should"。

Exercises

1. **Decide whether each of the following statements is true (T) or false (F) according to the passage.**

(1) In the 1980s, health practitioners found it easy to get specific information and to distinguish critical information from less important issues in the package insert.

(2) As far as the function of the package insert is concerned, the FDA finds that it is usually time-intensive and clinically inefficient for many practitioners to get the information they need, because the package insert format disproportionately stressed the occurrence of extremely rare clinical events.

(3) For the drugs that received the FDA's approval more than 5 years before the final ruling in June 2006, the pharmaceutical companies may elect either to continue the old format of the package insert or to reformat it.

(4) The "Recent Major Changes" section lists only major changes in the boxed warning, indications and usage, dosage and administration, contraindications and warnings, and precautions sections.

(5) The FPI contains cross-references to the Highlights, which contains the full explanatory text for the bulleted summaries and is easily accessed by practitioners to encourage its use and discourage use of the Highlights section as the sole source of information.

(6) In the FPI text, both the sections dealing with risk information and the sections not dealing with risk are grouped, but separately. But clinical pharmacology and patient counseling information are not included in this section.

2. **Questions for oral discussion.**

(1) What is "black box warning"? In what situation should it be indicated?

(2) Are length, detail and complexity the criteria to judge a package insert? How to comment on a package insert?

(3) What is included in "Highlights of prescribing information"?

(4) What are observed ADRs and expected ADRs in a drug insert?

3. **Choose the best answer to each of the following questions.**

(1) Which of the following statements is true according to the passage?

　　A. The first drug insert appeared in 1968, with the two lines of warning placed in the isoproterenol inhaler package.

　　B. Since a separated drug insert is required by the FDA, the drug insert has become more lengthy and detailed.

　　C. "Boxed warning" can help health practitioners distinguish critical information from less important information.

　　D. The drug insert is compiled and distributed by drug manufacturers, providing detailed drug information to health practitioners.

(2) Why did FDA decide to reformat drug insert in the 1980s?

　　A. Because the information the health professional need in drug insert is not accessible.

　　B. "Boxed warning" was not included in the drug insert.

　　C. The occurrence of rare clinical events is not proportionately included in the drug insert.

　　D. None of the above.

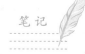
笔记

(3) According to the passage, the new format of a drug insert issued by the FDA in 2000 _____.

    A. was made up of three major sections

    B. was more convenient for the users to get access to the critical information

    C. excluded the less important clinical event disproportionately

    D. became less lengthy, detailed and complex

(4) Which of the following statements is true according to the passage?

    A. The Highlights of Prescribing Information section contains the most prominent risk and warning information in detail.

    B. Warning information can be put in either Black Box Warning section or Highlights of Prescribing Information section.

    C. Some prescribers find that Black Box Warning can help them to avoid the risk of being accused.

    D. The information in Black Box Warning is the most important in a drug insert.

(5) According to the passage, information that has implication usually occurs in_____ section.

    A. Highlights of Prescribing Information   B. Contraindication

    C. Recent Major Changes   D. Black Box Warning

(6) Which of the following statements is right according to the passage?

    A. Both known dangers and theoretical possibilities should be listed in "Contraindications".

    B. Adverse reaction is usually included in Highlights of Prescribing Information section.

    C. There is a relationship between the significance of the contraindications and the likelihood of occurrence and the size of population.

    D. That there are no known contraindications for a drug means therapeutical benefits outweigh risks.

(7) In a drug insert, pharmacokinetic effects are included in _____ section.

    A. Drug Interaction   B. FPI Contents

    C. Contraindications   D. Recent Major Changes

(8) Some information in FPI Contents section is cross-referenced in _____ section.

    A. Black Box Warning   B. Highlights of Prescribing Information

    C. Contraindications   D. Warnings and Precautions

(9) When the ADR requires adjusting drug dosage or regimen, discontinuing the drug and evaluating the patient for medication compliance, it means that the ADR associated with use of the drug is _____.

    A. clinically insignificant   B. clinically insufficient

    C. clinically significant   D. clinically sufficient

(10) Which of the following statements is right according to the passage?

    A. Expected ADRs refer to the average events that have happened before with a drug of similar class.

    B. The new drug insert format has decreased $3.5 billion in hospital expenses.

    C. Some hospital-based medication errors are due to the insufficient information in drug insert.

    D. The purpose of the FDA's developing a new drug insert format is to make drug insert contain more information.

4. Fill in the blanks of the following incomplete sentences with the words given.

笔记

(1) But infection with H. pylori alone does not lead to stomach cancer; other factors, like

genetic _____ (susceptibility/sensibility) of the stomach, are also necessary for the condition to develop.

(2) Annual worldwide deaths from asthma have been estimated at 250,000, but the _____ (mortality/ morbidity)does not appear to correlate well with prevalence.

(3) The effect of constant and _____(intermittent/independent) hyperglycemia on the membrane deformation of endothelial cells and the internal mechanism were investigated in the study.

(4) The SARS did great harm to them physically and mentally. Most of them have kinds of _____(consequence/sequelae), like lung disease, especially the mental maladjustment, caused by people's discrimination

(5) A researcher at the University of Nebraska looked at chicken soup and its effect on _____ (inflammatory/ inflammable) cells in a petri dish.

(6) The reprogrammed cells showed the defining characteristics of induced _____ (pluripotent/ multi-patent) stem cells, and they could both differentiate into various cell types and generate more of themselves.

(7) These microorganisms assist us in absorbing nutrients from our food and also occupy valuable real estate so that pathogens cannot _____ (expand/proliferate) and make us sick.

(8) Although this diet is not physically harmful, and can be helpful in reducing the weight in some instances, it's generally not wise to adopt this _____. (regimen/recipe)

(9) Pharmaceutical _____ (excess/excipient) is the important part of pharmaceutical preparations. It plays a key role in the improvements of the performance of drug form, bioavailability and reducing the side effect.

(10) There is little if any legal regulation of _____ (dietary/nutrient) supplements, which comprise a basket of herbs and teas as botanical supplements and weight loss supplements containing herbs and various substances.

5. Translate the following sentences and paragraphs into Chinese.

(1) In 1968, a two line warning placed on the isoproterenol inhaler package is considered as the first patient package insert.

(2) There is an adverse reaction so serious in proportion to the potential benefit from the drug that it is essential that it be considered in assessing the risks and benefits of using the drug.

(3) The studies conducted by the FDA documented that many practitioners usually find the information they need, but that the process was often time-intensive and clinically inefficient.

(4) A drug is classified as contraindicated in the clinical situation for which the risks outweigh any possible therapeutic benefit of the drug.

(5) Hospital-based medication errors and preventable ADR occur at a rate of 400,000 per year according to a recent Institute of Medicine study. These errors are reported to translate into an annual cost of $3.5 billion in extra hospital expense.

(6) A black box warning has implications for the manufacturer, health care provider, and patients. From the provider's and patients' perspective, the substitution of a drug without a black box warning may actually entail greater expense and exposure to another set of side effects than the use of the drug with a black box warning. Further, in the absence of patients' awareness of the potential dangers of a drug, when untoward events are precipitated by the drug, there is also an increased risk of litigation.

(7) Observed ADRs are those events that have been observed in association with use of the drug

笔记

and are serious or are otherwise clinically significant. Expected ADRs are events that can be anticipated to occur with a drug, based on observations from other members of the drug class or animal studies. Expected ADRs are appropriate for warnings and precautions if the reaction is clinically serious, indicating it could have an outcome of death, life-threatening illness, or require hospitalization to treat.

Text B
The Package Insert and Prescription

In 1937, sulfanilamide, the first sulfa antimicrobial drug, was marketed. The diluent for this sulfa preparation was diethylene glycol, a chemical analog of antifreeze. More than 100 people, many of whom were children, died after receiving the drug. As a result, the US Congress enacted the 1938 Federal Food, Drug and Cosmetic Act, which required proof of safety before the introduction of a new drug into clinical practice. This act also changed the focus of the FDA from a policing agency, with an emphasis on confiscation of adulterated drugs, to a regulatory agency supervising the evaluation of new drugs.

In the practice of pediatrics, drugs which are not approved by the Food and Drug Administration (FDA) as safe and effective in children are prescribed daily. This is due in part to the fact that many drugs released since 1962 carry an "orphaning clause" in the package insert such as, "not to be used in children, since clinical studies have been insufficient to establish recommendations for its use." What is the status of the package insert? Is it a legal directive to the physician, or is it intended as a guide for the physician in prescribing a drug?[1]

The package insert, by legal definition of the Federal Food, Drug and Cosmetic Act, is the official information piece for a drug. The information it contains is derived from data supplied by investigators and submitted by the pharmaceutical firm to the FDA. The insert is written and printed by the drug manufacturer, but its contents must be approved by the FDA. The Food, Drug and Cosmetic Act, as amended in 1962, requires full disclosure of all known facts pertaining to the use of the drug. Therefore, a great deal of information is included in the insert, including the chemical structure of the drug, a summary of its pharmacological and toxicological action, its clinical indications and contraindications, precautions, reported adverse reactions, dosage recommendations, and available dosage forms.

Many drugs have package inserts approved by the FDA before the Drug Amendments of 1962 when manufacturers were required to show the safety but not the effectiveness of their products. On the basis of evaluations of the efficacy of these older drugs by panels of experts selected by the National Academy of Sciences-National Research Council, the FDA is now requiring revision of these package inserts to eliminate unsupported claims and thus to make them more useful to the practitioner.

Is the pediatrician breaking the law when he prescribes drugs for his patients which carry the "orphaning clause?" No, he is not. The physician may exercise his professional judgment in the use of any drug. However, if he deviates from the instructions in the package insert and adverse reactions occur, he must be prepared to defend his position in court if there is a malpractice suit.

Many drugs are used by clinicians in the treatment of conditions not listed in the package insert. The FDA cannot require a pharmaceutical firm to include a new use for the drug product in the insert

笔记

even if it has been clinically tested and found useful for a given problem. Economic considerations are among a number of factors that may influence such a policy on the part of the company. If a new use for a drug is not yet included in the package insert, the manufacturer cannot advertise his product for that particular use. The package insert is legally binding on the manufacturer in limiting the conditions under which he can promote the use of the drug.

Another fact not generally recognized is that a physician's failure to use a drug approved as effective treatment for a specific disease might be construed as malpractice. In regard to this, it is important that the physician be informed about the availability of the drug and bases his decision to use it or not to use it on rational grounds. It would be unlikely that information taken from the package insert could be used successfully as evidence against the physician in a liability suit.

The dilemma facing the physician is illustrated by imipramine (Tofranil) when used in the treatment of enuresis. In 1965, a controlled study was published showing that this drug was useful in "training enuretic children to be dry." Its mechanism of action was not defined, but it appeared to be effective when given to children between the age of 5 and 12 years in a dosage up to 50 mg at bedtime. Following publication of this paper, imipramine became widely used for the treatment of enuresis. A straw poll of 15 pediatricians in the Cleveland area showed that 12 had prescribed imipramine for this condition. When one examines the package insert supplied with imipramine, two points are clear: ① the treatment of enuresis is not listed under conditions for the use of this drug; and ② there is a clear statement that the drug is not recommended for use in patients under 12 years of age. If a severe reaction occurred and litigation followed, how would a court react if a physician admitted to the use of this drug for the treatment of enuresis in view of the prohibitions in the package insert? Possibly, if other physicians made themselves available to give expert medical testimony and if other physicians in the community used the drug for this purpose, would the published clinical study, plus the physician's judgment in prescribing the drug, suffice?

The purpose of the FDA control of the package insert is not to legislate for the practice of medicine. As in the past, the physician is the individual prescribing the drug. The fact that he followed the recommendations in the package insert does not absolve him from responsibility for harm resulting to his patient, nor does failure to follow the recommendations in the package insert necessarily render him legally culpable.

The statements made in the package insert and approved by the FDA are not in themselves legally binding on the physician in his practice of medicine. Furthermore, no physician should rely on the package insert as his sole source of drug information. Drug dosages, as given in the insert, are guides for instituting therapy. The dose may have to be increased or decreased, depending on the patient's response. And, each time a drug is used, the question of benefit versus risk to the patient must be considered.

American Academy of Pediatrics Committee on Drugs has taken the view that the insert should be viewed as a useful guide to the physician; its recommendations should be judged on an equal footing with other publications and research reports. The package insert contains useful information, but the physician's decision on therapy should be based on cumulative knowledge derived from many sources. When sound scientific data exist which have shown that a drug is reasonably safe and effective in the treatment of a specific disease in adults, it should not necessarily be withheld from a sick child with the same disease just because its use has not been studied in children.[2] However, if used under these circumstances the physician should be cautious, and the use of the drug should be reported

笔记

to the manufacturer, the FDA, or in the medical literature to add to the knowledge concerning such use. The foregoing situation must be distinguished from use of the drug when the package insert states that the drug is contraindicated in infants or children on the basis of studies showing it to be unsafe or ineffective in these age groups.

The Committee feels that the pediatrician is likely to ignore the "orphan clause" in the insert if, in his judgment, his patient requires a particular medication for optimal treatment. Whether or not this places him in unusual legal jeopardy is a question not yet resolved by the courts. It is the opinion of the Committee that this practice should not be a problem if the physician is well informed on the pharmacology and toxicology of the drugs he uses and closely follows his patient's response to treatment.

Changing the directives in the package insert, except to disclose pertinent new data, will not solve the problem of "therapeutic orphans." Echoing Dr. Harry Shirkey's stand, the Committee believes that the ultimate solution requires the development of programs in pediatric clinical pharmacology to ensure that all drugs used in infants and children are adequately tested for safety and efficacy.

According to an FDA poll, the majority of physicians use the package insert compiled in the "Physicians Desk Reference". To them,

1. "The labeling shall contain the essential scientific information needed for the safe and effective use of the drug.

2. The labeling shall be informative and accurate without being promotional, false, or misleading.

3. The labeling shall be based on data providing substantial evidence of safety and effectiveness."

Today, the FDA's regulatory scope and authority include ensuring the safety and purity of foods, drugs, medical devices, nutritional supplements, vaccines, and cosmetics. Of particular concern to the anesthesiologist is the timely access to drug evaluation, pharmacologic and medical device data.[3] With the dramatic upsurge in the number of new prescription drugs and over-the-counter supplements, the need for up-to-date drug information has never been more crucial.[4]

Word Study

1. amend [əˈmend] v. 修正，改进
2. analog [ˈænəlɔːg] adj. 模拟的，类比的
3. anesthesiologist [ˌænəs,θiːziˈɔːlədʒist] n. 麻醉师
4. antifreeze [ˈæntifriːz] n. 防冻剂，防冻液
5. confiscation [ˌkɔnfisˈkeiʃən] n. 没收，把……充公
6. construe [kənˈstruː] v. 理解，解释，识解
7. culpable [ˈkʌlpəbl] adj. 该负责任的；应受处罚的，有罪的
8. deviate ˈdiːvieit] v. 背离，偏离
9. diethylene [diəˈθiliːn] n. 二次乙基，   diethylene glycol [ˈglaikəul] n. 二甘醇
10. diluent [ˈdiljuənt]adj. 稀释的 (=diluting) n. 稀释剂
11. disclosure [disˈkləuʒə] n. 揭发，透露，公开（秘密等）
12. efficacy [ˈefikəsi] n. 功效，效能
13. enact [iˈnækt] v. 制定（法律），通过（法案），颁布
14. enuresis [ˌenjuˈriːsis] n. 遗尿症
15. footing [ˈfutiŋ] n. 立场，基础
16. foregoing [ˈfɔːrgəuiŋ] adj. 前面的，上述的

笔记

17. glycol ['glaikəul] *n.* 二醇、乙二醇；

18. imipramine [i'miprə,mi:n] *n.* 丙米嗪（一种抗抑郁剂）

19. institute ['institu:t] *v.* 创立，制定；开始，着手

20. jeopardy ['dʒepədi] *n.* 危险

21. legislate ['ledʒisleit] *v.* 立法，制定法律

22. liability [,laiə'biləti] *n.* （赔偿等）责任，义务

23. malpractice [,mæl'præktis] *n.* 医疗失当，医疗差错，行为不当

24. optimal ['ɔptiməl] *adj.* 最理想的，最佳的

25. panel ['pænl] *n.* 座谈小组，全体陪审员

26. pediatrician [,pi:diə'triʃn] *n.* 儿科医生

27. pediatrics [,pi:di'ætriks] *n.* 儿科学

28. pertain [pə'tein] *v.* 从属，pertaining to 与……有关系，关于，固有的

29. pertinent ['pə:tnənt] *adj.* 相关的，有关的

30. rational ['ræʃnəl] *adj.* 理性的，合理的

31. suffice [sə'fais] *v.* 足够，使满足

32. sulfa ['sʌlfə] *adj.* 磺胺的 sulfa drug 磺胺药物

33. sulfanilamide [,sʌlfə'nilə,maid] *n.* 氨苯磺胺，磺胺

34. testimony ['testiməuni] *n.* （法庭上的）证词

35. upsurge ['ʌpsə:dʒ] *n./v.* （突然）增长

36. withhold [wið'həuld] *v.* (…from…) 把……扣着，压住，隐瞒

Notes

1. 在"Is it a legal directive…, or is it intended as a guide for the physician in prescribing a drug?"中，be intended for 意为："打算供……用""是为……而准备的"。

2. 在理解"When sound scientific data exist which have shown that a drug is reasonably safe and effective in the treatment of a specific disease in adults, it should not necessarily be withheld from a sick child with the same disease just because its use has not been studied in children."句子时，要注意两点：①"which have shown that a drug is reasonably safe and effective in the treatment of a specific disease in adults"是一个定语从句修饰前面的"data"，放在动词"exist"后面是为了平衡。②"a sick child with the same disease"意思是"患有同样疾病的儿童"，这里"with 结构"作定语，修饰"a sick child"。

3. 在 Of particular concern to the anesthesiologist is the timely access to drug evaluation, pharmacologic and medical device data. 中，"of concern to sb"意思是"某人关注的"，"access to"的基本意思是"进入……"，在这里引申为"接近或取得……的方法、手段、权利等"，这个句子的意思是"对麻醉师而言特别关注的是能够及时了解药品评估、药理学数据以及医疗装置数据。"

4. With the dramatic upsurge in the number of new prescription drugs and over-the-counter supplements, the need for up-to-date drug information has never been more crucial. 这个句子的意思是"随着新的处方药和非处方药数量的急剧增加，对最新药品信息的需求从来没有现在这样迫切。""with the dramatic upsurge in the number of…"意思是"随着……数量的急剧增加"；"has never been more crucial"，是强调结构：never...more...，意思是"没有比这再迫切的了""非常关键 / 迫切"。再如"I can't agree with you any more."意思是"我非常同意你的观点。"

笔记

Supplementary Parts

1. Medical and Pharmaceutical Terms Made Easier (14): Common Morphemes in English Terms for Human Anatomy

Morpheme	Meaning	Example
spir/o	呼吸	respiration 呼吸
nas/o	鼻	oronasal 口鼻的
rhin/o	鼻	rhinitis 鼻炎
pharyng/o	咽	pharyngotomy 咽切开术
laryng/o	喉	laryngophony 喉听诊音
trache/o	气管	tracheostomy 气管造口术
bronch/o	支气管	bronchogenic 支气管原的
pulm/o	肺	pulmometry 肺容量测定法
pulmon/o	肺	pulmonary 肺的
pneum/o	气，肺	pneumococci 肺炎球菌
pneumon/o	气，肺	pneumonia 肺炎
pleur/o	胸膜	pleural 胸膜的
muc/o	黏液	mucosal 黏膜的
diaphragm/o	膈	diaphragmitis 膈炎
phren/o,phrenic/o	膈神经	phrenicectomy 膈神经切除术
-pnea	呼吸	eupnea 呼吸正常
atel/o	不完全的，有缺陷的	atelectasis 肺不张
myc/o	真菌	mycoplasmas 支原体
or/o	口，嘴	oral 口的
stomat/o	口，嘴	stomatopathy 口（腔）病
labi/o	唇	labial 唇的
cheil/o	唇	cheilostomatoplasty 唇口成形术
dent/i	牙齿	dentalgia 牙痛
odont/o	牙齿	periodontal 牙周的
lingu/o	舌	sublingual 舌下的
gloss/o	舌	glossitis 舌炎
aden/o	腺	adenoid 腺样的
saliv/a	涎，吐液	salivation 流涎
sial/o	涎，吐液	sialoangitis 涎管炎
pharyng/o	咽	pharyngolaryngitis 咽喉炎
esophag/o	食管	esophageal 食管的
gastr/o	胃	gastric 胃的
pylor/o	幽门	pylorospasm 幽门痉挛
lapar/o	腹壁	laparotomy 剖腹术
enter/o	小肠	parenteral 胃肠外的
duoden/o	十二指肠	duodenostomy 十二指肠造口术
jejun/o	空肠	jejunitis 空肠炎
ile/o	回肠	ileal 回肠的

笔记

续表

Morpheme	Meaning	Example
col/o	结肠	colitis 结肠炎
append/o	阑尾	appendectomy 阑尾切除
rect/o	直肠	rectal 直肠的
an/o	肛门	anal 肛门的
proct/o	肛门和直肠	proctalgia 肛部痛
hepat/o	肝	hepatitis 肝炎
cholecyst/o	胆囊	cholecystotomy 胆囊切开术
bil/i	胆	bilirubin 胆红素
chol/e	胆	cholemia 胆血症
pancreat/o	胰	pancreatic 胰的
peritone/o	腹膜	intraperitoneal 腹膜内的
succ/o	汁,分泌,分泌物	succagogue 促分泌的
pept/i	消化	peptic 消化(性)的
peps/i	消化	dyspepsia 消化不良
chlorhydr/o	盐酸	achlorhydria 胃酸缺乏
gluc/o	糖	glucatonia 血糖极度降低
glyc/o	糖	glycemia 糖血
sacchar/o	糖	polysaccharide 多糖
amyl/o	淀粉	amyloid 淀粉样的
lip/o	油,脂肪	lipemia 脂血(症)
steat/o	油,脂肪	steatolysis 脂肪分解
fec/a	粪便	fecal 粪便的
-lithiasis	结石	cholelithiasis 胆石病
-helcosis	溃疡形成	gastrohelcosis 胃溃疡
herni/o	疝	herniorrhaphy 疝修补术
gingiv/o	齿龈	gingivitis 齿龈炎
dentin/o	牙本质	dentinoma 牙质瘤
cement/o	牙骨质	cementoblast 成牙骨质细胞
orth/o	直的	orthodontics 畸齿矫正术
py/o	脓	pyorrhea 脓溢
ren/o	肾	renal 肾的
nephr/o	肾	nephromegaly 肾肥大
pyel/o	肾盂	pyelolithotomy 肾盂石切除术
ureter/o	输尿管	ureterolith 输尿管结石
vesic/jo	膀胱	vesicotomy 膀胱切开术
cyst/o	囊、膀胱	cystitis 膀胱炎
urethr/o	尿道	urethropexy 尿道固定术
ur/o	尿,尿道	diuretic 利尿剂
hydr/o	水	hydronephrosis 肾盂积水
lith/o	石,结石	lithonephrotomy 肾石切除术
staphyl/o	一束	staphylococcus 葡萄球菌
cocc/o	球菌	micrococcus 微球菌
retro-	向隔,在后	retroperitoneal 腹膜后的
test/o	睾丸	testosterone 睾酮

笔记

续表

Morpheme	Meaning	Example
orchi/o	睾丸	orchiocele 睾丸突出，睾丸瘤
andr/o	男性，雄性的	androgen 雄激素
epididym/o	副睾	epididymovasostomy 输精管附睾吻合术
prostat/o	前列腺	prostatectomy 前列腺切除术
pen/o	阴茎	penile 阴茎的
genit/o	生殖器	genital 生殖的，生殖器的
gon/o,gonad/o	性腺，生殖腺	gonorrhea 淋病
sperm/o	精子	spermicide 杀精子剂
zo/o	生物	spermatozoon 精子
gamet/o	配子	gametogenesis 配子发生
ov/o	卵，卵子	ovulation 排卵
oo/o	卵，卵子	oophoritis 卵巢炎
uter/o	子宫	uteritis 子宫炎
hyster/o	子宫	hysterectomy 子宫切除术
cervic/o	颈，宫颈	cervicectomy 子宫颈切除术
vagin/o	阴道	intravaginal 阴道内的
men/o	月经	menorrhagia 月经过多
gynec/o	妇女，女性	gynecologist 妇科专家
embry/o	胎儿，胚胎	embryonic 胚胎的
par(t)/o	娩出	postpartum 产后的
umbilic/o	脐	umbilical 脐的
mamm/o	乳房	mammography 乳房 X 线照相术
mast/o	乳房	mastectomy 乳房切除术
pseud/o	假的，伪的	pseudohermaphrodite 假两性体
crypt/o	隐藏的	cryptorchidism 隐睾
-plasia	形成	hyperplasia 增生
cardi/o	心	electrocardiogram 心电图
coron/o	冠，心脏	coronary 冠状的
aort/o	主动脉	aortic 主动脉的
angi/o	血管	angiogram 血管造影照片
vas/o	血管	vasoconstrictor 血管收缩剂
arteri/o	动脉	arteriostenosis 动脉狭窄
ven/o	静脉	venous 静脉的
phleb/o	静脉	phlebitis 静脉炎
capill/o	非常小的血管	capillary 毛细血管
steth/o	胸	stethoscope 听诊器
sphygm/o	脉搏	sphygmomanometer 血压计
hemat/o	血	hematuria 血尿
granul/o	小结节，颗粒	agranulocyte 无粒细胞
plasm/o	血浆	plasmapheresis 血浆去除术
thromb/o	凝块，血块	thrombosis 血栓形成
-poiesis	产生	hemopoiesis 造血，血细胞生成
fibr/o	纤维，纤维组织	fibrous 纤维性的
reticul/o	网	reticular 网状的

笔记

续表

Morpheme	Meaning	Example
agglutin/o	凝块，凝集	agglutinogen 凝集原
glob/o	圆的，球	globin 球蛋白
ser/o	血清	serous 血清的，血浆的
nucle/o	核	mononuclear 单核的
kary/o	核	megakaryocyte 巨核细胞
phag/o	吃，吞噬	phagocyte 吞噬细胞
immun/o	安全，免疫	immunology 免疫学
lymph/o	淋巴	lymphadenitis 淋巴结炎
nod/o	结	nodal 结的，节点的
splen/o	脾	splenocyte 脾细胞
thym/o	胸腺	thymic 胸腺的
tonsill/o	扁桃腺	tonsillectomy 扁桃体切除术
ather/o	脂肪堆积	atherosclerosis 动脉粥样硬化
necr/o	死亡	necrosis 坏死
angin/o	阻塞	anginal（心）绞痛的
tach/o	快速	tachycardia 心动过速
brachy	短的	brachycardia 心动过缓
ster/o	固体	cholesterol 胆固醇
coll/o	胶	colloid 胶质
somat/o	身体	somatotropin 生长激素
thyr/o	甲状腺	thyrocele 甲状腺肿
adren/o	肾上腺	adrenal 肾上腺
neur/o	神经	neuroblast 成神经细胞
myelin/o	髓磷脂	myelinic 髓磷脂的
myel/o	脊髓	myelocele 脊髓突出
gangli/o	神经节	ganglionic 神经节的
cerebr/o	大脑	cerebral 大脑的
encephal/o	脑	encephalomeningocele 脑脑膜膨出
ventricul/o	室	ventricular 脑室的，心室的
thalam/o	丘脑	thalamic 丘脑的
menin/o, meningi/o	脑膜	meningitis 脑膜炎 meningioma 脑（脊）膜瘤
spin/o	脊髓	spinocerebellar 脊髓小脑的
sympath/o	自主神经系统交感部分	sympathoblast 成交感神经细胞
cut/i	皮肤	subcutaneous 皮下的
derm/o	皮肤	epidermis 表皮
kerat/o	角质的,硬的	keratonosis 皮肤角质层病
trich/o	毛发	trichosis 毛发病
pil/o	毛发	pilous 毛的
hidr/o	汗	hidropoiesis 汗生成
hol/o	整个，全部	holocrine 全分泌的

笔记

续表

Morpheme	Meaning	Example
mer/o	部分	merocrine 部分分泌的
oste/o	骨	osteoblast 成骨细胞
chondr/o	软骨	chondral 软骨的
cran/o	颅骨	craniotome 开颅器
cervic/o	颈	cervical 颈的，子宫颈的
thorac/o	胸	thoracic 胸的
lumb/o	腰、背下部	lumbar 腰的
spondyl/o	椎骨	spondylosyndesis 脊柱制动术
vertebr/o	椎骨	intervertebral 椎间的
myel	脊髓，骨髓	myelitis 脊髓炎，骨髓炎
pelv/o	骨盆	pelvic 骨盆的
my/o, myos/o	肌肉	myitis (myositis) 肌炎
muscul/o	肌肉	muscular 肌肉的
sarc/o	肉	sarcolemma 肉膜
arthr/o	关节	arthritis 关节炎
articul/o	关节	articulation 关节
synovi/o	滑液	synovial 滑液的
fibr/o	纤维组织	fibroblast 成纤维细胞
tend/o	腱	tendotome 腱刀
ophthalm/o	眼	ophthalmologist 眼科专家
ocul/o	眼	ocular 眼的
phac/o	晶体	phacomalacia 晶状体软化
pupill/o	瞳孔	pupillary 瞳孔的
core/o	瞳孔，虹膜	corectopia 瞳孔异位
corne/o	角性的，角膜	corneal 角膜的
kerat/o	角膜	keratomalacia 角膜软化
scler/o	巩膜	sclerectasia 巩膜膨胀
retin/o	视网膜	retinoscopy 视网膜镜检查
lacrim/o	眼泪，泪小管	lacrimal 泪的，泪管的
dacry/o	眼泪	dacryoadenitis 泪腺炎
conjunctiv/o	结膜	conjunctivitis 结膜炎
audi/o	听觉	audiometer 听力计
acou/o	听觉	acoustic 听觉的
aur/o	耳	aural 耳的
ot/o	耳	otitis 耳炎

(1) Write down the Latin or Greek affixes according to the same Chinese meaning.

1) 鼻   ＿＿＿＿＿＿＿   ＿＿＿＿＿＿＿

2) 口，嘴   ＿＿＿＿＿＿＿   ＿＿＿＿＿＿＿

3) 牙齿   ＿＿＿＿＿＿＿   ＿＿＿＿＿＿＿

4) 胆   ＿＿＿＿＿＿＿   ＿＿＿＿＿＿＿

5) 肾   ＿＿＿＿＿＿＿   ＿＿＿＿＿＿＿

6) 子宫　　　　　＿＿＿＿＿＿＿＿＿＿＿＿　　＿＿＿＿＿＿＿＿＿＿＿＿

7) 血管　　　　　＿＿＿＿＿＿＿＿＿＿＿＿　　＿＿＿＿＿＿＿＿＿＿＿＿

8) 核　　　　　　＿＿＿＿＿＿＿＿＿＿＿＿　　＿＿＿＿＿＿＿＿＿＿＿＿

9) 皮肤　　　　　＿＿＿＿＿＿＿＿＿＿＿＿　　＿＿＿＿＿＿＿＿＿＿＿＿

10) 毛发　　　　＿＿＿＿＿＿＿＿＿＿＿＿　　＿＿＿＿＿＿＿＿＿＿＿＿

11) 眼　　　　　＿＿＿＿＿＿＿＿＿＿＿＿　　＿＿＿＿＿＿＿＿＿＿＿＿

12) 听觉　　　　＿＿＿＿＿＿＿＿＿＿＿＿　　＿＿＿＿＿＿＿＿＿＿＿＿

(2)　Word-matching 1.

1) eupnea	A. 食管的
2) esophageal	B. 气管造口术
3) succagogue	C. 输尿管结石
4) intraperitoneal	D. 呼吸正常
5) laparotomy	E. 胸膜的
6) tracheostomy	F. 咽切开术
7) pleural	G. 畸齿矫正术
8) ovulation	H. 排卵
9) pharyngotomy	I. 促分泌的
10) ureterolith	J. 肺炎球菌
11) orthodontics	K. 腹膜内的
12) pneumococci	L. 剖腹术

(3)　Word-matching 2.

1) coronary	A. 神经节的
2) atherosclerosis	B. 结膜炎
3) thrombosis	C. 淋巴结炎
4) brachycardia	D. 毛细血管
5) ganglionic	E. 血栓形成
6) lymphadenitis	F. 软骨的
7) chondral	G. 冠状的
8) conjunctivitis	H. 动脉粥样硬化
9) capillary	I. 视网膜镜检查
10) retinoscopy	J. 胸的
11) corectopia	K. 瞳孔异位
12) thoracic	L. 心动过缓

(4)　Complete the following expression according to its Chinese meaning in the brackets.

1) （不良）＿＿＿＿＿＿reactions

2) （分子）＿＿＿＿＿＿weight

3) （肝）＿＿＿＿＿＿function

4) （过敏）＿＿＿＿＿＿reaction

5) （缓解）＿＿＿＿＿＿effect

6) （降压）＿＿＿＿＿＿action

7) （尿常规）＿＿＿＿＿＿examination

8) （失效）＿＿＿＿＿＿date

9) （胃肠道）＿＿＿＿＿＿disorder

笔记

10) significant_____effect（疗效）

11) cardiac_____（不全）

12) （兴奋）_____effect

(5) Translate the following passage into Chinese.

Dosage & Administration:

Usual dosage: Adult: two capsule to be taken three times daily or as directed by the physician.

Children 6 to 12 years of age; one capsule to be taken three times daily or as directed by the physician.

Complete the whole treatment course even if the condition seems to be improved.

Acute urethritis: 3 grams daily in 2 divided doses.

Gonorrhoea: 3 grams in a single dose.

Side effects: As with other penicillin, AMOXYCILLIN may cause occasionally gastrointestinal disturbances, urticaria, rash and hypersensitivity reactions which may occur in patients with history of asthma, hay fever and urticaria. However, such side effect may disappear after cease of the treatment.

Precaution: Caution use in penicillin–sensitive patients.

2. English-Chinese Translation Skills: 药学英语翻译中的语篇意识

药学英语翻译直接目标是篇章翻译，单个句子翻译是很少的。系统功能语法认为语篇是由一组相互连贯的句子所体现的意义单位，或称为语言运用单位。根据语言学理论，判断一系列句子是否构成了一个篇章取决于句内与句间的连贯关系。判断语篇的完整性有七个标准，包括"衔接性"(cohesion)、"连贯性"(coherence)、"意图性"(intentionality)、"可接受性"(acceptability)、"信息性"(informativity)、"情境性"(situationality) 和"互文性"(intertextuality)。在这七个标准中，衔接性和连贯性最为重要，语篇没有衔接性和连贯性，其他几个标准在一定程度上很难实现。药学英语翻译中的语篇意识可以从衔接手段和主位结构来分析。

功能语法将衔接分为五种：指称、替代、省略、连接和词汇衔接，词汇衔接包括重复、同义词/反义词以及上下义词等。衔接是语篇表层结构上的有形网络，当语篇中一个成分的含义依赖于另一个成分的解释时，便产生了衔接与连贯关系。由于英语和汉语语言结构存在差异，在翻译语篇时，要注意两种语言中衔接表达方式上的差异。如：

例 1：Traditional Chinese herbal medicine draws on ancient practice. Herbal medicine is as old as humanity itself. Early human beings were hunter-gatherers whose survival depended on their knowledge of their environment. Direct experience taught them which plants were toxic, which ones imparted strength and sustained life, and which had special healing qualities.

Thousands of medicinal substances are used in China today. Indeed, more than a million tons of herbs are used each year in China. Thirty herbs, mostly tonics, account for more than 50 percent of this figure, with *Gancao* topping the list at 86,000 tons.

参考译文：中药源于古代社会实践，和人类历史一样久远。古人靠狩猎和采集为生，生存与否取决于他们对环境的了解。直接的经验教会他们哪些植物有毒，哪些可以助长力气、延年益寿，哪些有特殊的治疗作用。

今天中国有数千种中药仍在使用。实际上，中国每年消耗的中药材超过百万吨。其中 30 种中药，主要是补药，使用量超过总量的 50%。甘草消耗量最大，每年用量八万六千吨。

说明：在第一小段中，前两个小句主语分别是 traditional Chinese herbal medicine，和 herbal medicine，两个意义重复的主语表明这两个句子之间的衔接。但是在翻译成汉语时，如果按照原文将两个重复主语翻译出来就显得啰嗦，汉语译文省略一个主语，符合汉语表达习惯也保留了两个小句的意义衔接。第二小段第一句中主语"thousands of medicinal substances"与第一段中的"traditional Chinese herbal medicine"以及本段中下面两句中的"herbs"形成重复，构成意义上的衔接，但是如果按照字面翻译将"thousands of medicinal substances"译成"数千种药物"，则明显破坏了整个语篇意义上的衔接。

例2：[1] Another form of transmucosal **delivery** takes advantage of the superior absorptive properties of (the respiratory tract, nose, and bronchial tree). [2] *Drugs* can be **delivered** to (these tissues) via **sprays**. [3] The level at which the *drug* acts in (the respiratory system) can be controlled by the particle size. [4] Smaller particles penetrate further into (the lung) before they are filtered out.

[5] **Spray delivery** has already been used to deliver two *peptides*, gonadotrophin-releasing factor, a potential male contraceptive, and vasopressin, a pituitary hormone being tested for memory enhancement. [6] **Spray delivery** is now being tested with *insulin*. [7] **Sprays** are preferred for *peptides* because peptides, like proteins, are hydrolyzed in the stomach. [8] **Respiratory delivery** would also be advantageous for *antibiotics* used to treat pneumonia and for anticancer drugs for (lung) cancer. [9] *Vaccines* might ideally be administered **this way**. [10] And *cardiovascular drugs* should be more effective by **this route** since **delivery** to the highly vascular (lung) is equivalent to an intra-arterial injection.

参考译文：[1] 另一种经黏膜给药法利用了呼吸道、鼻子和支气管卓越的吸收特性，[2] 药物可以通过喷射进入这些组织，[3] 颗粒的大小可控制作用于呼吸道的药物水平，[4] 小颗粒在被滤出之前就可渗入肺的深处。

[5] 喷剂已用于两种肽给药，一种是潜在的男性避孕药，促性腺激素释放因子，另一种是正在测试其增强记忆功能的脑垂体激素加压素。[6] 喷剂也在试用于胰岛素的给药。[7] 喷剂更适用于肽，因为肽和蛋白质一样，可在胃中水解。[8] 呼吸道给药法对治疗肺炎的抗生素和治疗肺癌的抗癌药都有其优越性，[9] 也是服用疫苗的最佳途径，[10] 心血管药物通过这一途径服用会更有效，因为心血管密布的肺部送药与动脉内注射是一样的。

说明：该句是关于药物给药系统中的"呼吸道给药法"，共有两个小段，10 个小句，为了便于说明分别给每个小句标上 [1] 到 [10] 的编号。在第 [1] 句中 another form 与前文中的 one form 构成连接，形成语篇上下文整体连贯。其他衔接关系有：

(1) 第 [1]、[2]、[5]、[6]、[7]、[8] 句中的 delivery、spray deliver、spray 等构成重复关系；

(2) 第 [1]、[2]、[3]、[4]、[8]、[10] 句中的 the respiratory tract, nose, and bronchial tree、these tissues、the respiratory system、lung 等构成上下义词关系，其中 tissues，respiratory system 是上义词，其他名词则是下义词；

(3) 第 [9]、[10] 句中的 this way，this route 与前文中的 delivery 等构成指代关系；

(4) 第 [2]、[3]、[5]、[6]、[7]、[8]、[9]、[10] 中的 drug、peptides、insulin、antibiotics、anticancer drugs、vaccines、cardiovascular drugs 等构成重复和上下义词关系；

(5) 第 [3]、[4] 句中的 the particle size 和 smaller particles、they 等构成重复和指代关系。

从这些衔接关系分析中可见，(1)、(2) 和 (4) 表示的关系是本语篇的主要衔接关系，说明此语篇的主要内容是关于"给（药）"(delivery)、"呼吸"(respiratory) 和"（给）药"(drug)。

语法衔接关系构成语篇意义上的连贯，但是英汉两种语言差异要求在翻译时要注意不同语言在衔接与连贯关系表达上的差别，在翻译过程中不能够将源语言的衔接关系完全移植到目的语中。分析参考译文，第 [4] 句中的指代词 they 和第 [9] 句中的指导词 this way 都省略了，翻译过程中通过英汉语不同的衔接手段实现译文的语篇连贯。

功能语法将小句分为主位和述位两个部分，主位就是句子谓语动词前面的部分，除了主位，句子的其他成分就是述位。主位是话题，小句信息的出发点；述位是目标，小句信息传递的核心内容。英语和汉语主位结构相似，都是主位在前，述位在后；主位往往都是已知信息，述位都是新信息。英汉两种语言在主位结构上的相似性应用在翻译中可以采取顺着原句顺序保留原文的主位结构的直译方式，实现源语语篇和目的语语篇的结构对应。

在上面例 2 中的第一段，源语语篇有 4 个小句，其中小句 [3] 和小句 [4] 是复合小句，因此第一段中共有 6 个主位，它们分别是：[1] another form of transmucosal delivery, [2] drugs, [3] the level (…) 和定语从句中的 the drug, [4] smaller particles 和时间状语从句中的 they。分析这第一段的译文可见，小句 [1] 和小句 [2] 的翻译中保留了英语小句的主位结构；小句 [3] 的译文将原英语小句中的述位"the particle size"变成了主位，这里就值得商榷。按照语言学的理论，主位是已知信息，是小句信息的出发点，而译文中的主位"颗粒大小"确是前文中没有出现的，是"新信息"，这样处理破坏了原英语小句的信息结构。如果将小句 [3] 翻译成："药物作用于呼吸道的水平可由颗粒大小控制"，则可以较好地表述原句的信息，虽然原小句的主位 the level 和 drug 的位置发生了变化，但这是由英汉两种语言的结构差异所致。在小句 [4] 中，原英语小句中的一个主位 they 被省略了，但是原句的信息结构没有改变，这些语言上的变化属于必要性转变（obligatory shifts）。

完整语篇中，连续小句的主位构成"主位 - 述位"推进。英语中"主位 - 述位"按照一定规律推进，小句间主位、述位交替，环环相扣，构成衔接有序的语篇。

再看例 2：

第一段中：小句 [2] 的述位中的 delivered 是小句 [1] 中的主位，小句 [3] 中的主位 drug 对应小句 [2] 的主位，小句 [4] 的主位是小句 [3] 的述位。在第二段中：小句 [5]、[6]、[7]、[8] 主位相同，而小句 [9]、[10] 的主位则是前面 4 个小句的述位（上下义关系或同义、并列关系）。再将第一段和第二段联合分析可见这段语篇中 10 个小句的主位推进模式构成了意义连贯的语篇。

药学英语属于科技英语语篇，语言结构严谨，内容丰富，专业性强。在药学英语翻译过程中，除了必须掌握基本的翻译技巧以外，更要注重英汉两种语言在构成语篇衔接性与连贯性上的异同性，使译文能够更好地传递原文的语篇信息。

笔记

28